Common Toxicologic Issues in Small Animals: An Update

Editors

STEPHEN B. HOOSER
SAFDAR A. KHAN

VETERINARY CLINICS OF NORTH AMERICA: SMALL ANIMAL PRACTICE

www.vetsmall.theclinics.com

November 2018 • Volume 48 • Number 6

ELSEVIER

1600 John F. Kennedy Boulevard • Suite 1800 • Philadelphia, Pennsylvania, 19103-2899
http://www.vetsmall.theclinics.com

**VETERINARY CLINICS OF NORTH AMERICA: SMALL ANIMAL PRACTICE Volume 48, Number 6
November 2018 ISSN 0195-5616, ISBN-13: 978-0-323-64270-5**

Editor: Colleen Dietzler
Developmental Editor: Meredith Madeira

Veterinary Clinics of North America: Small Animal Practice (ISSN 0195-5616) is published bimonthly by Elsevier Inc., 360 Park Avenue South, New York, NY 10010-1710. Months of issue are January, March, May, July, September, and November. Business and Editorial Offices: 1600 John F. Kennedy Blvd., Ste. 1800, Philadelphia, PA 19103-2899. Customer Service Office: 3251 Riverport Lane, Maryland Heights, MO 63043. Periodicals postage paid at New York, NY and additional mailing offices. Subscription prices are $325.00 per year (domestic individuals), $622.00 per year (domestic institutions), $100.00 per year (domestic students/residents), $430.00 per year (Canadian individuals), $773.00 per year (Canadian institutions), $469.00 per year (international individuals), $773.00 per year (international institutions), and $220.00 per year (international and Canadian students/residents). To receive student/resident rate, orders must be accompanied by name of affiliated institution, date of term, and the *signature* of program/residency coordinator on institution letterhead. Orders will be billed at individual rate until proof of status is received. Foreign air speed delivery is included in all *Clinics* subscription prices. All prices are subject to change without notice. **POSTMASTER:** Send address changes to *Veterinary Clinics of North America: Small Animal Practice*, Elsevier Health Sciences Division, Subscription Customer Service, 3251 Riverport Lane, Maryland Heights, MO 63043. Customer Service (orders, claims, online, change of address): Elsevier Periodicals Customer Service, Elsevier Health Sciences Division Subscription **Customer Service 3251 Riverport Lane Maryland Heights, MO 63043. Tel: 1-800-654-2452 (U.S. and Canada); 314-447-8871 (outside U.S. and Canada). Fax: 314-447-8029. E-mail: journalscustomerservice-usa@elsevier.com (for print support); journalsonlinesupport-usa@elsevier.com (for online support).**

Reprints. For copies of 100 or more of articles in this publication, please contact the Commercial Reprints Department, Elsevier Inc., 360 Park Avenue South, New York, NY 10010-1710. Tel.: 212-633-3874; Fax: 212-633-3820; E-mail: reprints@elsevier.com.

Veterinary Clinics of North America: Small Animal Practice is also published in Japanese by Inter Zoo Publishing Co., Ltd., Aoyama Crystal-Bldg 5F, 3-5-12 Kitaaoyama, Minato-ku, Tokyo 107-0061, Japan.

Veterinary Clinics of North America: Small Animal Practice is covered in *Current Contents/Agriculture, Biology and Environmental Sciences, Science Citation Index, ASCA, MEDLINE/PubMed (Index Medicus), Excerpta Medica, and BIOSIS.*

Contributors

EDITORS

STEPHEN B. HOOSER, DVM, PhD
Diplomate, American Board of Veterinary Toxicology; Head, Toxicology Section,
Indiana Animal Disease Diagnostic Laboratory, Professor, Department of Comparative
Pathobiology, College of Veterinary Medicine, Purdue University, West Lafayette, Indiana

SAFDAR A. KHAN, DVM, MS, PhD
Diplomate, American Board of Veterinary Toxicology; Associate Director, Global
Pharmacovigilance, Zoetis Animal Health, Kalamazoo, Michigan; Adjunct Toxicology
Instructor, University of Illinois, ASPCA Animal Poison Control Center, Urbana, Illinois

AUTHORS

KARYN BISCHOFF, DVM, MS
New York State Animal Health Diagnostic Center, Department of Population Medicine
and Diagnostic Sciences, Cornell University, Ithaca, New York

AHNA BRUTLAG, DVM, MS
Diplomate, American Board of Toxicology; Diplomate, American Board of Veterinary
Toxicology; Director, Veterinary Services and Senior Veterinary Toxicologist, Pet Poison
Helpline and SafetyCall International, Bloomington, Minnesota; Adjunct Assistant
Professor, Department of Veterinary and Biomedical Sciences, College of Veterinary
Medicine, University of Minnesota, St Paul, Minnesota

CAMILLE DeCLEMENTI, VMD
Vice President, ASPCA Animal Hospital, New York, New York; ASPCA Animal Poison
Control Center, Urbana, Illinois

ERIC K. DUNAYER, VMD
Diplomate, American Board of Toxicology; Diplomate, American Board of Veterinary
Toxicology; Associate Professor, Department of Clinical Veterinary Sciences,
St. Matthew's University School of Veterinary Medicine, Grand Cayman, Cayman
Islands; Senior Toxicologist, ASPCA Animal Poison Control Center, Urbana, Illinois

PAUL A. EUBIG, DVM, MS, PhD
Diplomate, American Board of Toxicology; Lecturer, Department of Physiology and
Pharmacology, College of Veterinary Medicine, University of Georgia, Athens, Georgia

PATTI GAHAGAN, DVM
Novartis Animal Health US, Inc, Greensboro, North Carolina

SHARON GWALTNEY-BRANT, DVM, PhD
Diplomate, American Board of Veterinary Toxicology; Diplomate, American Board of
Toxicology; Veterinary Information Network, Mahomet, Illinois

CRISTINE L. HAYES, DVM
Diplomate, American Board of Toxicology; Diplomate, American Board of Veterinary Toxicology; Senior Toxicologist, Team Leader, ASPCA Animal Poison Control Center, Urbana, Illinois

HOLLY HOMMERDING, DVM
Consulting Veterinarian, Clinical Toxicology, Pet Poison Helpline and SafetyCall International, Bloomington, Minnesota

STEPHEN B. HOOSER, DVM, PhD
Diplomate, American Board of Veterinary Toxicology; Head, Toxicology Section, Indiana Animal Disease Diagnostic Laboratory, Professor, Department of Comparative Pathobiology, College of Veterinary Medicine, Purdue University, West Lafayette, Indiana

SAFDAR A. KHAN, DVM, MS, PhD
Diplomate, American Board of Veterinary Toxicology; Associate Director, Global Pharmacovigilance, Zoetis Animal Health, Kalamazoo, Michigan; Adjunct Toxicology Instructor, University of Illinois, ASPCA Animal Poison Control Center, Urbana, Illinois

MARY KAY McLEAN, DVM, MS
Veterinary Corps Officer, US Army, Fort Benning, Georgia

IRINA MEADOWS, DVM
Diplomate, American Board of Toxicology; ASPCA Animal Poison Control Center, Urbana, Illinois

CHARLOTTE MEANS, DVM, MLIS
Diplomate, American Board of Veterinary Toxicology; Diplomate, American Board of Toxicology; Director of Toxicology, ASPCA Animal Poison Control Center, Urbana, Illinois

VALENTINA M. MEROLA, DVM, MS, MPH
Diplomate, American Board of Veterinary Toxicology; Diplomate, American Board of Toxicology; Public Health Officer, 78th Medical Group, United States Air Force, Robins AFB, Warner Robins, Georgia

LISA A. MURPHY, VMD
Diplomate, American Board of Toxicology; Associate Professor of Toxicology, Department of Pathobiology, University of Pennsylvania School of Veterinary Medicine, PADLS New Bolton Center Toxicology Laboratory, Kennett Square, Pennsylvania

BIRGIT PUSCHNER, DVM, PhD
Diplomate, American Board of Veterinary Toxicology; Professor and Chair, Department of Molecular Biosciences, School of Veterinary Medicine, University of California, Davis, California

WILSON K. RUMBEIHA, BVM, PhD
Veterinary Diagnostics and Production Animal Medicine, College of Veterinary Medicine, Iowa State University, Ames, Iowa

MARY SCHELL, DVM
Diplomate, American Board of Veterinary Toxicology; Diplomate, American Board of Toxicology; ASPCA Animal Poison Control Center, Urbana, Illinois

BRANDY R. SOBCZAK, DVM
Consulting Veterinarian in Clinical Toxicology, ASPCA Animal Poison Control Center, Urbana, Illinois

LAURA STERN, DVM
Diplomate, American Board of Veterinary Toxicology; ASPCA Animal Poison Control Center, Urbana, Illinois

COLETTE WEGENAST, DVM
ASPCA Animal Poison Control Center, ASPCA Midwest Office, Urbana, Illinois

CHRISTINA R. WILSON-FRANK, PhD
Head Analytical Chemist, Clinical Associate Professor of Toxicology, Indiana Animal Disease Diagnostic Laboratory, Department of Comparative Pathobiology, College of Veterinary Medicine, Purdue University, West Lafayette, Indiana

TINA WISMER, DVM, MS
Diplomate, American Board of Veterinary Toxicology; Diplomate, American Board of Toxicology; Medical Director, ASPCA Animal Poison Control Center, Urbana, Illinois

Contents

Each year the Animal Poison Control Center of the American Society for the Prevention of Cruelty to Animals receives thousands of reports of suspected animal poisonings. By using an electronic medical record database maintained by the Animal Poison Control Center, data on current trends in animal poisoning cases are mined and analyzed This article explores recent trends in veterinary toxicology including the types of animals and breeds that are most commonly exposed to different toxicants, seasonal and geographic distribution of poisoning incidents, the therapies that are most commonly administered, and trends in agents that are most frequently involved in poisonings.

Although most commercial pet foods are safe, there have been a few instances in which chemical or bacterial contamination have caused outbreaks of illness in animals. Because of concerns regarding cases of contaminated commercial pet food that have been reported over the past several years, some pet owners may be choosing to feed noncommercial, home-prepared diets. When pet food contamination is suspected, pet owners often seek advice from their veterinarian regarding its health impact and subsequent diagnosis. This article addresses the role of the veterinarians in pet food contamination and highlights recommended approaches to handling pet food outbreaks or recalls.

Commercial pet foods are usually safe, but incidents of contamination can have a devastating impact on companion animals and their owners. There are numerous possible contaminants ranging from natural contaminants to nutrient imbalances to chemical adulteration, making it impossible to predict what will cause the next pet food recall. Veterinarians involvement with pet food recalls includes examining and treating affected animals, documentation and sample collection, and communicating with pet food manufacturers and regulatory agencies.

on the classification, uses, pharmacokinetics, mechanisms of action, and treatment of the most commonly encountered NSAIDs in dogs and cats.

Lisa A. Murphy and Eric K. Dunayer

Xylitol ingestions in dogs may result in severe hypoglycemia followed by acute hepatic failure and associated coagulopathies. Aggressive treatment may be needed, but the prognosis is generally expected to be good for dogs developing uncomplicated hypoglycemia. Because of increased availability of xylitol-containing products in the market and in the dog's environment, it is likely that there will continue to be increased exposures and toxicity in dogs.

Valentina M. Merola and Paul A. Eubig

Overdoses of macrocyclic lactones in dogs and cats can result in such signs as tremors, ataxia, seizures, coma, and blindness. Dogs with the ABCB1-1Δ gene defect are predisposed to macrocyclic lactone toxicosis at lower dosages than dogs without the defect. Intravenous lipid emulsion therapy has been suggested for treatment of macrocyclic lactone toxicosis but evidence of efficacy is limited. Initial decontamination and supportive care remain the mainstays of therapy for macrocyclic lactone toxicosis.

Tina Wismer and Charlotte Means

In the broadest definition, a pesticide (from fly swatters to chemicals) is a substance used to eliminate a pest. Newer insecticides are much safer to the environment, humans, and nontarget species. These insecticides are able to target physiologic differences between insects and mammals, resulting in greater mammalian safety. This article briefly reviews toxicity information of both older insecticides such as organophosphates, carbamates, permethrins, and pyrethroids, as well as some newer insecticides.

Camille DeClementi and Brandy R. Sobczak

This article focuses on the 3 most commonly used rodenticide types: anticoagulants, bromethalin, and cholecalciferol. It is important to verify the active ingredient in any rodenticide exposure. Many owners use the term D-con to refer to any rodenticide regardless of the brand or type of rodenticide. The Environmental Protection Agency released their final ruling on rodenticide risk mitigation measures in 2008 and all products sold had to be compliant by June 2011, changing to consumer products containing either first-generation anticoagulants or nonanticoagulants, including bromethalin and cholecalciferol. These regulations have caused an increase in the number of bromethalin and cholecalciferol cases.

increasing in conjunction with greater accessibility. Cannabis products are even sold for use in pets. In addition, exposure to illegal synthetic cannabinoids remains concerning. Veterinarians need to be able to recognize associated clinical signs and understand when cases have the potential for severity. This article provides a brief history of cannabis along with a review of the endocannabinoid system, common cannabis products, expected clinical signs, and medical treatment approaches associated with cannabis exposure in pets.

Stephen B. Hooser

Exposure of dogs and cats to clinically significant amounts of ionizing radiation is unlikely. However, accidental release of radiation has occurred and nuclear terrorism is possible. If an incident occurs, early reaction will be by first responders, followed by state and federal emergency personnel. It is possible that veterinarians will be called upon to assist to evaluate animals for contamination and/or exposure, perform initial life-saving tasks, and decontaminate people's pets. Therefore, veterinary professionals should understand radiation exposure, what is happening, the possible effects on animals, and how to provide veterinary care and assistance in a radiation emergency.

VETERINARY CLINICS OF NORTH AMERICA: SMALL ANIMAL PRACTICE

SERIES OF RELATED INTEREST

Veterinary Clinics of North America: Exotic Animal Practice
https://www.vetexotic.theclinics.com/

THE CLINICS ARE NOW AVAILABLE ONLINE!
Access your subscription at:
www.theclinics.com

Preface

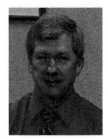 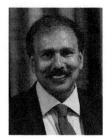

Stephen B. Hooser, DVM, PhD Safdar A. Khan, DVM, MS, PhD
Editors

ACKNOWLEDGMENTS FROM STEPHEN B. HOOSER

As always, I would like to express my appreciation, gratitude, and many thanks to my wife, daughter, and son for their support and patience without which I could not have accomplished all that I have. I would also like to acknowledge the support of our papillons and Border terrier, whose energy and fluffiness invigorate my day except when they piddle on the floor.

Veterinary medicine is a dynamic profession that continually advances the body of scientific knowledge, diagnostics, therapeutics, and patient care in all species, even the one species for which we leave clinical care to those single animal specialists, the physicians. This issue of *Veterinary Clinics of North America: Small Animal Practice* continues the dissemination of knowledge in Common Toxicologic Issues in Small Animals. The articles herein provide updates on the toxicants to which dogs and cats are exposed, the latest understanding of pathophysiology of those toxicants, and current diagnostics and treatments. Since the previous issue in 2012, the sale of marijuana and products containing marijuana has been legalized in several states. Not surprisingly, exposure to, and intoxication by, marijuana has also increased in dogs. The addition of a new article on marijuana provides basic information to help identify, diagnose, and treat marijuana intoxication. Another new article offers background information concerning response to incidents involving exposure of small animals to nuclear radiation. Through updates such as this issue of *Veterinary Clinics of North America: Small Animal Practice*, we continue augmenting our pool of knowledge so that rather than becoming Masters of Mediocrity, we continue to learn and progress throughout our careers in this ever-rewarding profession.

ACKNOWLEDGMENTS FROM SAFDAR KHAN

I would like to thank my wife and four boys for their untiring support in completing this issue. Without their endearing love and support, it would not have been possible to complete this project.

Vet Clin Small Anim 48 (2018) xiii–xiv
https://doi.org/10.1016/j.cvsm.2018.08.011
0195-5616/18/© 2018 Published by Elsevier Inc.

vetsmall.theclinics.com

It is hard to believe that more than six years have passed since the last issue of Common Toxicologic Issues in Small Animals was published. Because of rapid changes occurring in our field, it is necessary to frequently update these changes so that all stakeholders stay current and benefit from these updates. The focus of the updated issue remains the same, and that is, the clinical and diagnostic aspect of veterinary toxicology. All of the articles in the current issue have been updated with the most recent information available by the experts in their respective areas. We hope this updated resource will be beneficial to veterinary clinicians, diagnosticians, students, researchers, and academicians.

Stephen B. Hooser, DVM, PhD
Toxicology Section
Animal Disease Diagnostic Laboratory
Department of Comparative Pathobiology
College of Veterinary Medicine
Purdue University
West Lafayette, IN 47907, USA

Safdar A. Khan, DVM, MS, PhD
Global Pharmacovigilance
Zoetis Animal Health
Kalamazoo, MI 49007, USA

University of Illinois at Urbana-Champaign
Urbana-Champaign, IL, USA

E-mail addresses:
shooser1@purdue.edu (S.B. Hooser)
Safdar.Khan@zoetis.com (S.A. Khan)

An Overview of Trends in Animal Poisoning Cases in the United States: 2011 to 2017

Charlotte Means, DVM, MLIS*, Tina Wismer, DVM, MS

KEYWORDS

- Veterinary • Toxicology • Toxicants • Animal poisoning incidents/trends

KEY POINTS

- Dogs are the species most commonly exposed to potentially toxic substances, and exposures are more often reported during summer months in the mid-afternoon.
- Current trends show that human medications continue to be a common risk for pets and that there has been an increase in the number of vitamin D exposures reported.
- Decontamination remains an important therapy to lessen the risk for signs after an exposure, and although its effectiveness remains debatable, the experimental use of intravenous lipid fat emulsion has risen.
- The continued monitoring of medical record databases ensures clinicians are up-to-date and well informed of emerging trends in toxicology.
- It is only by monitoring trends that toxicities, such as lily exposures in cats, or grape and raisin toxicosis in dogs, were discovered, and through which other new toxicities will be recognized.

Each year the American Society for the Prevention of Cruelty to Animals Animal Poison Control Center (APCC) receives thousands of reports of suspected animal poisonings. By using AnTox, an electronic medical record database maintained by the APCC, data on current trends in animal poisoning cases are mined and analyzed. This article explores recent trends in veterinary toxicology including the types of animals and breeds that are most commonly exposed to different toxicants, seasonal and geographic distribution of poisoning incidents, the therapies that are most commonly administered, and trends in agents that are most frequently involved in poisonings.

MATERIALS AND METHODS

The APCC is a 24-hour service that receives calls from the United States and Canada regarding animal exposures to a variety of man-made and natural substances. When a

The authors have nothing to disclose.
ASPCA Animal Poison Control Center, 1717 South Philo Road, Suite 36, Urbana, IL 61802, USA
* Corresponding author.
E-mail address: charlotte.means@aspca.org

call is received, the APCC veterinary staff collects information about the animal's signalment, medical history, exposure history, onset time, types and duration of clinical signs, treatment information, and laboratory findings. If needed, follow-up calls are made to track the progression of clinical signs, the animal's response to and the effectiveness of treatments implemented, laboratory changes, and the final outcome. The electronic medical records from more than 3 million animal poisoning cases reported to the APCC were reviewed. Data collected from January 1, 2012, to December 31, 2017, were retrieved and analyzed.

WHERE AND WHEN EXPOSURES/POISONINGS OCCUR

Suspected animal exposures/poisonings occur year round across the country. The data collected from 2012 to 2017 show that calls regarding animal exposures to various agents are distributed throughout the year evenly. The highest number of calls (26.9%) was reported in summer months followed by Fall (24.6%) and Spring (25.47%). A total of 22.9% of calls were received during winter months (**Box 1**). The largest volume of calls occurs in July (9.2% of calls) and the least number of calls occurs in February (7%).

Exposures/poisonings occur at all hours of the day. A review of 2017 case data shows that the highest number of calls occurs from 2 to 3 PM CST with 6.89% of exposures being reported during that hour (**Table 1**). The slowest call volume occurs overnight from 4 to 5 AM CST with only 0.51% of the cases being reported at that time. This is a change from highest call volumes occurring in the early evening. The reason behind this change is not clear, although it may indicate changes in work day hours, or parents bringing children home from school. Although poisoning cases also occur overnight, the owner's may not know about it until the morning when they wake up and then call the APCC about it.

Information on the state (geographic information) from which a poisoning report originated was collected from 2015 cases (**Table 2**). This information could be dependent on a variety of factors including the public's awareness of the APCC, and because the APCC is a fee-based, cost-recovery service, many poisoning incidents may go unreported. Other factors can include a veterinarian's familiarity with various toxins, decreasing the need to call about common toxins.

TYPES OF ANIMALS INVOLVED IN POISONING CASES

The species of animals involved in poisonings reported to the APCC has remained consistent over the past 5 years. In 2016 and 2017, canines accounted for 64.69% (2016) and 63.22 (2017). Cats represented 7.78% of cases in 2016 and 6.74% of cases in 2017 (**Table 3**).

Labradors and Labrador mixes, golden retrievers, chihuahuas, Yorkshire terriers, shih tzus, German shepherds, beagles, mixed breeds, and pit bulls have consistently

---

Box 1
Seasonal distribution of exposure reports from 2012 to 2017

Winter, 22.9%

Spring, 25.47%

Summer, 26.9%

Fall, 24.6%

Table 1
Hourly distribution of exposure reports from 2010

Time of Day	Total Calls for Year	Percentage of Calls
12 AM	4657	2.02
1 AM	3254	1.41
2 AM	1738	0.76
3 AM	1221	0.53
4 AM	1164	0.51
5 AM	1719	0.75
6 AM	2920	1.27
7 AM	5619	2.44
8 AM	9023	3.92
9 AM	10,413	4.52
10 AM	14,121	6.13
11 AM	14,457	6.28
12 PM	14,369	6.24
1 PM	14,666	6.37
2 PM	15,818	6.87
3 PM	14,625	6.35
4 PM	14,872	6.46
5 PM	15,027	6.52
6 PM	14,766	6.41
7 PM	13,715	5.96
8 PM	13,087	5.68
9 PM	11,470	4.98
10 PM	10,105	4.39
11 PM	7386	3.21
Total	230,192	

topped the list of dog breeds involved in poisonings. Pit bulls and mixed breeds may be climbing in numbers because there have been many programs by shelters to encourage adopting these dogs. Mixes also are increasing because of increases of designer dogs (**Table 4**).

When compared with American Kennel Club registration statistics, in 2015 to 2017 Labrador retrievers topped the list of the most registered dogs followed by German shepherds, and golden retrievers. In 2017, French bulldogs reached fourth most popular dog breed by registrations, and were sixth in 2015 and 2016. Of other breeds on the APCC top 10 list, chihuahuas dropped from 28th in 2015 to 32nd in 2017. Yorkshire terriers remained steady at ninth place in 2016 and 2017. Beagles dropped to sixth place in 2017 from fifth place in 2015 and 2016.

TRENDS IN THE TYPES OF TOXICANTS INVOLVED

As a result of curiosity and indiscriminate eating habits, animals are exposed to a variety of agents in their environment. Although many exposures occur accidentally, some exposures occur maliciously, or when owners administer agents with good intentions not knowing they can actually cause harm. Consistently, human medications have topped the list accounting for 17.5% of exposures in 2017 and 17% in 2016.

Table 2
State (geographic information) from which a poisoning report originated

State	% of Calls
California	12
New York	7.9
Pennsylvania	6.5
Texas	6.1
New Jersey	5.9
Virginia	5.4
Massachusetts	5.3
Florida	4.8
Illinois	4.3
Connecticut	3.7
North Carolina	3.5
Ohio	3.5
Maryland	3
Arizona	2.7
Michigan	2.3
Colorado	2.3
Wisconsin	2.2
Washington	2
Georgia	1.5
Indiana	1.3
Oregon	1.3
Tennessee	1.3
South Carolina	1.2
Minnesota	1
Nevada	0.8
Missouri	0.8
New Hampshire	0.7
Kentucky	0.6
Louisiana	0.6
Rhode Island	0.6
New Mexico	0.5
Delaware	0.5
Maine	0.5
Kansas	0.5
Iowa	0.4
West Virginia	0.4
Oklahoma	0.4
Hawaii	0.4
Alaska	0.3
Alabama	0.3
Idaho	0.2
Vermont	0.2

(continued on next page)

Table 2 (continued)	
State	**% of Calls**
Nebraska	0.2
Utah	0.2
Arkansas	0.2
Mississippi	0.1
Montana	0.1
South Dakota	0.1
Wyoming	0.1
North Dakota	0.05

Other top categories included over-the-counter products (OTC); insecticides, such as flea control spot-ons; rodenticides; human food; veterinary medications; chocolate; household toxicants, such as bleach and cleaning supplies; plants; herbicides; and outdoor products, such as antifreeze and ice melts.

The most common human medication exposures represent a wide range, but pain medications, antidepressants, and heart medications are the most common medications for which the APCC received calls in 2017. In 2016, the top three classes of human prescription medications included heart medications, antidepressants, and attention-deficit/hyperactivity disorder medications. OTC drugs are an enormous class, encompassing nearly 7000 products. Of these, ibuprofen is the number one

Table 3 Species of animals involved in poisonings reported to the APCC in 2017	
Species	**%**
Canine	63.22
Feline	6.74
Equine	0.25
Bird	0.14
Lagomorph	0.119
Ferret	0.033
Bovine	0.31
Rodent	0.06
Fish	0.89
Caprine	0.052
Porcine	0.07
Lizard	0.01
Ovine	0.0013
Poultry	0.18
Turtle	0.004
Snake	0.004
Nonhuman primate	0.007
Marsupial	0.007
Canine wild	0.004
Feline wild	0.001

Percentage of species reported by total number of reports.

Table 4
Yearly distribution (percentage) of the top 10 dog breeds reported in 2015, 2016, and 2017

2015		2016		2017	
Breed	**%**	**Breed**	**%**	**Breed**	**%**
Labrador retriever	8.83	Labrador retriever	8.96	Labrador retriever	8.63
Mixed breed	4.65	Mixed breed	4.68	Mixed breed	4.65
Golden retriever	3.18	Golden retriever	3.43	Golden retriever	3.55
Chihuahua	3.06	Chihuahua	3.09	Chihuahua	3.15
American pit bull terrier	2.52	American pit bull terrier	2.6	American pit bull terrier	2.74
German shepherd dog	2.27	German shepherd dog	2.32	German shepherd dog	2.29
Yorkshire terrier	2.23	Yorkshire terrier	2.19	Yorkshire terrier	2.02
Shih tzu	1.96	Beagle	1.91	Beagle	1.8
Beagle	1.94	Shih tzu	1.85	Shih tzu	1.79
Boxer	1.69	Boxer	1.67	Maltese	1.5

Data from American Kennel Club. AKC most popular dog breeds-full ranking list. Available at: https://www.akc.org/expert-advice/news/most-popular-dog-breeds-full-ranking-list/. Accessed June 1, 2018.

OTC drug that the APCC received calls on in 2016. Ibuprofen is a nonsteroidal anti-inflammatory drug inhibiting cyclooxygenase (COX)-1 and COX-2 isoenzymes. Among other functions, COX-1 promotes the production of the natural mucus lining of the stomach, so even at therapeutic doses the inhibition of COX-1 can cause gastrointestinal ulcerations. At higher doses, ibuprofen can cause renal damage and/or failure.

Human food is the third most common category the APCC received calls on in 2016 and 2017. Food dangers include garlic and onions, grapes and raisins, alcohol, and xylitol. These cases accounted for 10.9% of calls in 2017. Chocolate (which has its own category) was number 6 in 2016 and number 5 in 2017. Chocolate accounted for 8.8% of calls in 2017 and 7.9% in 2016.

In 2017, veterinary products were fourth on the list with 8.9% of cases. With many chewable pills available, dogs are willing to take their own medication, and then ingest the entire bottle if it is accessible. Sixth place in 2017 belongs to household items, including glue, art supplies, cleaning supplies, laundry detergents and dish soap, and shampoos and conditioners. Laundry pods are increasing in popularity enabling dogs and other pets to have access to them. When ingested, animals often have mild to moderate vomiting, anorexia, upper respiratory irritation, and coughing. Aspiration pneumonia is also a risk.

Insecticide calls have been decreasing. In 2017, only 6.3% of cases involved insecticides. Granular bifenthrin lawn products primarily cause mild vomiting and diarrhea, but larger ingestions can cause tremors. Other clinical signs include ataxia, lethargy, trembling, hyperesthesia, and seizures. Newer insecticides are discussed further in Tina Wismer and Charlotte Means' article, "Toxicology of Newer Insecticides in Small Animals," in this issue.

Rodenticide exposures accounted for 6.3% of cases in 2017. Anticoagulant and bromethalin rodenticides are still the most common rodenticides, but in 2018 cholecalciferol cases are increasing. Discussions of clinical signs, decontamination, and treatment recommendations are found in Camille DeClementi and Brandy R. Sobczak's article, "Common Rodenticide Toxicoses in Small Animals," in this issue.

Plants consisted of 5.4% of cases in 2017. Determining the toxicity of a plant before it is purchased remains sound advice. Some of the most common toxic plants include lilies (*Lilium* and *Hemerocallis sp*), sago palms (*Cycas revoluta*), and oleander (*Nerium oleander*). Lilies can cause renal failure in cats, sago palms cause liver failure, and oleander is a cardiotoxin.

Garden products accounted for 2.6% of cases. These include fertilizers, herbicides, soil enhancements, and root stimulators. Many dogs find fertilizers (organic and inorganic) irresistible because many contain bone meal, fish meal, blood meal, manure, and other appealing substances. In most cases, only mild, self-limiting gastrointestinal upset is seen. Larger ingestions can cause impaction or abdominal pain (boarded abdomen), hind limb weakness, or tremors. Treatment is generally symptomatic and supportive.

Over the past few years, there have been some notable trends in animal exposures most likely caused by regulatory changes, new product availability, and the increase or decrease of popularity of certain agents. New Environmental Protection Agency guidelines may increase the availability of cholecalciferol-based rodenticides, contributing to the increase in reports of exposures in animals (**Table 5**). On May 28, 2008, the Environmental Protection Agency released their final ruling on rodenticide risk mitigation measures. These measures required all products on the market to satisfy the new guidelines by June 2011.[1,2] The purpose of the regulatory changes is to reduce ecologic effects and exposure risk of children, wildlife, and pets to second-generation anticoagulant rodenticides, such as brodifacoum, bromadiolone, difethiolone, and difenacoum, by eliminating them from consumer products and requiring the use of bait stations for agricultural products. Although anticoagulant rodenticides continue to be used and the number of cases reported has increased (**Table 6**), the APCC has seen a slight increase in bromethalin-based rodenticide exposures. In 2002, bromethalin accounted for only 0.07% of cases, and that number increased to 0.16% in 2010 (**Table 7**).

Other noticeable trends in exposures come from the increased popularity of dark chocolates containing high percentages of cocoa and therefore greater methylxanthine content, and the increased availability of synthetic cannabinoids or K2. As marijuana becomes legalized, the number of cases increases. At this time, there are nine states and the District of Columbia that have legalized recreational marijuana, and 30 states with legal medical marijuana. Canada will make marijuana legal across the entire country in the Fall of 2018. Edibles frequently contain chocolate, and many products are using cannabutter or oil, which increases the amount of tetrahydrocannabinol in a product. Clinical signs noted after ingestion of edibles, oils, butter, waxes, or shatter are frequently much more intense than clinical signs noted after ingestion of joints or plant material.

TRENDS IN THERAPIES

Although there have been some recent additions to the therapies used to treat different toxicities, common mainstay medications and treatment recommendations

Table 5
Yearly cholecalciferol exposures from 2012 to 2018

Year	Cholecalciferol Exposures (Total Number of Cases)
2012	56
2013	59
2014	27
2015	20
2016	19
2017	21
2018 (Jan 1–May 31)	102

Table 6
Total number of anticoagulant cases (chlorphacinone, diphacinone, warfarin, brodifacoum, bromadiolone, difenacoum, difethialone) per year

Year	Anticoagulant Exposures (Total Number of Cases)
2012	4326
2013	4083
2014	3412
2015	3846
2016	4108
2017	5214

have included methocarbamol, use of fluids (intravenous and subcutaneous), omeprazole (Prilosec), sucralfate, acepromazine, monitoring of blood work profiles (blood chemistries and complete blood counts), and cyproheptadine. Decontamination with activated charcoal and induction of emesis also remain effective, especially in the dog. The use of activated charcoal in dogs and cats has decreased over the years. The decrease in the use of activated charcoal may be because of the potential of hypernatremia developing after the administration of activated charcoal in some dogs. Clearly, the use of activated charcoal in appropriate exposures is beneficial but, as with all therapies, clinicians must weigh risk versus benefit before using it.

The use of intravenous lipid fat emulsion in veterinary toxicology has become popular in recent years. The benefits and mechanism of action are still being studied, but there have been many anecdotal reports and some published data on efficacy when treating patients acutely exposed to lypophilic substances. It has been proposed that lipid emulsion therapy may be effective because small lipid particles have a high binding capacity, allowing them to trap highly lipid soluble substances; the lipids may activate calcium channels reversing intoxications from calcium channel blocking agents; or lipids can help overcome a decrease in fatty acid transport.[3] However, clinicians must remember it does not work in all cases, including some involving lipophilic substances. Lipids are discussed in Sharon Gwaltney-Brant and Irina Meadows' article, "Intravenous Lipid Emulsions in Veterinary Clinical Toxicology," in this issue.

Cholestyramine is the chloride salt of a basic anion exchange resin. It binds with bile acids in the intestine preventing reabsorption and producing a complex that is excreted in the feces. Cholestyramine was originally designed to help lower serum cholesterol in patients with primary hypercholesterolemia. It has also been used to treat toxicosis, particularly caused by overdose of amiodarone, digitoxin, chlordane, piroxicam, or vitamin D. In veterinary medicine, it is used particularly for vitamin D (or cholecalciferol) overdose, sago palm, Amanita mushroom ingestions, and

Table 7
Bromethalin exposures from 2012 to 2017

Year	Bromethalin Exposures (Total Number of Cases)
2012	1541
2013	1615
2014	2112
2015	2791
2016	3819
2017	4835

nonsteroidal anti-inflammatory drugs (particularly diclofenac, piroxicam, naproxen, or indomethacin).

SUMMARY

Veterinary toxicology is constantly evolving. Although the demographics of animals exposed to different toxicants remains steady, changes in society norms have an effect on the potential substances to which animals are exposed. Dogs are the species most commonly exposed to potentially toxic substances, and exposures are more often reported during summer months in the mid-afternoon. Current trends show that human medications continue to be a common risk for pets and that there has been an increase in the number of vitamin D exposures reported. As veterinary medicine advances, new and more effective therapies will continue to affect how suspected exposures to toxic substances are treated. Decontamination remains an important therapy to lessen the risk for signs after an exposure, and although its effectiveness remains debatable, the experimental use of intravenous lipid fat emulsion has risen. The continued monitoring of medical record databases ensures clinicians are up-to-date and well informed of emerging trends in toxicology. It is only by monitoring trends that such toxicities as lily exposures in cats, or grape and raisin toxicosis in dogs were discovered, and through which other new toxicities will be recognized.

REFERENCES

1. US Environmental Protection Agency. Risk mitigation decision for ten rodenticides. Washington, DC: United States Environmental Protection Agency; 2008.
2. AnTox Database. Risk mitigation decision for ten rodenticides. Urbana (IL): ASPCA Animals Poison Control Center 2001–2011.
3. O'Brien T, Clark-Price S, Evans E, et al. Infusion of a lipid emulsion to treat lidocaine intoxication in a cat. J Am Vet Med Assoc 2010;237:1455–8.

Investigative Diagnostic Toxicology and the Role of the Veterinarian in Pet Food–Related Outbreaks: An Update

Christina R. Wilson-Frank, PhD[a,b,*], Stephen B. Hooser, DVM, PhD[a,b]

KEYWORDS

- Food-related illness • Pet food • Outbreak • Pet food recall • Diagnostic testing

KEY POINTS

- The veterinarian plays a crucial role in recognizing and helping diagnose pet food–related outbreaks.
- Because of the potential local and global implications of pet food contamination associated outbreaks, proper reporting and consultation with the government and state agencies are crucial.
- Accurate diagnoses and identification of the source of illness in these outbreaks are promising when thorough case histories are documented, appropriate samples are collected, and resources available at the state and federal agencies, such as veterinary diagnostic laboratories and the Food and Drug Administration Center for Veterinary Medicine, are used effectively.

PET FOOD–RELATED OUTBREAKS AND RECALLS

Contaminated pet food, resulting in animal illness, can be due to several factors, such as incorrect formulation of the nutritional components in the food, insufficiencies in analytical testing of food for toxins or toxicants, mixing errors during the production process, or incorporation of contaminated raw materials (eg, grains, meats, or other feed components) into the product.[1] Although industry quality control measures and

This article is an update of the previously published article in the March 2012 issue of *Veterinary Clinics of North America: Small Animal Practice*.

The authors have nothing to disclose.

[a] Indiana Animal Disease Diagnostic Laboratory, College of Veterinary Medicine, Purdue University, 406 South University, West Lafayette, IN 47907-1175, USA; [b] Department of Comparative Pathobiology, College of Veterinary Medicine, Purdue University, 725 Harrison Street, West Lafayette, IN 47907-1175, USA

* Corresponding author. Indiana Animal Disease Diagnostic Laboratory, Department of Comparative Pathobiology, Purdue University, 406 South University, West Lafayette, IN 47907-1175.

E-mail address: wilsonc@purdue.edu

voluntary recalls by pet food manufacturers usually preclude incidents of adverse health events in animals, there have been a few instances in which pet food contamination has been associated with significant morbidity or mortality in dogs and cats. For example, in 2006 and 2010, feed mixing errors resulted in incorrect formulations of vitamin D in a pet food product. In the 2010 incident, the ingredient supplier for the pet food manufacturer produced a vitamin D supplement immediately before preparing ingredients for the pet food. Residual vitamin D in the manufacturing process carried over into the pet food ingredients caused cross-contamination of the product. According to the Food and Drug Administration (FDA), the 2010 recall resulted in 36 reported cases of nephrotoxicity nationwide.[2,3]

Adulteration of pet food products has also occurred due to contamination during general food processing. In 2006, *Salmonella enterica* serotype Schwarzengrund was responsible for widespread recalls of dry dog and cat food.[4] The number of affected animals in this outbreak, which was reported in 19 states, totaled 79. Contamination was thought to be due to the presence of the *Salmonella* strain in a flavoring room where the manufacturer sprayed the product to enhance palatability. In 2018, a recall was issued for approximately 4000 pounds of ground turkey–containing pet food products due to potential *Salmonella* contamination in which 2 children became ill and several pets also died or became ill when exposed to the product.[5] *Salmonella* bacteria–contaminated raw or undercooked meat products were thought to be the source of the adulteration in this case. Voluntary recalls due to suspect *Salmonella* contamination in pig ear products, pet treats, and canned or dry dog and cat food happen occasionally and are usually initiated before food-borne illness is reported.

Another example of pet food–related illness occurred in 2005 when approximately 19 varieties of dog food were recalled due to contamination with aflatoxin.[6] Various animals in 23 different states in the United States and 29 other countries to which the product was exported were affected. It was later discovered that corn and corn products contaminated with aflatoxin were inadvertently incorporated into commercial dog food. This error was likely due to the company not adhering to its own quality control guidelines for aflatoxin testing in shipments of corn to be used in the product.

Possibly the most notable pet food–related outbreak was the occurrence of renal failure in dogs and cats exposed to food adulterated with melamine and cyanuric acid, which resulted in a massive recall of pet food in the United States in 2007. In this incident, it was discovered that wheat and rice gluten incorporated into pet food was artificially contaminated with melamine and cyanuric acid in order to increase the apparent protein concentration of the product. Exposure to toxic amounts of these chemicals caused formation of yellow-brown melamine-cyanuric acid crystals in renal tubules, resulting in proximal tubular epithelial damage, necrosis leading to nephrotoxicity in exposed cats and dogs.[7] More than 1000 commercial pet foods were recalled due to this widespread adulteration.[8] Approximately 450 cases of renal failure were reported in cats and dogs, of which approximately 100 animals died.[9,10]

THE ROLE OF THE VETERINARIAN AND THE HUMAN ELEMENT

It is evident that the veterinarian plays a crucial role in recognizing adverse events associated with pet food adulteration and the severity of animal health risk. Although these occurrences have a tremendous impact on animal health, the veterinarian must also be cognizant of the potential human health risks. For example, human exposure to *Salmonella* Schwarzengrund–contaminated pet food (through handling) resulted in the first case of human salmonellosis linked to the use of dry cat and dog food.[10] In this outbreak, 79 people were infected. Of these 79 people, 48% were children under the age of 2 years. This case emphasizes the importance of the veterinarian in educating pet households on the proper handling and storage of pet foods. It also underscores the need for veterinarians to have an awareness of potential human exposure in pet client households, in addition to being attentive to animal health effects.

Also, highlighting the importance of the role of the veterinarian is the fact that animals can serve as sentinels for human exposure to various toxins or toxicants. An example of this was highlighted when nephrotoxicity had occurred in dogs and cats due to melamine-cyanuric acid–contaminated pet foods in 2007. Recognition of this pet food contamination event seems to have expedited the relationship between the development of nephrolithiasis and acute kidney injury in children likely due to the consumption of melamine-cyanuric acid–contaminated infant formula in 2008. Because of this unfortunate event, an estimated 53,000 children were affected and 6 deaths were reported in China.[11–13] Therefore, the potential for human health risk and the global implications of these incidents emphasize the significance of the role of veterinarian with respect to both animal and human health.

ESTABLISHING A CAUSAL RELATIONSHIP BETWEEN CLINICAL SIGNS AND SUSPECT FOODSTUFF
Obtaining a Thorough Case History

Recent changes in pet's food or treats that coincide chronologically with changes in the animal's eating behavior or with onset of health-related problems can be an early indication of a food contamination issue. Documenting a thorough case history is the most crucial, initial step in successfully establishing a causal relationship between the animal's clinical signs and the suspect food source. Being thorough in taking the case history helps ascertain whether other differentials should be considered during the diagnostic workup for the case. Working in collaboration with the pet owner, the veterinarian should begin the case history at a point in time preceding the owner's first discovery that there was a problem and then progress chronologically from that point. A thorough case history should include detailed information about the animal or animals exposed as well as the pet food product in question. **Boxes 1** and **2** include important information that should be considered when taking the case history.

Box 1
Information regarding the animal exposed

1. Signalment (sex, breed, age, weight of animal)

2. Animal's complete medical history (including vaccinations, current and previous medications, and treatments given)

3. Results of any diagnostic testing or clinical pathology tests performed (eg, complete blood count, chemistries, urinalysis, serology)

4. Description of the progression of clinical signs (onset time, duration, and types of clinical signs exhibited by the pet)

5. Timeframe between feeding product and onset of clinical signs/change in behavior

6. Duration of exposure and approximate amount of food product animal consumed

7. Number of animals affected in the household

8. Number of animals and humans potentially exposed

9. Description of how the owner stored/handled the pet food

10. Other potential sources of exposures to other toxins/toxicants/drugs in pet's environment

---

Box 2
Information regarding the pet food product in question

1. Brand name and product's description from the label

2. Types of food (kibble, moist, semi-moist, frozen, freeze dried, raw)

3. Prescription types of food (renal, dermatologic, gastroenteric, overweight management, and other)

4. Purchase date, purchase location, and total amount purchased

5. Type of product container (can, pouch, bag, other)

6. Name of the manufacturer of the product

7. Lot number and expiration date (best by or best before date)

8. UPC code (barcode)

9. Product date and product code

10. Amount of food product used and the amount unused owner still has

11. Where and how the product was stored (storage conditions)

The case information obtained by the veterinarian must be documented in case records with time and date. Once the case history and the information regarding the pet food in question have been completed, the veterinarian can use the pet food product information to query the FDA Center for Veterinary Medicine (CVM) pet food recall products list. Accessing the pet food recall products list will help to establish whether the pet food product in question has already been recalled due to contamination or other adulteration. The pet food recall products list can be accessed at their Web site at https://www.fda.gov/AnimalVeterinary/SafetyHealth/RecallsWithdrawals. Other useful resources regarding pet food recalls, case consultation, or information include contacting a state veterinarian, the Veterinary Information Network, the ASPCA Animal Poison Control Center, the Pet Poison Helpline, or veterinary diagnostic laboratories.

Effective Use of Veterinary Diagnostic Laboratories

Collecting appropriate samples for diagnostic testing
After the case history is thoroughly documented, establishing differential diagnoses will likely begin with performing diagnostic tests. Therefore, collecting the appropriate samples from the affected animals and saving as much of the suspect pet food product as possible will be the key to arriving at an accurate diagnosis. After doing some fact finding, particularly if a recall has been initiated, the veterinarian may already have knowledge of the contaminant/adulterant of concern. In this case, the veterinarian can query the American Association of Veterinary Laboratory Diagnosticians' Web site (http://www.aavld.org/) to investigate which veterinary diagnostic laboratory would be appropriate for consulting regarding information about appropriate sample collection and diagnostic testing, if necessary. The information provided at this website will direct the veterinarian to which veterinary diagnostic laboratory can perform analytical testing for that specific analyte and obtain guidance regarding which sample or samples are recommended for submission. In addition, the FDA CVM or the manufacturer of the pet food product can be contacted regarding guidance for analytical testing. It is likely that the FDA CVM or the manufacturer of the product will also perform follow-up testing on the foodstuff in question.

As part of the diagnostic investigative toxicology workup, it is imperative that the client or veterinarian retains as much of the food product as possible. Retaining these samples includes storing the product in its original packaging (no subsampling from the bag, can, pouch, or so forth). There are some adulterants or contaminants for which diagnostic testing of biological samples is limited. For example, aflatoxin M_1 was detected in 7 out of 8 submitted livers from one of the feed-related aflatoxin outbreaks in dogs.[5] Although aflatoxin M_1 was detected in this case, diagnostic methods for testing aflatoxins in tissues have not been developed or validated to the extent that veterinary diagnostic laboratories could offer it as a routine diagnostic test. However, there are sensitive, accurate methods for quantitating aflatoxins in foodstuffs. Therefore, it is imperative to save as much of the pet food product because this may be the only sample that can be analyzed for the case in question. Approximately 1 kg of dry food or 4 cans of food should be saved for analysis, and some should be saved for future reference. Food should be properly identified and labeled (date and time of collection; sample type and site of collection) and stored frozen or at room temperature in an airtight bag or jar. Other source material can be collected, such as water (eg, from their water bowl) and other foodstuffs the animal has eaten within the timeframe of onset of clinical signs.

In addition to saving the suspect food source, collecting biological samples from affected animals is also essential. Antemortem samples should be collected as soon as possible after exposure and stored at the appropriate conditions. A list of recommended, antemortem samples to collect is described in **Table 1**. Whole blood collected should be stored refrigerated until analysis. Although the other antemortem samples listed in **Table 1** can be stored refrigerated for several days, it is recommended that they be stored frozen until analysis.

In circumstances in which animal mortality has occurred, performing a complete necropsy on the animal is highly recommended. Although the practitioner can perform a necropsy and collect the appropriate tissue samples for testing, submitting the animal for a complete necropsy to a veterinary diagnostic laboratory would be optimal. At the diagnostic laboratory, a thorough gross and histopathologic examination can be performed by a veterinary pathologist. Pathology results can help refine the differential diagnoses or direct further testing. If the practitioner performs the necropsy, the postmortem samples recommended for collecting are listed in **Table 1**. It is important to

Table 1	
Antemortem and postmortem samples to collect for diagnostic testing	
Antemortem	**Postmortem**
Suspect pet food product[a]	Suspect pet food product[a]
Whole blood (EDTA)	Brain (half in 10% formalin and the other half frozen)
Serum or plasma	Eyeball or ocular fluid[b]
Vomitus or ingesta[b]	Ingesta[b]
Urine[b]	Liver (one piece in 10% formalin and one piece frozen)
Samples for infectious disease testing	Kidney (one piece in 10% formalin and one piece frozen)
Other source material[c]	Intestinal contents Urine[b] Samples for infectious disease testing Other source material[c]

[a] Save entire suspect pet food product in the original package (eg, bag, can, pouch).
[b] Store chilled or frozen.
[c] Collect other source material such as other food sources or water.

document any remarkable, gross anatomic observations noted during the necropsy. After fixing representative tissue samples in 10% formalin for histopathology, the remaining samples procured by the practitioner can be refrigerated; however, for long-term storage, samples should be kept frozen. Ideally, 2 sets of tissue samples should be prepared. One set should be composed of thinly sliced tissues stored in 10% formalin for histologic examination. The other set should include large, frozen tissues (50–100 g each if possible) for toxicology testing.

Toxicology testing is often limited by inadequate sample size or submission of an inappropriate sample; therefore, it is important to collect as much of each sample as possible to maximize diagnostic testing efforts, particularly if testing in multiple laboratories is warranted. Being cognizant of the fact that the causative agent or contaminant may not be toxicologically relevant (ie, an infectious agent) is another reason to be thorough and complete in collecting samples from affected animals for diagnostic testing.

REPORTING A PET FOOD COMPLAINT
Agencies Regulating Commercial Pet Foods

The Association of American Feed Control Officials (AAFCO) works in collaboration with the FDA to ensure the safety of commercial pet foods. The AAFCO regulations on pet food products are intended to address the nutrient content of pet foods and label claims on the product to guarantee uniform consistency and enforcement of these claims.[12] The FDA's role involves regulating health claims on pet food products, particularly regarding the safety of new ingredients or food additives. In 2007, the FDA Amendments Act was passed, giving the FDA more jurisdiction for taking action against pet food contamination or safety issues.[12] The FDA CVM is the primary authority for regulating health claims on pet food labels.

How to Report a Pet Food Complaint

Veterinarians should not wait for diagnostic testing to be completed before reporting a pet food–borne illness. If the practitioner has reasonable suspicion that the adverse health event was due to pet food contamination, he or she should initially contact the manufacturer of the food product. The manufacturer may be able to provide insight into the potential issue and will also need that information to trace increased occurrences associated with a particular product or ascertain if there is an outbreak associated with a specific geographic location. If there is heightened suspicion that a contaminant in pet food is the source of illness (eg, diagnostic tests are completed or most differentials are eliminated), then the veterinarian should report a pet food complaint to the FDA CVM. A complaint can be reported electronically through the FDA's "Safety Reporting Portal" or it can be reported by calling the FDA Consumer Complaint Coordinator in that state. By opening the FDA CVM Web site (https://www.safetyreporting.hhs.gov/), the "Safety Reporting Portal" can be accessed electronically and information regarding the clinical case history and pet food product can be entered. If reporting by telephone, the FDA CVM Web site (http://www.fda.gov/Safety/ReportaProblem/ConsumerComplaintCoordinators/) has an "FDA Consumer Complaint Coordinators" directory that lists the telephone number for the coordinators in each state. The practitioner can also contact their state veterinarian, the Office of the State Chemist, or its equivalent in that state or notify state veterinary diagnostic laboratories to make them aware of the issue. If human exposure is suspected, then the state department of human health should be notified.

SUMMARY

Although pet food products are generally safe and incidences of contamination are rare given the enormous quantities of pet foods manufactured and sold, there are still some instances in which pet food–borne illness occurs in dogs and cats. The veterinarian plays a crucial role in recognizing and helping diagnose these adverse events, including assessing the severity of animal and human health risks. Because of the potential local and global implications of pet food contamination associated outbreaks, proper reporting and consultation with the government and state agencies are crucial. Accurate diagnoses and identification of the source of illness in these outbreaks are promising when thorough case histories are documented, appropriate samples are collected, and resources available at the state and federal agencies, such as veterinary diagnostic laboratories and the FDA CVM, are used effectively.

REFERENCES

1. Remillard RL. Homemade diets: attributes, pitfalls, and a call for action. Top Companion Anim Med 2008;23(3):137–42.
2. Press release. Blue Buffalo Company, Ltd. Recalls limited production code dates of dry dog food because of possible excess vitamin D. http://www.fda.gov/AnimalVeterinary/default.htm. Accessed December 6, 2011.
3. Refsal K, Schenck P. Pet food illness in dogs results in a national recall. Q Newsl DCPA Health News 2010;4:2.
4. Centers for Disease Control and Prevention. Update: recall of dry dog and cat food products associated with human Salmonella Schwarzengrund infections: United States. Morb Mortal Wkly Rep 2008;57:1200–2.
5. Raws for Paws recalls turkey pet food because of possible *Salmonella* health risk. 2018. Available at: https://www.fda.gov/Safety/Recalls/ucm596043.htm. Accessed June 09, 2018.
6. Stenske KA, Smith JR, Newman SJ, et al. Aflatoxicosis in dogs dealing with suspected contaminated commercial foods. J Am Vet Med Assoc 2006;228: 1686–91.
7. Brown CA, Jeong K, Poppenga RH, et al. Outbreaks of renal failure associated with melamine and cyanuric acid in dogs and cats in 2004 and 2007. J Vet Diagn Invest 2007;19:525–31.
8. Rumbeiha WK, Agnew D, Maxie G, et al. Analysis of a survey database of pet food-induced poisoning in North America. J Med Toxicol 2010;6:172–84.
9. Puschner B, Reimschuessel R. Toxicosis caused by melamine and cyanuric acid in dogs and cats: uncovering the mystery and subsequent global implications. Clin Lab Med 2011;31:181–99.
10. Behravesh CB, Ferraro A, Deasy M, et al. Human Salmonella infections linked to contaminated dry dog and cat food, 2006-2008. Pediatrics 2010;126:477–83.
11. Bhalla V, Grimm PC, Chertow GM, et al. Melamine nephrotoxicity: an emerging epidemic in an era of globalization. Kidney Int 2009;75:774–9.
12. Xin H, Stone R. Chinese probe unmasks high-tech adulteration with melamine. Science 2008;322:1310–1.
13. Chase LP, Daristotle L, Hayek MG, et al. History and regulation of pet foods. In: Canine and feline nutrition: a resource for companion animal professionals. 3rd edition. Maryland Heights (MO): Mosby; 2011. p. 121–9.

Pet Food Recalls and Pet Food Contaminants in Small Animals: An Update

Karyn Bischoff, DVM, MS[a,b,*], Wilson K. Rumbeiha, BVM, PhD[c]

KEYWORDS

- Aflatoxin • Cholecalciferol • Cyanuric acid • Melamine • Thiamine • Vitamin B_1
- Vitamin D

KEY POINTS

- Commercial pet foods are usually safe, but incidents of contamination can have a devastating impact on companion animals and their owners.
- There are numerous possible contaminants ranging from natural contaminants to nutrient imbalances to chemical adulteration, making it impossible to predict what will cause the next pet food recall.
- Veterinarians involvement with pet food recalls includes examining and treating affected animals, documentation and sample collection, and communicating with pet food manufacturers and regulatory agencies.

Most pet foods are safe. Only 1.7% of reported poisonings in dogs and cats are attributed to pet foods.[1] Incidents of contamination occur through microbial action, mixing error, or intentional adulteration. Although rare, the effects of pet food contamination can be physically devastating for companion animals and emotionally devastating and financially burdensome for their owners. Whereas most people consume a diet from various sources, for companion animals a single bag of food or cans from a single brand and lot will likely be the major or sole source of nutrition until that food has been completely consumed. Thus, the effects of food contaminants in people is diluted by the varied diet, but the uniform diet of most dogs and cats, although

This article is an update of the previously published article in the March 2012 issue of *Veterinary Clinics of North America: Small Animal Practice*.

The authors have nothing to disclose.

[a] New York State Animal Health Diagnostic Center, PO Box 5786, Room A2, 232, Ithaca, NY 13081, USA; [b] Department of Population Medicine and Diagnostic Sciences, Cornell University, PO Box 5786, Room A2 232, Ithaca, NY 14853-5786, USA; [c] Veterinary Diagnostics and Production Animal Medicine, College of Veterinary Medicine, Iowa State University, 2659 Vet Med, Ames, IA 50011, USA

* Corresponding author. Department of Population Medicine and Diagnostic Sciences, Cornell University, PO Box 5786, Room A2 232, Ithaca, NY 14853-5786.

E-mail address: KLB72@cornell.edu

preferred for nutritional reasons, increases the risk of adverse effects if a contaminant is present. As the companion animal veterinarian is aware, many animal owners consider their dog or cat to be a vulnerable family member that needs to be protected.[2] Based on the authors' experiences, pet owners often experience seemingly disproportionate guilt when pets become sickened or die after they have been unknowingly fed contaminated pet foods. Some owners have described feeling responsible for poisoning their pet during pet food contamination incidents.

When pet food is contaminated or adulterated, there is usually a food recall. There are 3 types of recalls involving chemical contaminants: class I—reasonable probability that the contaminated food will cause adverse health consequences or death; class II—the contaminated food can cause temporary or medically reversible adverse health consequences but is unlikely to cause serious adverse health effects; and class III—the contaminated food is unlikely to cause adverse health consequences. There were 22 class I and II pet food recalls in the United States over a 12-year period (1996–2008), and 6 were due to chemical contaminants.[3] Of these 6, 2 were due to aflatoxin (a mycotoxin), 3 were due to feed mixing or formulation errors (2 excess vitamin D_3 and 1 excess methionine), and 1 was due to adulteration of food ingredients with melamine and related compounds.[3]

Since 2008, there have been cat foods and dog foods recalled due to mixing or formulation errors (inadequate thiamine in the cat foods, excessive vitamin D_3 in dog food), due to contamination with aflatoxin, and due to contamination with pentobarbital. There have also been warnings in the United States, Canada, and Australia concerning a Fanconi-like renal syndrome in dogs after ingestion of large amounts of chicken jerky treat products, manufactured in China.[4–6] Despite extensive testing, the cause of the adverse health effects associated with consumption of chicken jerky has not been discovered.

Pet food contamination incidents due to adulteration are rare but occurred with melamine and cyanuric acid. The melamine contamination investigation in 2007 led to the discovery that other cases of melamine poisoning had happened in companion and agricultural animals in the Republic of Korea, Japan, Thailand, Malaysia, Singapore, Taiwan, the Philippines, South Africa, Spain, China, and Italy.[7–11]

There have been several other international pet food contamination incidents. There have been occasional news reports of aflatoxin contamination of dog food in South Africa and Israel since 2006. The use of sulfur dioxide, which destroys thiamine, in pet foods has been associated with repeated outbreaks of polioencephalomalacia in dogs and cats in Australia.[12–14] Also in Australia, there was a unique recall of irradiated cat food in 2008 to 2009, after it was found to cause severe central nervous system damage to cats. The proximate cause of the neurologic disorder that afflicted cats fed irradiated pet food in Australia has not been determined to date. More recently, there was an Australian recall of cat food associated with neurologic effects, although a diagnosis was not definitively made.

The Food and Drug Administration (FDA) is charged with ensuring the wholesomeness of pet foods. The US Congress passed the FDA Amendments Act of 2007 (FDAAA) to improve responsiveness to contamination of pet foods and other products after the adulteration of pet food with melamine and related compounds was identified that year. The FDAAA requires manufacturers to report incidents of possible contamination to the FDA within 24 hours, investigate the cause, and report findings of the investigation. When contamination is confirmed, the pet food is recalled. Recall initiation is usually voluntary by the manufacturer at the request of the FDA. The FDA can secure a court order to issue a recall if the manufacturer is reluctant, but this is rare because of the bad publicity and increased potential for litigation should a manufacturer refuse to initiate a recall.[1]

Veterinarians must be involved for the FDAAA to work properly. The veterinarian must examine and treat animals when adverse effects from pet foods are suspected, document their findings, collect appropriate samples, advise pet owners, and contact the FDA and pet food manufacturers. Samples for laboratory analysis include the suspected food and its packaging (or, if unavailable, lot numbers, manufacturing codes, and other identifying information), and samples from the pet such as blood, serum, urine, vomitus or gastric lavage fluids, and feces. A full necropsy with postmortem sample collection for histopathology and analytical chemistry includes fresh urine, adipose tissue, and heart blood, fresh and fixed brain, liver, and kidney, and fixed lung, spleen, and bone marrow. These samples are often required to rule in or out toxins when the affected animal dies or is euthanized. Often the pet food manufacturer will help with associated costs of treatment and testing; thus, it is in the interests of the pet owner and veterinarian to contact them as soon as contamination is suspected. Manufacturer contact information is usually found on product packaging. Consumer complaints can be reported to local FDA consumer complaint coordinators or online (http://www.fda.gov/cvm/petfoods.htm). Local government agriculture or food safety agencies should also be alerted when contamination of a commercial product is suspected.

The rest of this text gives some details concerning major pet food contamination or formulation errors that have been associated with morbidity and mortality in pets in the United States, with mention of some minor contaminants and formulation errors. The most common natural contaminant of pet food is aflatoxin, a fungal metabolite. Common conditions that have been associated with misformulation include hypervitaminosis D and polioencephalomalacia. Last, included in the category of adulterants are melamine and related cyanuric acid, as well as pentobarbital.

NATURAL AND ACCIDENTAL CONTAMINANTS

The most common natural contaminants in pet foods are mycotoxins (fungal metabolites). Aflatoxins are the most common mycotoxins to cause pet food recalls in the United States, but other mycotoxin contaminants have been reported. There was a recall of dog food due to contamination with the mycotoxin deoxynivalenol (DON) in 1995. DON is produced on grain by *Fusarium* spp under temperate conditions. Pet food DON concentrations of greater than 4.5 ppm and 7.7 ppm were associated with feed refusal in dogs and cats, respectively, and concentrations of 8 ppm or greater caused vomiting in both species.[15,16] Animals recover quickly once the food is replaced, although supportive care is needed if gastroenteritis is severe.[16]

Mercury contamination is also considered here. Mercury bioaccumulates in seafood and elevated mercury concentrations in dogs and cats on fish-based diets have historically been reported.[17,18] The authors have noted a recent increase in interest among veterinarians and the industry in pet food mercury content. Cats are considered one of the most susceptible species to mercury toxicosis.[19] A study by Ganther and Sunde[20] determined that cats could tolerate dietary mercury concentrations of up to approximately 3 ppm (presumably on a wet-weight basis) for 21 weeks without evidence of toxicosis, but they reported significant morbidity and mortality in cats fed diets containing 2 ppm mercury for more than 29 weeks. Blood mercury concentrations were approximately 100 μg/dL in unaffected cats and 600 μg/dL in affected cats. Because clinical signs of mercury toxicosis in cats, which include ataxia, proprioceptive deficits, incoordination, and muscle weakness, can resemble those associated with polioencephalomalacia,[19] thiamine deficiency should be ruled out before making the diagnosis of mercury toxicosis.

Aflatoxin

Aflatoxicosis in dogs was first described in 1952 as "hepatitis X" and reproduced in experimental dogs using contaminated feed in 1955, then by dosing with purified aflatoxin B_1 in 1966. Moldy corn poisoning in swine in the 1940s and turkey X disease in turkeys fed peanut meal were also linked to aflatoxin.

Aflatoxins are a group of related compounds *sometimes* produced as metabolites of various fungi, *Aspergillus parasiticus*, *Aspergillus flavus*, *Aspergillus nomius*, some *Penicillium* spp, and others. Names of common aflatoxins are derived from the colors that fluoresce: aflatoxins B_1, the most common and potent form, and B_2 fluoresce blue. Aflatoxins B_1 and B_2 both fluoresce green. High-energy foods, such as corn, peanuts, and cottonseed, are most often affected. Rice, wheat, oats, sweet potatoes, potatoes, barley, millet, sesame, sorghum, cacao beans, almonds, soy, coconut, safflower, sunflower, palm kernel, cassava, cowpeas, peas, and various spices can also be affected.[21,22] Aflatoxin production can occur on field crops or in storage. Temperature, humidity, drought stress, insect damage, and handling techniques influence mycotoxin production.[21] Use of aflatoxin-contaminated food commodities in the manufacture of pet foods has caused intoxication in pets. Improper storage of dog food and ingestion of moldy garbage have been implicated in aflatoxicosis.[23]

Dogs and cats are very sensitive to aflatoxin.[22] The oral median lethal dose (LD_{50}) for aflatoxin in dogs is between 0.5 and 1.5 mg/kg.[24] The experimental oral LD_{50} for cats is 0.55 mg/kg, although field cases in cats are rare.[22] It is difficult to determine the total dose of aflatoxin received in field cases, where the period of exposure and amount fed are not always available. Aflatoxin concentrations of 60 ppb in dog food have been implicated in aflatoxicosis.[24] Factors associated with increased susceptibility to aflatoxicosis include genetic predisposition, concurrent disease, age, and sex, with young males and pregnant females considered particularly susceptible.[24,25]

Aflatoxin is highly lipophilic and absorbed rapidly and almost completely, particularly in young animals, mostly in the duodenum. Aflatoxin entering the portal circulation is highly protein bound in the blood. The unbound fraction is distributed to the tissues, with highest concentrations accumulating in the liver.[21] The liver is the primary site of metabolism, although some takes place in other tissues, including the kidneys and small intestine. Phase I metabolism of aflatoxin B_1 by cytochrome P450 enzymes produces the reactive intermediate aflatoxin B_1 8,9-epoxide. Some aflatoxin B_1 is eventually metabolized to aflatoxin M_1.[25] During phase II metabolism, aflatoxin B_1 8,9-epoxide is conjugated to glutathione in a reaction catalyzed by glutathione S-transferase.[26] Metabolites of aflatoxin are excreted in the urine and bile, primarily as M_1 in dogs. More than 90% of metabolized aflatoxin detected in canine urine is excreted within the first 12 hours, and urine aflatoxin is below detectable concentrations within 48 hours.[27] Conjugated aflatoxin is excreted mostly in bile.[21]

Aflatoxin B_1 8,9-epoxide is a potent electrophile and binds readily to cellular macromolecules such as nucleic acids, proteins, and constituents of subcellular organelles.[28] Formation of DNA adducts modifies the DNA template and the ability of DNA polymerase to bind, affecting cellular replication. Binding to ribosomal translocase effects protein production.[24,29] These changes can lead to necrosis of hepatocytes and other metabolically active cells such as renal tubular epithelium.[25] Coagulopathy results from synthetic hepatic failure and decreased prothrombin and fibrinogen.[30] No carcinogenic effects have been reported in cats and dogs, although aflatoxins are known to cause cancer in some species, including rats, ferrets, ducks, trout, swine, sheep, and rats, and are classified by the International Agency for Research on Cancer as class I human carcinogens.[22,29]

The presentation of aflatoxicosis in small animals may be acute or chronic. Exposure to contaminated foods can occur for weeks or months before dogs become clinically affected; indeed, in one author's experience, contaminated food was removed from the diet of a dog approximately 3 weeks before clinical aflatoxicosis was evident. Many dogs die within a few days of initial clinical signs, but illness can be protracted for up to 2 weeks.[25] Early clinical signs of aflatoxicosis in dogs include feed refusal or anorexia, weakness and obtundation, vomiting, and diarrhea. Later, dogs become icteric, often with melena or frank blood in the feces, hematemesis, petechia, and epistaxis.[22,31] Experimentally poisoned cats died within 3 days of onset of signs.[22]

Complete blood cell count, serum chemistry, including bile acids, and urinalysis are helpful to support the diagnosis of aflatoxin poisoning and rule out other causes of liver failure. Total bilirubin is increased in aflatoxicosis and hepatic enzyme concentrations, including alanine aminotransferase, aspartate aminotransferase, alkaline phosphatase, and gamma-glutamyl transpeptidase, can be variably elevated.[24,25] Liver function tests are often more helpful in supporting the diagnosis. Prothrombin time increases due to decreased synthesis of clotting factors, and serum albumin, protein C, antithrombin III, and cholesterol concentrations decrease.[31]

Diagnosis of aflatoxicosis is usually based on history, clinical signs, clinical pathology findings, and postmortem changes. Differential diagnoses for dogs in food contamination–related cases of aflatoxicosis have included leptospirosis, parvovirus, and anticoagulant rodenticide toxicosis based on the severe gastrointestinal hemorrhage, and a variety of hepatotoxic agents including acetaminophen, xylitol, microcystin from cyanobacteria (blue-green algae), amanitin and phalloidin from mushrooms, toxins associated with cycad palms, phosphine, and iron.[24,31,32] Necropsy is helpful in ruling out other conditions and confirming the diagnosis. Common gross findings include icterus, hepatomegaly with evidence of lipidosis (**Fig. 1**), ascites, gastrointestinal hemorrhage, and multifocal petechia and ecchymosis.[24,30,31] The primary histologic changes of canine aflatoxicosis are associated with the liver, although pigmentary nephrosis and necrosis of the proximal convoluted renal tubules have been reported.[24,30] Liver lesions in acute aflatoxicosis include fatty degeneration of hepatocytes with one to numerous lipid vacuoles. Centrilobular necrosis and canalicular cholestasis with mild inflammation are commonly reported.[23,30,31] Dogs with

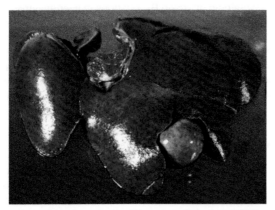

Fig. 1. Liver from a dog with aflatoxicosis. (*Courtesy of* Prof. S.P. McDonough, DVM, PhD, DAVCP, Ithaca, NY.)

subacute toxicosis still have fatty degeneration, canalicular cholestasis, and multifocal to locally extensive necrosis, often with neutrophilic inflammation and evidence of regeneration. Fibrosis is more prominent in subacute and chronic toxicosis, with bridging of portal triads, bile ductule proliferation, and obfuscation of the central vein by dilated sinusoids. Chronic aflatoxicosis is characterized by less fatty degeneration, marked fibrosis, and regenerative nodules, causing disruption of the normal hepatic architecture.[30] Experimental cats with aflatoxicosis had hepatomegaly with petechiation, minimal hepatocystic glycogen storage, and, in cats surviving more than 72 hours, bile duct hyperplasia was also present.[22]

Laboratory testing of dog food or other implicated material helps to confirm the diagnosis, but due to the extended time between exposure and onset of aflatoxicosis, the contaminated food is often unavailable. Before the 2005 dog food recall, a veterinarian submitted dog food from each of 3 households, only 2 of which had dogs with clinical aflatoxicosis, to a laboratory. The single sample that contained aflatoxin in toxicologically significant concentrations was from the household of the dog that had no clinical signs of toxicosis at the time of submission.

Commercial grain is routinely screened for aflatoxin, but sampling error is possible due to the uneven distribution of mold within grain and other commodities. Current analytical techniques use enzyme-linked immunosorbent assays, high-performance liquid chromatography, and liquid chromatography/mass spectrometry to detect aflatoxin. Some laboratories can test for aflatoxin M_1 in the urine, but urinary excretion is very rapid in dogs.[27] Urine may be useful for a period of up to 48 hours after exposure. Serum or liver can be analyzed, but due to the rapid metabolism and excretion of aflatoxin, this testing is often of limited usefulness.[24]

The prognosis for dogs with clinical aflatoxicosis is guarded. Early intervention improves the prognosis, but many cases fail to respond to treatment.[23,24] Patient assessment and stabilization are the first steps in management. Remove access to contaminated food and replace it with a high-quality protein-containing diet if the dog continues to eat. Supportive care includes hydration and electrolyte corrections with intravenous fluids, which can be supplemented with B vitamins, vitamin K, and dextrose.[25] Plasma transfusions improve coagulation ability.[24] Sucralfate, famotidine, and sometimes parenteral nutrition have been used for anorexic dogs and those with severe gastroenteritis.[24,29]

Liver protectants, such as silymarin (a mix of silybin and other flavolignans from milk thistle), have been used clinically and experimentally. When silymarin was given to chickens fed diets containing aflatoxin B_1, changes in liver enzyme profiles and histologic lesions were diminished compared with controls on clean diets.[28] A proposed mechanism of action for silybin is inhibition of phase I metabolism of aflatoxin B_1, thus decreasing epoxide production.[24,29] S-Adenosylmethionine, which can act as a sulfhydryl donor, has been used as a hepatoprotectant in aflatoxicosis.[24,31] N-Acetylcysteine, a commonly used sulfhydryl donor, is given parenterally rather than orally for severely affected dogs. Experimentally, N-acetylcysteine (Mucomyst) enhanced elimination of aflatoxin B_1 and prevented liver damage in poultry.[26]

MISFORMULATION

As noted earlier, misformulation is a common cause of adverse reactions to pet foods in cats and dogs. Hypervitaminosis D and thiamine deficiency are discussed in detail later. Other misformulations have involved methionine, which caused a US recall, and excessive vitamin A in Thailand. Excessive methionine was associated with anorexia and vomiting.[3] Misformulation of a feline research diet in Thailand in 2009 resulted in evident hypervitaminosis A (Dr Rosama Pusoonthornthum, personal communication, 2009). Hypervitaminosis A in cats and dogs causes osteopathy, commonly affecting the axial skeleton, and often presents as lameness, paresis, or paralysis due to entrapment of spinal nerves.[33,34] Some animals with hypervitaminosis A, even those severely affected, recover in the long term after they are placed on a new diet.

Hypervitaminosis D

Of the essential vitamins, vitamin D is the one that has been most frequently involved in pet food recalls. Vitamin D serves many physiologic roles, and regulation of calcium and phosphorous metabolism is one of the major roles. Other physiologic roles include immunomodulation and improved reproduction in animals. There are 2 major active forms of vitamin D in mammals. These forms are ergocalciferol (vitamin D_2) and chole-calciferol (vitamin D_3). There is also increasing use of 1,25-dihhydroxy vitamin D_3 in animal feeds, particularly poultry and swine feeds. Oversupplementation and unintentional cross-contamination have caused vitamin D_3 excess in pet food.

There have been multiple pet food recalls triggered by excessive vitamin D_3 in recent decades. In 1999, a dog food was recalled due to excessive amounts of cholecalciferol. In 2006, 4 products from the same manufacturer were recalled also due to excessive amounts of cholecalciferol. More recently, in 2010, a dog food was recalled due to contamination with 25-hydroxy vitamin D. Apparently this vitamin ingredient was intended for livestock feed, because it is not supposed to be used in the manufacture of dog food. This incident led to the discovery of a new phenomenon, the apparent physiologic interaction between 25-hydroxy vitamin D and cholecalciferol. The latter was present at recommended concentrations in the recalled dog food and yet clinically affected dogs had elevated serum ionized calcium and 25-hydroxy vitamin D and suppressed intact parathyroid hormone (PTH), all hallmarks of vitamin D toxicosis. In all these cases involving pet food, hypervitaminosis D occurred following prolonged ingestion of the contaminated food, usually weeks of exposure.

Following ingestion, cholecalciferol is rapidly absorbed and transported to the liver, where it is rapidly broken down to 25-hydroxy vitamin D_3, then further metabolized primarily to 1,25-dihydroxy vitamin D_3 (calcitriol) and 24,25-dihydroxy vitamin D_3 in renal proximal convoluted tubular epithelium. Calcitriol is the vitamin D metabolite most important in calcium-phosphorus metabolism; thus, imbalances in these macrominerals are important to the pathophysiology of vitamin D toxicosis.

Commonly reported clinical signs of vitamin D poisoning in pets include depression, weakness, anorexia polyuria, and polydipsia. Often these are the only clinical signs noticed but are significant enough to prompt pet owners to seek veterinary care for their pets. Diagnosis of vitamin D poisoning is based upon clinical signs consistent with vitamin D poisoning and serum vitamin D profile: serum intact PTH, total and ionized serum calcium, and serum 25-hydroxy vitamin D_3. In animals with vitamin D toxicosis, a significant increase in serum calcium and phosphorus concentrations occurs and intact PTH is suppressed. In pets that have died, finding elevated 25-hydroxy vitamin D_3 in the kidney, on top of histopathology characterized by metastatic soft tissue mineralization, is usually sufficient to confirm vitamin D poisoning.

In episodes of hypervitaminosis D triggered by pet food contaminxation, switching diets is often sufficient to correct the problem. Patience is required, though, as recovery takes weeks. Aggressive therapy includes use of pamidronate disodium, corticosteroids, and furosemide diuretic among others. Treatment of vitamin D poisoning has been discussed more extensively elsewhere.

Thiamine Deficiency

As noted in the introduction, there have been cat food recalls due to inadequate thiamine. Thiamine is a required B vitamin (B_1). Monogastric animals like cats and dogs cannot synthesize thiamine, and because it is a water-soluble vitamin, there is no long-term storage in the body. Factors such as age and diet affect the thiamine requirements for dogs and cats.[12] Thiamine is absorbed predominantly in the small intestine via a carrier molecule.[35] The vitamin is required as a coenzyme for pyruvate dehydrogenase, alpha-ketoglutarase, translocase, and other enzymes required for carbohydrate metabolism and energy production.[12] Pet foods should contain at least 5 mg/kg and 1 mg/kg thiamine on a dry matter basis, for cats and dogs, respectively.[13,36] Thiamine deficiency in cats has been associated with a food containing 0.56 mg thiamine/kg dry matter.[37]

Thiamine is found in meat, liver, and some cereal grains. Causes of thiamine deficiency in small animals include feeding of meat preserved with sulfur compounds that cleave thiamine, cooking and processing, which destroys 40% to 50% of thiamine, and natural thiaminases found in raw fish.[12,14,37] Absence of thiamine impairs cerebral energy metabolism, producing focal lactic acidosis and neuronal ischemia.[35,36]

Polioencephalomalacia describes the lesion associated with thiamine deficiency. Clinical signs described in experimental cats studied by Everett[38] began after 2 to 4 weeks on the deficient diet and included anorexia, which is responsive to thiamine injection, and weight loss. Progressive neurologic signs seen soon after included ataxia with a wide-based stance, circling, dilated pupils, positional ventroflexion of the head, and seizures, which may be spontaneous or secondary to stimulus. These signs remain responsive to thiamine supplementation. Eventually (after a month or more) cats become unable to walk and exhibit extensor tone in all limbs, which fails to respond to thiamine supplementation, followed eventually by coma and death.[38] Positional ventroflexion of the head, sometimes termed "the praying sign," is active and caused by vestibular dysfunction rather than muscle weakness. This sign can be observed when the cat is held by the hindquarters and the front end is moved toward the tabletop. The chin will drop to near the sternum.[39] Cats presented during the 2009 recall had similar clinical signs, including anorexia, head tilt, dilated pupils, apparent blindness, circling, ataxia, extensor rigidity of the front legs and positional ventral flexion of the head, and seizures. All cats in the 2009 case were responsive to thiamine treatment except one with marked extensor rigidity. A study of puppies found that the first clinical signs occurred after nearly 2 months on a thiamine-deficient diet and included inappetence, poor growth or weight loss, coprophagia, and neurologic signs similar to those seen in cats, although some puppies died before the abrupt onset of neurologic signs.[40]

Bilaterally symmetric changes have been observed in affected dogs and cats using MRI, with lesions documented in the cerebellar nodulus, caudal colliculi, and periaqueductal gray matter, and in dogs the red nuclei and vestibular nuclei, and in cats the facial nuclei and medial vestibular nuclei.[14,36] Diagnostic testing is infrequently used to confirm thiamine deficiency. However, functional tests are considered sensitive indicators of thiamine deficiency.[35] The most common is erythrocyte transketolase activity, which has been used in humans and dogs, but no reference values are available for cats.[12,35–37] The reported thiamine pyrophosphate concentration is 32 µg/dL in feline blood and 8.4 to 10.4 µg/dL in blood from healthy canines.[40,41] Cats in the 2009 outbreak had blood thiamine pyrophosphate concentrations ranging from 2.1 to 3.9 µg/dL, but no samples from unaffected cats were analyzed.

Postmortem lesions associated with thiamine deficiency-induced polioencephalo-malacia in cats and dogs include bilaterally symmetric areas of petechia in the brainstem and elsewhere, corresponding to the areas seen on MRI. Histologically, lesions include spongiform degeneration with reactive changes, including vascular hypertrophy, macrophage infiltrate, and gliosis.[12,40]

As noted, most animals respond to therapy with thiamine hydrochloride, given parenterally at a dose of 100 to 250 mg for cats and 5 to 250 mg/d for dogs.[42] After 5 days of parenteral dosing in a cat, oral thiamine at 25 mg/d was continued for 1 month.[36] Improvement is usually rapid, with significant improvement observed within a few days and often complete within 1 to 12 weeks.[14,35,37,43] However, persistent, ataxia, hearing loss, and positional nystagmus are reported.[35,43]

ADULTERATION

Adulteration of pet foods is rare but was responsible for the largest pet food recall in US history. Melamine was intentionally added to pet food ingredients to enhance the apparent protein content. Protein in pet foods is estimated based on the nitrogen content, which can be measured using the Kjeldahl method. Because melamine is 67% nitrogen based on the molecular weight, its addition to foodstuff increases the nitrogen content and thus the estimated protein content.

More recently, the FDA has recalled several pet food products due to pentobarbital contamination,[44,45] which occured when euthanized livestock were illegally used in the production of pet food.

Melamine and Cyanuric Acid

Melamine, or 1,3,5-triazine-2,4,6-triamine, has found numerous uses in manufacturing. It can be used in yellow pigments, dyes, and inks or can be polymerized with formaldehyde to produce a variety of durable resins, adhesives, cleansers, and flame-retardants. Cyanuric acid is an intermediate produced during melamine manufacture or degradation and is used to stabilize chlorine in swimming pools.

Early in 2007, there were several reports of renal failure in cats and dogs consuming commercial pet foods in the United States. Clinical signs included inappetence, vomiting, polyuria, polydipsia, and lethargy. A large number of affected cats were on feeding trials at a laboratory.[46] A recall was initiated on March 15, and melamine was detected in the cat food 2 weeks later, but at the time melamine was thought to have low oral toxicity based on early studies in rodents and dogs. Later, cyanuric acid, ammelide, and ammeline, which are intermediates in the production of melamine from urea, were detected in the food. An FDA investigation determined that wheat gluten and rice protein concentrates used in pet food production were intentionally mislabeled by Chinese exporters and actually contained wheat flour and poor quality rice protein mixed with melamine.[10] Eventually, more than 150 pet food products were identified, containing up to 3200 ppm melamine and 600 ppm cyanuric acid, and recalled.[46,47] Samples of imported wheat gluten contained 8.4% melamine, 5.3% cyanuric acid, and 2.3% and 1.7% ammelide and ammeline, respectively.[3] Estimates of the numbers of pets affected range from hundreds to thousands.

Many consider the 2007 pet food recall a sentinel event.[10,48] A year later, contamination of Chinese baby formula and other milk-based products was detected. Melamine concentrations ranged from 2.5 to 2563 ppm in 13 commercial brands of milk powder.[7] More than 52,000 Chinese children were hospitalized, and 6 died. There is evidence that children in Taiwan, Hong Kong, and Macau were also affected.[47,49,50]

Due to global marketing of food products and ingredients, melamine-contaminated foods were found in almost 70 countries, including the United States.

The oral LD_{50} of melamine is 3200 mg/kg in male rats, 3800 mg/kg in female rats, 3300 mg/kg in male mice, and 7000 mg/kg in female mice. Long-term dietary administration of melamine to laboratory rats at concentrations ranging from 0.225% to 0.9% produced urolithiasis and urinary bladder lesions, including transitional cell carcinoma and, in females, lymphoplasmacytic nephritis and fibrosis.[51] Sheep were given single (217 mg/kg) or multiple (200–1351 mg/kg/d for up to 39 days) doses of melamine. Clinical signs, including anorexia, anuria, and uremia, developed after 5 to 31 days after the first exposure in a dose-dependent manner.[52] A study involving dogs fed 125 mg/kg melamine reported crystalluria, but no other adverse effects were identified.[53] Cyanuric acid by itself has similarly low toxicity but is known to produce degenerative changes in the kidneys in guinea pigs at doses of 30 mg/kg body weight for 6 months, rats fed 8% monosodium cyanurate in the diet for 20 weeks, and dogs fed 8% monosodium cyanurate in the diet. Lesions included ectasia of the distal collecting tubules and multifocal epithelial proliferation.[54] The combination of melamine and cyanuric acid is markedly more toxic to most animals than either compound alone. Cats fed diets containing up to 1% melamine or cyanuric acid had no evidence of clinical abnormalities, but cats fed diets containing 0.2% each of melamine and cyanuric acid had evidence of acute renal failure within 48 hours. Lesions were typical of those associated with the recalled pet food.[55] A pig fed 400 mg/kg melamine and 400 mg/kg cyanuric acid daily had transient bloody diarrhea within 24 hours. Necropsy revealed perirenal edema and round golden-brown crystals with radiating striations in the kidneys. Similar lesions were present in tilapia, rainbow trout, and catfish dosed with 400 mg/kg each of melamine and cyanuric acid daily for 3 days, although most survived the renal damage.[56]

Melamine and cyanuric acid form crystals in distal convoluted tubules of the kidney when given together by binding to form a lattice structure at pH 5.8.[7,10] Renal pathologic condition most likely results from intratubular obstruction and increased intrarenal pressure. Interestingly, cyanuric acid did not contribute to the formation of melamine-containing urinary calculi in children.[57] Calculi in children were produced by a similar interaction between melamine and uric acid. Infants and many primates lack uricase, an enzyme that converts uric acid to allantoin, and thus excrete uric acid via the kidneys.[57] Urinary pH less than 5.5 is associated with the formation of urate crystals, and children with melamine/urate renolith formation were determined to have low urine pH.[57]

Melamine is minimally metabolized and does not accumulate in the animal body. It is about 90% eliminated within 1 day by the kidneys with a half-life for urinary elimination of 6 hours in dogs.[53] Therefore, melamine should be almost completely excreted within 2 days; however, crystals were seen microscopically in feline kidneys 8 weeks after dietary exposure to melamine and cyanuric acid.[46]

Cats and dogs had evidence of renal failure after ingesting recalled foods. Clinical signs included inappetence, vomiting, polyuria, polydipsia, and lethargy. Urine specific gravities less than 1.035 and elevated serum urea nitrogen and creatinine concentrations were seen in these cats. Circular green-brown crystals were observed in urine sediment (Fig. 2). Postmortem examinations of animals that died or were euthanized typically noted bilateral renomegaly and evidence of uremia. Microscopic lesions were primarily localized primarily to the kidneys: renal tubular necrosis, tubular rupture, and epithelial regeneration. In the distal convoluted tubules, there were large golden-brown birefringent crystals (15–80 μm in diameter) with centrally radiating striations, sometimes in concentric rings, and smaller amorphous crystals.[46,58] Crystals from

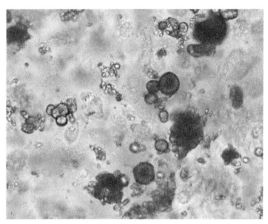

Fig. 2. Urine sediment with large, round, brown melamine and cyanuric acid crystals with radial striations. (*Courtesy of* R.E. Goldstein, DVM, DACVIM, DECVIM.)

kidneys and urine contained 70% cyanuric acid and 30% melamine based on infrared spectra.[10,58] The outbreak of melamine-induced nephropathy in children differed from that in domestic animals by the absence of cyanuric acid. Uroliths associated with nephrotoxicosis in infants contained melamine and uric acid at a molar ratio of 1:1 to 2, respectively.[47]

Treatment regimens for crystalluria and urolithiasis related to melamine ingestion in veterinary and pediatric patients included fluid therapy and supportive care.[59,60] Oral and parenteral fluid therapy increased urine output. Because low urinary pH is associated with crystal formation in infants, urine pH was maintained between 6.0 and 7.8 in affected children by adding sodium bicarbonate or potassium citrate to intravenous fluids. Most children recovered with conservative management.[57,60]

Analysis of 451 cases matching the definition of melamine toxicosis found that 65.5% were cats and 34.4% were dogs. The case mortalities were 73.3% and 61.5% for affected dogs and cats, respectively. Older animals and those with preexisting conditions were less likely to survive.[3] However, more than 80% of exposed cats during the original feeding trials survived with supportive care.[46]

Pentobarbital

Pentobarbital and phenytoin are common ingredients in veterinary euthanasia drugs. Between spring of 2017 and 2018, there were 2 pet food recalls related to pentobarbital contamination.[44,45] The first recall was associated with pet food contamination that had been reported previously, for example, in the United Kingdom in 1980.[61] Interestingly, this was accidental exposure to pentobarbital and phenytoin through ingestion, although the circumstances were not elucidated.[62] The FDA does not allow chemically euthanized animals to be used for pet food, and the presence of pentobarbital in pet food at any concentration renders the product adulterated by FDA standards.[44]

Pentobarbital sodium is a short-acting barbiturate with approximate oral LD_{50} doses of 85 mg/kg in dogs and 125 mg/kg in cats. Distribution across the blood-brain barrier and placenta is rapid.[63,64] Pentobarbital is metabolized by P450 enzymes and can affect the metabolism of other compounds, including endogenous steroids and xenobiotics.[64] Metabolism is relatively rapid in dogs compared with cats, and pentobarbital and metabolites are excreted in the urine.[63] The primary clinical effects of pentobarbital are due to potentiation at the γ-aminobutyric acid (GABA) receptor complex and effects on chemoreceptors.[63,64]

Onset of clinical signs due to pentobarbital contamination of pet food is somewhat variable based on gastrointestinal absorption, but usually occurs within 30 minutes. Duration is dependent on species, breed, dose, nutritional status, age, sex, and body composition.[63] Because GABA is an inhibitory neurotransmitter, clinical signs associated with pentobarbital overdose relate to depression of the central nervous system and anesthesia and can include ataxia, weakness, and loss of reflexes.[61,64,65] Hypothermia, respiratory depression, dysrhythmia, and weak pulses are also reported.[61,63–65]

Treatment is based on decontamination, monitoring, and supportive care. Emetics can only be given soon after ingestion in the asymptomatic patient.[65] Intubation and gastric lavage are more appropriate in the animal with central nervous system depression, and activated charcoal can decrease the biological half-life.[64] Monitoring of body temperature and respiratory and cardiac function and correction as needed are critical.[63] Intubation and assisted ventilation for respiratory depression and fluid therapy for cardiac function are recommended.[64,65] Intravenous lipid infusion has been used with varying success.[66]

Diagnosis is based on history, clinical signs, and analysis of contaminated products, urine, blood, or tissue. A positive barbiturate reaction on an over-the-counter urine drug test kit can give a presumptive diagnosis.[66]

SUMMARY

With myriad possible contaminants, ranging from fungal metabolites like aflatoxin and vomitoxin, to misformulations producing hypervitaminoses and other nutritional excesses and deficiencies, to adulteration with industrial chemical such as melamine and related compounds, it is impossible to predict the cause of the next pet food recall. Indeed, the definitive cause of Fanconi syndrome in dogs associated with consumption of jerky treats for dogs has also not been found. Vigilance is the major line of defense.

ACKNOWLEDGMENTS

The authors would like to thank Drs Sanderson and Gluckman for their work with the aflatoxin dogs, Dr McDonough for his pathology work and for contributing **Fig. 1**, Drs Woosley and Hubbard for their work with the polioencephalomalacia cats, Dr Kang for his thiamine analysis, Dr Rosama Pusoonthornthum for information about hypervitaminosis A, and Dr Goldstein for his work with melamine-poisoned cats and for contributing **Fig. 2**.

REFERENCES

1. Dzanis D. Anatomy of a recall. Top Companion Anim Med 2008;23:133–6.
2. Feng T, Keller LR, Wang L, et al. Product quality risk perception and decisions: contaminated pet food and lead-painted toys. Risk Anal 2010;30:1572–89.
3. Rumbeiha W, Morrison J. A review or class I and class II pet food recalls involving chemical contaminants from 1996 to 2008. J Med Toxicol 2011;7:60–6.
4. Anonymous. Jerky treats from China could be causing illness in pets. J Am Vet Med Assoc 2007;231:1183.
5. May K. Remain vigilant for illness possibly linked to chicken jerky treat consumption. Available at: http://atwork.avma.org/2011/06/17/remain-vigilant-for-illness

-possibly-linked-to-chicken-jerky-treat-consumption/. Accessed December 6, 2011.

6. Thompson MF, Fleeman LM, Arteaga A, et al. Proximal renal tubulopathy in dogs exposed to a common dried chicken treat: a retrospective study of 99 cases (2007–2009). Aust Vet J 2013;91(9):369–73.

7. Bhalla V, Grimm PC, Chertow GM, et al. Melamine nephrotoxicity: an emerging epidemic in an era of globalization. Kidney Int 2009;75:774–9.

8. Cocchi M, Vascellari M, Galina A, et al. Canine nephrotoxicosis induced by melamine-contaminated pet food in Italy. J Vet Med Sci 2010;72:103–7.

9. Gonzalez J, Puschner B, Perez V, et al. Nephrotoxicosis in Iberian piglets subsequent to exposure to melamine and derivatives in Spain between 2003 and 2006. J Vet Diagn Invest 2009;21:558–63.

10. Osborne CA, Lulich JP, Ulrich JL. Melamine and cyanuric acid-induced crystalluria, uroliths, and nephrotoxicity in dogs and cats. Vet Clin North Am Small Anim Pract 2008;39:1–14.

11. Yhee JY, Brown C, Yu CH, et al. Retrospective study of melamine/cyanuric acid-induced renal failure in dogs in Korea between 2003 and 2004. Vet Pathol 2009; 46:348–54.

12. Singh M, Thompson M, Sullivan N. Thiamin deficiency in dogs due to the feeding of sulphite-preserved meat. Aust Vet J 2005;85:412–7.

13. Steel R. Thiamin deficiency in a cat associated with the preservation of 'pet meat' with sulfur dioxide. Aust Vet J 1997;75:719–21.

14. Studdert VP, Lubac RH. Thiamin deficiency in cats and dogs associated with feeding meat preserved with sulfur dioxide. Aust Vet J 1991;68:54–7.

15. Hughs DM, Gahl MJ, Graham CH, et al. Overt signs of toxicity to dogs and cats of dietary deoxynivalenol. J Anim Sci 1999;3:693–711.

16. Puschner B. Mycotoxins. Vet Clin North Am Small Anim Pract 2002;32:409–19.

17. Boyer CI, Andrews EJ, deLahuta A, et al. Accumulation of mercury and selenium in tissues of kittens fed commercial cat food. Cornell Vet 1978;68:365–74.

18. Hansen JC, Danscher G. Quantitative and qualitative distribution of mercury in organs from arctic sledgedogs: an atomic absorption spectrophotometric and histochemical study of tissue samples from natural long-termed high dietary organic mercury-exposed dogs from Thule, Greenland. Pharmacol Toxicol 1995;77:189–95.

19. EFSA. Mercury as an undesirable substance in animal feed scientific opinion of the panel on contaminants in the food chain. The EFSA Journal 2008;654:1–76.

20. Ganther HE, Sunde ML. Factors in fish modifying methylmercury toxicity and metabolism. Biol Trace Elem Res 2007;119:221–3.

21. Meerdink GL. Mycotoxins. In: Plumlee KH, editor. Clinical veterinary toxicology. St Louis (MO): Mosby; 2004. p. 231.

22. Newbern PM, Butler WH. Acute and chronic effects of aflatoxin on the liver of domestic and laboratory animals: a review. Cancer Res 1969;29:236.

23. Liggett AD, Colvin BM, Beaver BW, et al. Canine aflatoxicosis: a continuing problem. Vet Hum Toxicol 1986;28:428–30.

24. Stenske KA, Smith JR, Shelly JN, et al. Aflatoxicosis in dogs and dealing with suspected contaminated commercial foods. J Am Vet Med Assoc 2006;228: 1686.

25. Hooser SB, Talcott PA. Mycotoxins. In: Peterson ME, Talcott PA, editors. Small animal toxicology. 2nd edition. St Louis (MO): Elsevier Saunders; 2006. p. 888–97.

26. Valdivia AG, Martinez A, Damian FJ, et al. Efficacy of N-acetylcysteine to reduce the effects of aflatoxin B_1 intoxication in broiler chickens. Poult Sci 2001;80:727.

27. Bingham AK, Huebner HJ, Phillips TD, et al. Identification and reduction of urinary aflatoxin metabolites in dogs. Food Chem Toxicol 2004;42:1851.
28. Tedesco D, Steidler S, Gallette S, et al. Effects of silymarin-phosphide complex in reducing the toxicity of aflatoxin B_1 in broiler chickens. Poult Sci 2004;83: 1839–43.
29. Miller DM, Wilson DE. Veterinary diseases related to aflatoxins. In: Eaton DL, Groopman JD, editors. The toxicology of aflatoxins. San Diego (CA): Academic Press; 1994. p. 347–64.
30. Bastianello SS, Nesbit JW, Willliams MC, et al. Pathological findings in a natural outbreak of aflatoxicosis in dogs. Onderspoort J Vet Res 1987;64:635.
31. Dereszynski DM, Center S, Randolph JF, et al. Clinical and clinicopathologic features of dogs that consumed foodborne hepatotoxic aflatoxins: 72 cases (2005-2006). J Am Vet Med Assoc 2008;232:1329–37.
32. Bischoff K, Ramiah SK. Liver toxicity. In: Gupta RC, editor. Veterinary toxicology basic and clinical principles. New York: Elsevier; 2007. p. 145–60.
33. Cho DY, Frey RA, Guffy MM, et al. Hypervitaminosis A in the dog. Am J Vet Res 1975;36:1597–603.
34. Polizopoulou ZS, Patsikas MN, Roubies N. Hypervitaminosis A in the cat: a case report and review of the literature. J Feline Med Surg 2005;7:363–8.
35. Garosi LS, Dennis R, Platt SR, et al. Thiamine deficiency in a dog: clinical, clinicopathologic, and magnetic resonance imaging findings. J Vet Intern Med 2003; 17:719–23.
36. Penderis J, McConnell JF, Calvin J. Magnetic resonance imaging features of thiamine deficiency in a cat. Vet Rec 2007;160:270–2.
37. Davidson M. Thiamin deficiency in a colony of cats. Vet Rec 1992;130:94–7.
38. Everett G. Observations on the behavior and neurophysiology of acute thiamin deficient cats. Am J Physiol 1944;141:439–48.
39. Malik R, Sibraa D. Thiamin deficiency due to sulfur dioxide preservative in 'pet meat': a case of deja vu. Aust Vet J 2005;83:408–11.
40. Read DH, Harrington DD. Experimentally induced thiamine deficiency in beagle dogs: clinical observations. Am J Vet Res 1981;42:984–91.
41. Rubin L. Atlas of veterinary ophthalmoscopy. Philadelphia: Lea & Febiger; 1974. p. 258.
42. Plumb D. In: veterinary drug handbook. 4th edition. White Bear Lake (MN): PharmaVet Publishing; 2002. p. 788–9.
43. Leow FM, Martin CL, Dunlop RH, et al. Naturally-occurring and experimental thiamin deficiency in cats receiving commercial cat food. Can Vet J 1970;11: 109–13.
44. US Food and Drug Administration. Questions and answers; Evanger's dog and cat food. Available at: https://www.fda.gov/animalveterinary/safetyhealth/product safetyinformation/ucm544348.htm#animals. Accessed April 10, 2018.
45. US Food and Drug Administration. FDA alerts pet owners about potential pentobarbital contamination in canned dog food manufactured by the J.M. Smuckers Company including certain Gravy Train, Kibbles 'N Bits, Ol' Roy, and Skippy products. Available at: https://www.fda.gov/AnimalVeterinary/NewsEvents/ucm597135.htm. Accessed April 10, 2018.
46. Cianciolo RE, Bischoff K, Ebel JG, et al. Clinicopathologic, histologic, and toxicologic findings in 70 cats inadvertently exposed to pet food contaminated with melamine and cyanuric acid. J Am Vet Med Assoc 2008;233:729–37.
47. Skinner CH, Thompson JD, Osterloh JD. Melamine toxicity. J Med Toxicol 2010;6: 50–5.

48. Lewin-Smith MR, Kalasinsky JF, Mullick FG, et al. Melamine containing crystals in the urinary tract of domestic animals: sentinel event? Arch Pathol Lab Med 2009; 133:341–2.
49. Hau AK, Kwan TH, Lee PK. Melamine toxicity in the kidney. J Am Soc Nephrol 2009;20:245–50.
50. Reimschussel R, Evans E, Andersen WC, et al. Residue depletion of melamine and cysnuric acid in catfish and rainbow trout following oral administration. Vet Pharmacol Ther 2009;33:172–82.
51. Melnick RL, Boorman GA, Haseman JK, et al. Urolithiasis and bladder carcinogenicity of melamine in rodents. Toxicol Appl Pharmacol 1984;72:292–303.
52. Clark R. Melamine crystalluria in sheep. J S Afr Vet Med Assoc 1966;37:349–51.
53. Lipschitz WL, Stokey E. The mode of action of three new diuretics: melamine, adenine, and formoguanamine. J Pharmacol Exp Ther 1945;82:235–49.
54. Canelli E. Chemical, bacteriological, and toxicological properties of cyanuric acid and chlorinated isocyanurates as applied to swimming pool disinfection, a review. Am J Public Health 1974;64:155–62.
55. Puschner B, Poppenga RH, Lowenstine LJ, et al. Assessment of melamine and cyanuric acid toxicity in cats. J Vet Diagn Invest 2007;19:616–24.
56. Reimschuessel R, Gieseker CM, Miller RA, et al. Evaluation of the renal effects of experimental feeding of melamine and cyanuric acid to fish and pigs. Am J Vet Res 2008;69:1217–28.
57. Gao J, Shen Y, Sun N, et al. Therapeutic effects of potassium sodium, hydrogen citrate on melamine-induced urinary calculi in China. Chin Med J 2010;123: 1112–6.
58. Thompson ME, Lewin-Smith MR, Kalasinsky VF, et al. Characterization of melamine-containing and calcium oxalate crystals in three dogs with suspected pet food-induced nephrotoxicosis. Vet Path 2008;55:417–26.
59. Anonymous. Specialists confer about the pet food recall. J Am Vet Med Assoc 2007;233:1603.
60. Wen JG, Li ZZ, Zhang H, et al. Melamine related bilateral renal calculi in 50 children: single center experience in clinical diagnosis and treatment. J Urol 2010; 183:1533–8.
61. Humphreys DJ, Longstaffe HA, Stodulski JBJ, et al. Barbiturate poisoning from pet shop meat: possible association with perivascular injection. Vet Rec 1980;5:517.
62. Forrester MB. Human exposure to pentobarbital-phenytoin combination veterinary drugs. Hum Exp Toxicol 2017;36:755–61.
63. Branson KR. Injectable anesthetics. In: Adams R, editor. Veterinary pharmacology and therapeutics. 8th edition. Ames (IA): Iowa State University Press; 2001. p. 213–67.
64. Vomer PA. "Recreational" drugs. In: Peterson ME, Talcott PA, editors. Small animal toxicology. 2nd edition. Philadelphia: Saunders; 2005. p. 273–311.
65. Kisseberth WC, Trammel HL. Illicit and abused drugs. Vet Clin North Am Small Anim Pract 1990;20:405–18.
66. Bischoff K, Jaeger R, Ebel JG. An unusual case of relay pentobarbital toxicosis in a dog. J Med Toxicol 2011;7:236–9.

Intravenous Lipid Emulsions in Veterinary Clinical Toxicology

Sharon Gwaltney-Brant, DVM, PhD[a],*, Irina Meadows, DVM[b]

KEYWORDS

- Poisoning • Antidote • Intravenous lipid emulsion • Intralipids
- Intravenous fat emulsion • Intoxication • Lipid resuscitation therapy

KEY POINTS

- Interest in the antidotal usage of ILE in human and veterinary medicine continues to expand, and further investigations continue to aid in elucidating the mechanisms of action of ILE when used to treat toxicoses.
- It is hoped the further investigation helps in identification of which toxicants best respond to ILE, and optimal infusion protocols for various toxicants.
- Although ILE provides a welcome tool to the veterinarian in the management of severe, life-threatening toxicoses, the judicious use of this treatment modality is imperative until the benefits versus risks have been fully defined.
- Further investigation is necessary to determine the true efficacy and safety of ILE when used as an antidote in the treatment of toxicoses.

INTRODUCTION

In 2006, the first successful resuscitation using intravenous lipid emulsion (ILE) was reported in a human with cardiac arrest secondary to bupivacaine toxicosis.[1] Since that time, the antidotal usage of ILE has expanded in human and veterinary medicine to the treatment of severe cardiotoxicity and neurotoxicity associated with intoxications from a variety of xenobiotics. Position statements released by the American College of Medical Toxicology and several national anesthesiology societies/associations have outlined basic recommendations for the antidotal use of ILE.[2,3] However, this treatment modality is not without controversy because of perceived reporting bias (ie, successful cases more likely to be reported), inconsistencies in clinical and experimental outcomes when ILE is used, and the fact that intoxicated patients receiving ILE are usually also receiving other treatments that may have impacted the outcome of the toxicoses.[4]

The authors have nothing to disclose.
[a] Veterinary Information Network, 501 North Dorchester Court, Mahomet, IL 61853, USA;
[b] ASPCA Animal Poison Control Center, 1717 South Philo Road, Suite 36, Urbana, IL 61802, USA
* Corresponding author.
E-mail address: sharon@vin.com

Vet Clin Small Anim 48 (2018) 933–942
https://doi.org/10.1016/j.cvsm.2018.07.006
0195-5616/18/© 2018 Elsevier Inc. All rights reserved.

vetsmall.theclinics.com

ILE is composed of neutral, medium- to long-chain triglycerides derived from combinations of plant oils (eg, soybean, safflower), egg phosphatides, and glycerin (**Table 1**). The lipid droplets, or liposomes, in ILE exist as single-layered spheres with phospholipid and phytosterol outer surfaces and inner hydrophobic triglyceride cores.[5] Formulated primarily as a source of essential fatty acids for patients requiring parenteral nutrition, ILE is available in preparations ranging from 10% to 30% lipid; the latter is for compounding use and is not labeled for direct infusion.[6] ILE is stored at room temperature, and an unopened container has a shelf-life of up to 2 years.[7] Once opened and/or mixed with other fluids, ILE should be refrigerated between uses and used within 24 hours. ILE is administered via peripheral or central venous catheter. ILE has a high margin of safety, with an estimated intravenous LD_{50} in rats of 67 mL/kg.[8] The most commonly reported ILE used in antidotal therapy is the soybean oil–based product, although positive results using formulations containing other lipid compositions have also been reported.[9,10]

MECHANISMS OF ACTION

Recent investigations into the mechanisms of action of ILE therapy have provided information on how this treatment modality may work, but the full picture on the antidotal effects of ILE in toxicoses has yet to be developed. Early theories into the effects of ILE on local anesthetic cardiotoxicity included alteration of myocardial cell metabolism; enhanced production of nitric oxide; redistribution of drug within the heart; and creation of a lipid phase in the plasma that acted as a "sink" that sequestered lipophilic drugs, preventing them from reaching their target sites.[5] Investigations into the antidotal use of ILE has resulted in refinement of the proposed mechanisms of action into scavenging and nonscavenging actions. The static "lipid sink" theory has been modified to a more dynamic "lipid shuttle" theory whereby the lipid phase within the plasma scavenges xenobiotic molecules from target tissues (eg, heart, brain) and shuttles them to tissues where they may be stored (eg, skeletal muscle, adipose tissue), metabolized (eg, liver), or excreted (eg, kidney).[5] Lipid solubility (as measured by LogP, the octanol-water partition coefficient) of a xenobiotic was initially thought to be the deciding factor in ILE scavenging activity, but the apparent efficacy of ILE

Table 1			
Food and Drug Administration–approved lipid emulsions for intravenous use			
Trade Name	**Composition**	**Total Lipid Content**	**Manufacturer**
Clinolipid	16% olive oil, 4% soybean oil	20%	Baxter Healthcare
Intralipid	30% soybean oil, 1.2% egg yolk phospholipids, 1.7% glycerin	30%	Baxter Healthcare
	20% soybean oil, 1.2% egg yolk phospholipids, 2.25% glycerin	20%	
	10% soybean oil, 1.2% egg yolk phospholipids, 2.25% glycerin	10%	
Nutrilipid	20% soybean oil, 1.2% egg yolk phospholipids, 2.5% glycerin	20%	B. Braun Medical
Smoflipid	6% soybean oil, 6% medium-chain triglycerides, 5% olive oil, 3% fish oil, 1.2% egg phospholipids, 2.5% glycerin, 0.3% sodium oleate, 0.016%–0.023% all-*rac*-α-tocopherol	20%	Fresenius Kabi USA

in management of intoxications from compounds with low lipophilicity, such as baclofen (which has a negative LogP) suggests that other physiochemical features of xenobiotics, such as ionization, may also be important. Proposed nonscavenging mechanisms of ILE include support of blood pressure via alteration of nitric oxide signaling, direct cardiotonic effects, and a postconditioning effect that minimizes reperfusion injury.[5]

EXPERIENCE WITH ANTIDOTAL INTRAVENOUS LIPID EMULSION

In 2009, the first case report on the successful use of ILE in the treatment of a puppy with moxidectin overdose was published.[11] Since that time, more than two dozen case reports or case series have been published on the use of ILE in management of toxicoses in a variety of veterinary species including cats, dogs, goats, horses/ponies, and a lion.[3,12–14] Most of these reports indicate a positive response to ILE therapy, but unsuccessful treatment with ILE was reported in clinical cases of lisdexamfetamine toxicosis in a cat, bromethalin toxicosis in dogs, disulfoton toxicosis in a dog, and ivermectin toxicosis in three dogs that were determined to be ABCB1-Δ mutants (ie, P-glycoprotein defective).[15–17] A randomized controlled clinical trial in cats with permethrin toxicosis demonstrated that use of ILE resulted in more rapid improvement of clinical signs compared with conventionally treated cats.[18]

Reports that have documented declining serum levels of toxicants following ILE therapy are intriguing, but they uniformly lack a control to demonstrate whether the declining serum levels were actually caused by the ILE intervention or whether they were caused by the normal distribution and elimination kinetics for those toxicants. One report of naproxen overdose ingestion by three dogs showed that the serum levels of naproxen declined within 3 hours following ILE therapy.[19] However, the maximum serum naproxen levels in the dogs (30–96 μg/dL) were 50 to 100 times lower than what is expected with a single oral dosage of 5 mg/kg (36–56 μg/mL)[20]; at these low serum concentrations (probably because of successful decontamination efforts), it is likely that the clearance of naproxen was largely caused by the normal pharmacokinetic processes of distribution and elimination. Similarly, a case report of bromethalin ingestion by a dog showed rapid reductions in serum concentrations of desmethylbromethalin (the active metabolite of bromethalin) following ILE therapy; however, no information is available on the normal plasma clearance of desmethylbromethalin, a highly lipid-soluble molecule that tends to distribute to adipose tissue.[21] Also, the dosage of bromethalin ingested by the dog (0.08–0.16 mg/kg) was much less than that expected to be toxic, and the maximum desmethylbromethalin serum level in the dog was very low (4 ppb) compared with levels in tissues that are associated with toxicosis (>60 ppb).[22,23]

Antidotal ILE has shown promise in treatment of veterinary clinical toxicoses from a variety of toxicants including amlodipine, amphetamines, baclofen, diltiazem, lamotrigine, local anesthetics, loperamide, macrocyclic lactones (eg, ivermectin, moxidectin), marijuana, minoxidil, permethrin, phenobarbital, Pieris japonica, synthetic cannabinoids, and tremorgenic mycotoxins.[3,12,16,18,24–28] Experimental studies in animals and human clinical cases have expanded the list of drugs whose toxicoses have responded to ILE therapy to include β-blockers, bupropion, bupivacaine, carbamazepine, clomipramine, doxepin, flecanide, hydrochloroquine, and verapamil.[10] Determining which toxicoses might best respond to ILE therapy is not as straightforward as determining the lipophilicity of the toxicant, because some toxicants that are poorly lipophilic (eg, baclofen, LogP of −1.32) have been reported to respond well to ILE therapy, suggesting that other physiochemical factors, such as electrostatic interactions, may influence the response of a toxicant to ILE administration.[5,29] Currently, gaps in knowledge on the mechanism of action of ILE make it difficult to determine if antidotal ILE failures are caused by incompatibility between toxicant and ILE, by inadequate dosing and/or rates of infusion, or by some other factor that has yet to be discovered. For the clinician managing a severe toxicosis and considering the use of ILE, consultation with an animal poison control center or veterinary toxicologist may be beneficial. **Table 2** includes general recommendations on the use of ILE therapy in toxicoses involving select toxicants.

Adverse effects reported with antidotal use of ILE have been infrequent. Pancreatitis has been reported in humans and veterinary patients, ostensibly related to hyperlipidemia.[7,30] Gross lipemia that persisted at least 48 hours and corneal lipidosis (identified on Day 3 of hospitalization and resolved within 1 week) were reported in a cat that received a high dose of ILE for permethrin toxicosis.[31] Hemolysis has been reported, perhaps related to high infusion rates.[7,24] Facial pruritus was reported in a cat receiving ILE, and hypersensitivity reactions have been reported as occurring frequently in pigs during experimental ILE infusion studies.[18,32] Pain associated with extravasation of ILE has been also reported.[33] The scavenging action of ILE is not highly selective, so the potential for ILE interacting with administered therapeutic drugs (eg, anticonvulsants) and potentially worsening the clinical signs of toxicosis must be considered when deciding whether or not ILE therapy is to be used.[7] Recrudescence of clinical signs may occur following initial improvement in toxicoses caused by toxicants with long half-lives; this phenomenon has been reported in humans but has yet to be noted in veterinary reports.[34] Other adverse effects reported in humans following antidotal use of ILE include acute kidney injury, acute lung injury, acute respiratory distress syndrome, cardiac embolism, fat overload syndrome, and increased susceptibility to infection.[30] Hyperlipidemia from ILE administration can interfere with several common clinical laboratory analyses, so blood samples for analysis should be collected before initiation of ILE infusion.[3,35] As with other intravenous fluid administrations, microbial contamination of ILE and administration sets must be avoided, and monitoring for development of hypersensitivity reactions is important. Patients should be monitored closely during infusion of ILE to avoid volume overload. The US Food and Drug Administration has established maximum dosing limits for ILE in humans of 12.5 mL/kg/d in adults and 15 mL/kg/d for pediatric patients.[36] In veterinary patients, a maximum dosage of 10 mL/kg/d has been recommended for parenteral nutrition, although higher rates are sometimes used.[10] However, these limits were established for nutritional rather than antidotal use, and humans have tolerated much higher acute dosages for treatment of toxicosis.[35]

CLINICAL APPLICATION OF INTRAVENOUS LIPID EMULSION IN VETERINARY TOXICOSES

Determination as to whether a toxicosis might be best treated with ILE requires careful evaluation of the individual situation in order for the veterinarian to make a reasoned assessment of the benefits versus risks of ILE administration. Because there are large gaps in understanding the mechanisms of action, appropriate dosages, appropriate dosing rates, and potential for adverse events, ILE therapy should be reserved for severe intoxications that are not responsive to standard medical therapy or where euthanasia is being considered because of poor prognosis or financial constraints.[3,10,24] ILE should not be the first-line treatment of toxicoses where

Table 2
Recommendations for use of ILE with select toxicants

Toxicant (LogP)	Case Reports and Response to Therapy	Recommendations
Amlodipine (LogP 3)	Improvement in 1 canine case ingesting 36.7 mg/kg.[16] APCC data showed little benefit*	Can attempt in life-threatening cases, but not recommended as first-line treatment.
Amphetamine (LogP 1.76) Methamphetamine (Log P 2.07)	Improvement in 2 canine cases (36.7 mg/kg).[16]	Can attempt in life-threatening cases, but not recommended as first-line treatment.
Baclofen (LogP −1.32)[29]	Positive results in several case reports and APCC data.[16,24,38,]* May take 2–3 doses for full response.[38]	Recommended for comatose, recumbent patients, especially those with respiratory depression.
Bromethalin (LogP 7.6)	No improvement noted in severely affected patients.[16,22]	Not recommended. At this time there is no solid evidence of improvement in severely affected cases.
Disulfoton (LogP 4.02) Methomyl (LogP 0.6)	No improvement in disulfoton case.[16] Time frame of recovery in methomyl case mirrors that of natural recovery from short-acting carbamate.[16,33]	Not recommended; symptomatic cases should be managed with atropine, benzodiazepines, and 2PAM.
Diltiazem (Log P 2.79)	Positive results in combination with high-dose insulin therapy in a dog.[39]	Can attempt severely affected patients, but not recommended as first-line or sole therapy.
Ibuprofen (LogP 3.97)	Improvement in neurologic status 3 h following ILE.[40]	Most neurologic signs expected to resolve within 4–5 h; consider if severe neurologic signs are not responding to supportive care.*
Ivermectin (LogP 4.1) Doramectin (LogP 4.5) Eprinomectin (LogP 3.5) Milbemycin (LogP 4.1) Moxidectin (LogP 4.3)	Several positive case studies in dogs and cats.[11,25,41] Treatment failures reported.[17] APCC data reveal unpredictable responses.*	May be considered as adjunctive treatment of severely affected animals. Dogs with ABCB1-Δ mutations may not respond as well as others.[17]
Lidocaine (LogP 2.44) Bupivacaine (LogP 3.41) Other local anesthetics	Positive results in a cat.[42] APCC data suggest most resolve with symptomatic care.*	Recommended use for cases with severe CNS and CV signs.
Loperamide (LogP 5.1)	Positive results in a dog with ABCB1-Δ mutation.[26]	Not recommended; CNS signs generally resolve with naloxone.
Marijuana Δ-9-tetrahydrocannabinol (LogP 7.6) Cannabidiol (LogP 8.0) Synthetic cannabinoids	Positive results in a dog.[27] Anecdotal reports from veterinary emergency clinics of positive results.*	May be used for severely affected patients (ie, comatose); not recommended for mild cases (ataxia, hyperesthesia, mild bradycardia).

(continued on next page)

Table 2 (continued)		
Toxicant (LogP)	Case Reports and Response to Therapy	Recommendations
Naproxen (LogP 3.18)	Declining serum naproxen concentrations but no control.[19]	Not recommended. Currently there is not enough data to support difference in outcome with standard treatment vs ILE.
Permethrin (LogP 6.5)	Generally positive results in several case reports, case series, and one randomized controlled study.[18,31,43,44]	Consider for cases refractory to methocarbamol and benzodiazepines. Not recommended as first-line or sole therapy for permethrin exposures, because most cases respond to treatment with methocarbamol and benzodiazepines.
Phenobarbital (LogP 1.47) Pentobarbital (LogP 2.1)	Moderate improvement has been seen in pentobarbital overdoses, whereas response in phenobarbital overdoses has been mild.*	Consider in severely affected patients especially those with respiratory compromise.
Tremorgenic mycotoxins (no LogP information available)	Review of 53 cases showed 96% positive response.[28]	Most cases respond well to methocarbamol and benzodiazepines; consider for refractory cases.

Abbreviations: APCC, Animal poison control center; CNS, central nervous system; CV, cardiovascular.
* ASPCA Animal Poison Control Center; AnTox Database unpublished data; 2018.

more established treatments hold reasonable likelihood of successful outcome. The antidotal use of ILE should be considered investigational, and informed consent from clients should be obtained after educating them on risks of adverse events and treatment failure. Patients should be stabilized as best as possible (ie, anticonvulsants, oxygen, correct electrolyte imbalances) before initiation of ILE infusions. Blood for serum chemistry, hematology, or other laboratory analyses should be taken before ILE administration.

For most toxicoses, 10% lipid emulsions are ineffective and 20% formulations are recommended, although 30% formulations may provide more rapid recovery from severe cardiotoxicity.[37] The use of in-line filters to remove particulates inherently present in ILE is advocated by some to minimize risk of adverse response to these particles.[16] In humans with oral drug overdoses, the recommended dosing is a 1.5 mL/kg intravenous bolus with an additional 0.25 mL/kg/min over 3 minutes, then 0.025 mL/kg/min × up to 6.5 hours.[36] The dosing and duration of the infusion in veterinary patients has varied considerably among different practitioners and institutions. **Table 3** lists some dosing regimens based on published reviews and cases. Patients should be monitored for signs of volume overload and pyrogenic or allergic reactions during infusion, and for several hours afterward for delayed allergic reactions. If there is concern for volume overload during constant rate infusion, a reduced rate of 0.07 mL/kg//min can be used.[3] When sufficient clinical improvement is seen following ILE infusion, patients should be monitored over at least 12 hours for return of clinical signs or delayed allergic response.

SUMMARY

Interest in the antidotal usage of ILE in human and veterinary medicine continues to expand, and further investigations continue to aid in elucidating the mechanisms of

Table 3
Dosing recommendations for management of severe toxicoses with 20% intravenous lipid emulsion

Bolus	Constant Rate Infusion	Comments	Reference
1.5 mL/kg	0.25–0.5 mL/kg/min × 30 min (do not exceed 10 mL/kg)	Dosing may be repeated if insufficient response	Ceccherini et al,[43] 2015
1.5 mL/kg over 1 min	0.25 mL/kg/min	*For cardiotoxicosis:* evaluate patient condition after 5 min; if necessary, second bolus of 1.5 mL/kg IV over 1 min and third similar bolus 5 min after second can be administered; if needed CRI can be increased to 0.25 mL/kg/min; as soon as heart function and circulation are restored, continue CRI for at least 10 min or until maximum dosage of 10–12 mL/kg for 30 min has been reached	Robben & Dijkman,[3] 2017
1.5 mL/kg over 1–2 min	0.25 mL/kg/min × 30–60 min	*For neurotoxicosis:* evaluate in 4–6 h after cessation of CRI; if insufficient or no improvement repeat dosing once or twice as soon as serum is no longer grossly lipemic and there are no signs of hemolysis; discontinue if no effect after 2–3 doses	Robben & Dijkman,[3] 2017
1.5–1.6 mL/kg	0.25 mL/kg/min × 30–90 min	Dosing may be repeated in 6 h if insufficient response to first dose	Becker & Young,[16] 2017
1.5–2.0 mL/kg over 1–15 min	0.25 mL/kg/min × 30–120 min	Dosing may be repeated in several hours if serum not lipemic	Gwaltney-Brant & Meadows,[24] 2012
1.5–4 mL/kg over 1 min	0.25 mL/kg/min × 30–60 min	Intermittent boluses q 4–6 h during initial 24 h as needed or CRI of 0.05 mL/kg/h not to exceed 24 h	Fernandez et al,[10] 2011

Abbreviations: CRI, constant rate infusion; IV, intravenous.

action of ILE when used to treat toxicoses. It is hoped the further investigation helps in identification of which toxicants best respond to ILE, and optimal infusion protocols for various toxicants. Although ILE provides a welcome tool to the veterinarian in the management of severe, life-threatening toxicoses, the judicious use of this treatment modality is imperative until the benefits versus risks have been fully defined. Further investigation is necessary to determine the true efficacy and safety of ILE when used as an antidote in the treatment of toxicoses.

REFERENCES

1. Rosenblatt MA, Abel M, Fischer GW, et al. Successful use of a 20% lipid emulsion to resuscitate a patient after a presumed bupivacaine-related cardiac arrest. Anesthesiology 2006;105(1):217–8.
2. American College of Medical Toxicology. ACMT position statement: interim guidance for the use of lipid resuscitation therapy. J Med Toxicol 2011;7(1):81–2.
3. Robben JH, Dijkman MA. Lipid therapy for intoxications. Vet Clin North Am Small Anim Pract 2017;47(2):435–50.
4. Forsberg M, Forsberg S, Edman G, et al. No support for lipid rescue in oral poisoning: a systematic review and analysis of 160 published cases. Hum Exp Toxicol 2017;36(5):461–6.
5. Fettiplace MR, Weinberg G. The mechanisms underlying lipid resuscitation therapy. Reg Anesth Pain Med 2018;43(2):138–49.
6. Intralipid 30% [package insert]. Deerfield (CT): Baxter Health Care; 2000.
7. Gwaltney-Brant SM. Intravenous lipid emulsions in veterinary toxicology: silver bullet or snake oil? Adv Small Anim Med Surg 2014;27(12):1–3.
8. Hiller DB, Di Gregorio G, Kelly K, et al. Safety of high volume lipid emulsion infusion: a first approximation of LD50 in rats. Reg Anesth Pain Med 2010;35(2): 140–4. Available at: http://www.ncbi.nlm.nih.gov/pubmed/20301820.
9. Cave G, Harvey M. Intravenous lipid emulsion as antidote beyond local anesthetic toxicity: a systematic review. Acad Emerg Med 2009;16(9):815–24.
10. Fernandez AL, Lee JA, Rahilly L, et al. The use of intravenous lipid emulsion as an antidote in veterinary toxicology. J Vet Emerg Crit Care 2011;21(4):309–20.
11. Crandell DE, Weinberg GL. Moxidectin toxicosis in a puppy successfully treated with intravenous lipids. J Vet Emerg Crit Care 2009;19(2):181–6.
12. Bischoff K, Smith MC, Stump S. Treatment of pieris ingestion in goats with intravenous lipid emulsion. J Med Toxicol 2014;10(4):411–4.
13. Bruenisholz H, Kupper J, Muentener CR, et al. Treatment of ivermectin overdose in a miniature Shetland Pony using intravenous administration of a lipid emulsion. J Vet Intern Med 2008;26(2):407–11.
14. Saqib M, Abbas G, Mughal MN. Successful management of ivermectin induced blindness in an African lion (Panthera leo) by intravenous administration of a lipid emulsion. BMC Vet Res 2015;11(1):1–7.
15. Akingbola OA, Singh D. Dexmedetomidine to treat lisdexamfetamine overdose and serotonin toxidrome in a 6-year-old girl. Am J Crit Care 2012; 21(6):456–9.
16. Becker MD, Young BC. Treatment of severe lipophilic intoxications with intravenous lipid emulsion: a case series. Vet Med Res Rep 2017;8(0):77–85.
17. Wright HM, Chen AV, Talcott PA, et al. Intravenous fat emulsion as treatment for ivermectin toxicosis in three dogs homozygous for the ABCB1-1Δ gene mutation. J Vet Emerg Crit Care 2011;21(6):666–72.

18. Peacock RE, Hosgood G, Swindells KL, et al. A randomized, controlled clinical trial of intravenous lipid emulsion as an adjunctive treatment for permethrin toxicosis in cats. J Vet Emerg Crit Care (San Antonio) 2015;25(5):597–605.

19. Herring JM, Mcmichael MA, Corsi R, et al. Intravenous lipid emulsion therapy in three cases of canine naproxen overdose. J Vet Emerg Crit Care 2015;25(5): 672–8.

20. Frey HH, Rieh B. Pharmacokinetics of naproxen in the dog. Am J Vet Res 1981; 42(9):1615–7. Available at: http://www.ncbi.nlm.nih.gov/pubmed/7325471.

21. Heggem-Perry B, McMichael M, O'Brien M, et al. Intravenous lipid emulsion therapy for bromethalin toxicity in a dog. J Am Anim Hosp Assoc 2016;52(4):265–8.

22. Romano MC, Loynachan AT, Bolin DC, et al. Fatal bromethalin intoxication in 3 cats and 2 dogs with minimal or no histologic central nervous system spongiform change. J Vet Diagn Invest 2018;30(4):642–5.

23. Dorman DC, Harlin KA, Buck WB, et al. Diagnosis of bromethalin toxicosis in the dog. J Vet Diagn Invest 1990;2(2):123–8.

24. Gwaltney-Brant S, Meadows I. Use of intravenous lipid emulsions for treating certain poisoning cases in small animals. Vet Clin North Am Small Anim Pract 2012;42(2):251–62.

25. Rawson-Harris P, Bates N, Edwards E. Lipid infusion: an analysis of cases reported to the Veterinary Poisons Information Service (VPIS). Clin Toxicol 2015;53(4):274–5. http://ovidsp.ovid.com/ovidweb.cgi?T=JS&PAGE=reference&D=emed13&NEWS =N&AN=71904114.

26. Long WM, Sinnott VB, Bracker K, et al. Use of 20% intravenous lipid emulsion for the treatment of loperamide toxicosis in a Collie homozygous for the ABCB1-1Δ mutation. J Vet Emerg Crit Care 2017;27(3):357–61.

27. Williams K, Wells RJ, McLean MK. Suspected synthetic cannabinoid toxicosis in a dog. J Vet Emerg Crit Care (San Antonio) 2015;25(6):739–44.

28. Kormpou F, O'Sullivan A, Troth L, et al. Use of intravenous lipid emulsion in dogs with suspected tremorgenic mycotoxicosis: 53 cases. Vet Evid 2018;3(2). Available at: https://www.veterinaryevidence.org/index.php/ve/article/view/166/240. Accessed August 3, 2018.

29. Abdel-Hafez AA, Abdel-Wahab BA. 5-(4-Chlorophenyl)-5,6-dihydro-1,3-oxazepin-7(4H)-one derivatives as lipophilic cyclic analogues of baclofen: design, synthesis, and neuropharmacological evaluation. Bioorg Med Chem 2008;16(17): 7983–91.

30. Hayes BD, Gosselin S, Calello DP, et al. Systematic review of clinical adverse events reported after acute intravenous lipid emulsion administration. Clin Toxicol 2016;54(5):365–404.

31. Seitz MA, Burkitt-Creedon JM. Persistent gross lipemia and suspected corneal lipidosis following intravenous lipid therapy in a cat with permethrin toxicosis. J Vet Emerg Crit Care 2016;26(6):804–8.

32. Bedocs P, Capacchione J, Potts L, et al. Hypersensitivity reactions to intravenous lipid emulsion in Swine: relevance for lipid resuscitation studies. Anesth Analg 2014;119(5):1094–101.

33. Bates N, Chatterton J, Robbins C, et al. Lipid infusion in the management of poisoning: a report of 6 canine cases. Vet Rec 2013;172(13):339.

34. Marwick PC, Levin AI, Coetzee AR. Recurrence of cardiotoxicity after lipid rescue from bupivacaine-induced cardiac arrest. Anesth Analg 2009;108(4):1344–6.

35. Cave G, Harvey M, Graudins A. Review article: intravenous lipid emulsion as antidote: a summary of published human experience. Emerg Med Australas 2011; 23(2):123–41.

36. Fettiplace MR, Akpa BS, Rubinstein I, et al. Confusion about infusion: rational volume limits for intravenous lipid emulsion during treatment of oral overdoses. Ann Emerg Med 2015;66(2):185–8.

37. Fettiplace MR, Akpa BS, Ripper R, et al. Resuscitation with lipid emulsion: dose-dependent recovery from cardiac pharmacotoxicity requires a cardiotonic effect. Anesthesiology 2014;120(4):915–25.

38. Butler J. Successful treatment of baclofen overdose with intravenous lipid emulsion. DVM360 2014;1-5.

39. Maton BL, Simmonds EE, Lee JA, et al. The use of high-dose insulin therapy and intravenous lipid emulsion to treat severe, refractory diltiazem toxicosis in a dog. J Vet Emerg Crit Care 2013;23(3):321–7.

40. Bolfer L, McMichael M, Ngwenyama TR, et al. Treatment of ibuprofen toxicosis in a dog with IV lipid emulsion. J Am Anim Hosp Assoc 2014;50:136–40.

41. Jourdan G, Boyer G, Raymond-Letron I, et al. Intravenous lipid emulsion therapy in 20 cats accidentally overdosed with ivermectin. J Vet Emerg Crit Care 2015; 25(5):667–71.

42. O'Brien TQ, Clark-Price SC, Evans EE, et al. Infusion of a lipid emulsion to treat lidocaine intoxication in a cat. J Am Vet Med Assoc 2010;237(12):1455–8.

43. Ceccherini G, Perondi F, Lippi I, et al. Intravenous lipid emulsion and dexmedetomidine for treatment of feline permethrin intoxication: a report from 4 cases. Open Vet J 2015;5(2):113–21. Available at: http://www.ncbi.nlm.nih.gov/pubmed/4663799.

44. Kaplan A, Whelan M. The use of IV lipid emulsion for lipophilic drug toxicities. J Am Anim Hosp Assoc 2012;48(4):221–7.

An Update on Calcium Channel Blocker Toxicity in Dogs and Cats

Cristine L. Hayes, DVM

KEYWORDS

- Calcium channel blocker • Verapamil • Diltiazem • Dihydropyridine • Amlodipine
- Toxicity • Dogs • Cats

KEY POINTS

- The most commonly encountered calcium channel blockers to which companion animals are exposed include verapamil, diltiazem, amlodipine, and nifedipine. Clinical signs of toxicosis may be seen even within a therapeutic dose range.
- Clinical signs can be delayed by several hours and may include lethargy, hypotension, cardiac rhythm changes, vomiting, and respiratory signs consistent with development of pulmonary edema.
- First-line therapies for exposure to calcium channel blockers include early decontamination, administration of intravenous crystalloid fluids, calcium, insulin-glucose, vasopressors, and/or atropine.
- If signs remain refractory to first-line therapies, subsequent treatment may include use of glucagon, intravenous lipid emulsion, inamrinone, or placement of a temporary pacemaker.

Calcium channel blockers (CCBs) are a commonly used group of drugs in both human medicine since the 1960s and in veterinary medicine since the 1980s.[1,2] They are defined by their ability to block the slow, or long-lasting (L-type), calcium channels, which are found primarily in cardiac and arterial smooth muscle tissues and to a much lesser extent in other tissues as well.[3] They have been commonly used for the treatment of hypertension, cardiac diseases (including hypertrophic cardiomyopathy and, in human medicine, angina and congestive heart failure), and cardiac arrhythmias, and they have also been suggested for other uses, such as premature labor in humans and acute renal failure in companion animals.[1,3,4]

This article originally appeared in *Veterinary Clinics of North America: Small Animal Practice*, Volume 42, Issue 2, March 2012.
The author has nothing to disclose.
ASPCA Animal Poison Control Center, 1717 South Philo Road, Suite 36, Urbana, IL 61802, USA
E-mail address: cristine.hayes@aspca.org

Several classes of CCB currently exist; of these, the most widely used are the phenylalkylamine verapamil (Calan, Verelan, Verelan PM, Isoptin, Isoptin SR, Covera-HS), the benzothiazepine diltiazem (Cardizem, Dilacor, Tiazac), and the dihydropyridines amlodipine (Norvasc), felodipine (Plendil), isradipine (Dynacirc), nicardipine (Cardine; Cardine SR), nifedipine (Adalat, Procardia, Afeditab, Nifediac), nimodipine (Nimotop), nitrendipine (not available in the United States), and nisoldipine (Sular). The only example of the diphenylpiperazine class, mibefradil (Posicor), was withdrawn from the market in 1998, and the only example of the diarylaminopropylamine class, bepridil (Vascor), was withdrawn in 2003.[5,6] Each class has a different affinity for the L-type calcium channels found in arterial smooth muscle and cardiac tissue.

Although there are no published data on the frequency of CCB toxicity in veterinary medicine, the American Society for the Prevention of Cruelty to Animals (ASPCA) Animal Poison Control Center (APCC) has consulted on approximately 7727 cases of CCB exposure between 2000 and 2017.[7] Overdose from CCBs can result in severe, life-threatening effects on cardiac conduction and blood pressure. In addition, there may also be effects on the digestive tract, pulmonary function, the nervous system, and pancreas. Treatment involves gastrointestinal decontamination (induction of emesis and administration of activated charcoal), stabilization of the cardiovascular system through blood pressure and cardiac rhythm regulation, and supportive care as needed to address other clinical signs.

PATHOPHYSIOLOGY

Calcium channels play a significant role in various cellular functions, particularly in the sinoatrial (SA) and atrioventricular (AV) nodes, myocardium, and arterial smooth muscle myocytes. In the normal physiologic state, there is a large concentration gradient of calcium across the cellular membrane, with high extracellular and low intracellular calcium concentrations.[1,3,4] Because calcium is unable to diffuse freely across the cellular membrane, this large concentration gradient is maintained by limiting calcium influx into the cell through specific calcium channels, sequestration of free intracellular calcium in the sarcoplasmic reticulum of myocytes, and maintaining an adenosine triphosphate (ATP)–driven calcium export pump.[1,3,4] When activated, the various calcium channels allow an intracellular influx of calcium, triggering a variety of responses depending on the tissue involved.[1,3,4,8]

There are several calcium channel types, including receptor-operated, stretch-operated, second messenger–operated, and voltage-sensitive calcium channels.[1,3] The various CCBs currently available act on the α_{1c} subunits of the L-type voltage-sensitive calcium channel, which are found primarily in the heart; vascular smooth muscle; skeletal muscle; and, to a lesser extent, pancreas, lung, brain, and other tissues.[3,8] The different classes of the CCBs have affinity for the various isoforms of the L-type calcium channel, which may account for the variability in their cardiovascular effects.[3,8]

In the heart, CCBs prevent the calcium influx in the nodal and myocardial cells, resulting in a slower sinus rate in the SA node and reduced AV conduction.[3,4] CCBs also affect muscular contraction by preventing the calcium influx into cardiomyocytes and vascular smooth muscles. This process results in reduced cytosolic calcium levels and reduced calcium-induced calcium release from the sarcoplasmic reticulum, leading to reduced cardiac inotropy and vascular tone.[1,3,4] For vascular beds with high resting tone (coronary and arterial smooth muscle), significant vasodilation occurs with reduced vascular tone.[3,4] For vascular beds with low resting tone (gastrointestinal and venous smooth muscle), little vasodilation occurs.[3,4]

The L-type calcium channels are also important systemically. In the pancreas, the L-type calcium channels influence insulin release from the pancreatic β cells. CCBs block the L-type calcium channels in these cells, resulting in reduced insulin release and hyperglycemia.[1] At the cellular level, the calcium influx through L-type calcium channels results in increased mitochondrial uptake of calcium, affecting intracellular ATP levels.[1,3] CCBs decrease mitochondrial calcium levels, resulting in reduced pyruvate dehydrogenase activity, leading to lactate accumulation.[1,3] Platelet aggregation may also be inhibited to some extent with CCBs.[3] Endothelin-mediated vasoconstriction is also dependent on L-type calcium channels. Acute renal failure secondary to endothelin-mediated vasoconstriction may be attenuated by CCBs.[3]

PHARMACOLOGY

There are currently only 3 classes of CCB available on the US market: the phenylalkylamine verapamil, the benzothiazepine diltiazem, and the dihydropyridines. These 3 types of CCB vary in the extent to which they affect the L-type calcium channels within vascular and cardiac tissues.

Verapamil

The representative drug of the phenylalkylamine class of CCB is verapamil. Verapamil is a nonspecific L-type CCB in that it has effects on both vascular and cardiac tissue, resulting in vasodilation, negative inotropy, and SA and AV node suppression.[3,4]

The pharmacokinetics for verapamil have been studied in dogs and humans (**Table 1**); however, little information regarding cats has been published. Verapamil is rapidly absorbed but has low bioavailability because of extensive first-pass metabolism. In dogs, verapamil is metabolized in the liver to several active and inactive metabolites.[9] Although no studies have been noted in dogs, in humans verapamil reaches the cerebrospinal fluid poorly, crosses the placenta, and passes into the milk.[10] Elimination of verapamil varies between dogs and humans, with biliary excretion as the primary route in dogs and renal excretion as the primary route of elimination in humans.[9,10] The onset of pharmacologic action and time to peak plasma concentration depend on the route of administration and formulation, with intravenous dosing fastest (1–5 minutes) and oral controlled-onset extended-release preparations longest at 11 hours in humans.[10]

Diltiazem

Diltiazem is the most commonly used drug of the benzothiazepine CCB class. Compared with verapamil, diltiazem has less significant effects on arterial vascular smooth muscle, cardiac contractility, and AV node suppression, although the SA node suppression is approximately the same between the two drugs.[3,4]

Diltiazem is formulated as a conventional immediate-release tablet or as a controlled-onset extended-release preparation.[11,12] The pharmacokinetics for diltiazem have been studied in cats, dogs, and humans (see **Table 1**).[3,9,13–16] In dogs and humans, systemic bioavailability is low because of a high first-pass effect; however, in cats, bioavailability is much higher.[3,13,14] This difference is hypothesized to be related to a reduced hepatic first-pass effect in the cat.[13] The time to reach the maximal plasma concentration for oral immediate-release/conventional diltiazem is 30 minutes in dogs and 45 minutes in cats, to an average of 5.7 hours following oral administration of the extended-release capsule Cardizem CD in cats.[12,13] Diltiazem is widely distributed through most tissues.[14] It can cross the placenta and can be found in milk as well, with one report suggesting that concentrations in human breast milk may approximate serum levels.[14] Diltiazem is metabolized in the liver through

Table 1
Pharmacokinetics of the different classes of calcium channel blocker

Class	Phenylalkylamine	Benzothiazepine	Dihydropyridine					
Representative Drug	Verapamil	Diltiazem	Amlodipine	Felodipine	Nifedipine	Nicardipine	Nisoldipine	Isradipine
Absorption (%)	Dog: 90 Human: 90	Dog: rapid Human: 98	60–65	10–25	30–60 (IR) 30–50 (ER)	35	87	15–24
Bioavailability (%)	Dog: 10–23 Human: 20–35	Dog: 17–24 Cat[a]: 71 (IR) 36 (ER)	Dog: 90 Human: 64–90	13–20 (ER)	30–60 (IR) 30–50 (ER)	35	4–8	14–24
Time to C_{max} (Oral) (h)	1–2 (IR) 7–11 (ER)[b]	Dog: 0.5 Cat[a]: 0.75 (IR) 5.7 (ER) Human: 2–4 (IR) 4–18 (ER)[b]	Dog: 6 Human: 6–12	2–6 (ER)	0.2–0.75 (IR) 6 (ER)	0.5–2 (IR) 1–4 (ER)	1–1.5 (IR) 4–13 (ER)	1.5 (IR) 7–18 (ER)
Time to Onset (Oral) (h)	0.5–1.5 (IR) 4–5 (ER)	0.25–1 (IR)	—	1 (IR) 5 (ER)	0.2 (IR) 0.5–1 (ER)	0.2	1–3 (IR)	1 (IR) 2 (ER)
Effect of Food	None	None	None	Increases rate of absorption	Variable	Reduced absorption	Slows absorption	?
Metabolism Site	Liver	Liver	Dog: liver Human: liver	Liver	Liver, gut wall	Liver	Liver, gut wall	Liver

Active Metabolites?	Dog: yes Human: yes	Yes	Yes	No	No	No	Yes	No
Excretion	Dog: mostly bile Human: kidney 70% Bile/feces 9%–16%	Bile/feces 65% Kidney 35%	Dog: feces 45%, kidney 45% as metabolites Human: kidney 70% as metabolites, 10% unchanged, bile/feces 20%–25%	Kidney 70%–80% Bile/feces <15%	Kidney 60% Bile/feces 35%	Kidney 60% Bile/feces 35%	Kidney 60%–80% Bile/feces 6%–12%	Kidney 60%–65% Bile/feces 30%
Elimination $T_{1/2}$ (h)	Dog: 1.8–3.8 Human: 8–12	Dog: 2–4 Cat[a]: 1.8 (IR) 6.8 (ER) Human: 3–6.6 (IR) 4–10 (ER)	Dog: 30–60	11–16 (IR) 27–33 (ER)	2–5	8.6	9–17	8

Data are for humans, unless otherwise specified.

There may be significant variability in pharmacokinetic data between species, and many of the listed medications have only been extensively studied in humans.

Abbreviations: C_{max}, peak plasma concentration; ER, non–immediate-release preparation (including extended-release, sustained-release, controlled-release, long-acting, and controlled-onset extended-release preparations); IR, conventional immediate-release preparation; $T_{1/2}$, half-life; XR, extended release.

[a] Cardizem IR and Cardizem CD have been studied in cats.[12]

[b] The time to peak plasma concentration (oral route) varies with the different extended-release preparations. The time listed is the range, including all extended-release, sustained-release, controlled-release, long-acting, and controlled-onset extended-release preparations.

Data from Refs.[3,9,10,12–22]

both deacetylation and demethylation in dogs and primarily through deacetylation in humans.[3,14,15] Diltiazem also undergoes enterohepatic recirculation in dogs and humans, with the second plasma peak in humans occurring 3 to 4 hours after ingestion.[3] Elimination of diltiazem in dogs and humans is blood flow dependent, whereas in cats it is suggested to be independent of blood flow.[13] It is primarily eliminated in the feces, although renal excretion accounts for approximately one-third of elimination in humans.[14] The terminal half-life depends on the formulation, with immediate-release preparations eliminated faster compared with extended-release formulations.[14]

Dihydropyridines

There are several drugs within the dihydropyridine CCB class, including amlodipine, felodipine, isradipine, nicardipine, nifedipine, nimodipine, nitrendipine, and nisoldipine.[7] Of these, the one most commonly involved in exposures reported to the APCC is amlodipine, which accounted for 83.2% of all dihydropyridine exposures from 2000 to 2017.[7] The dihydropyridines are most noted for their effects on vascular smooth muscle, whereas they have less effect on cardiac contractility or conduction.[3,4]

Dog and cat pharmacokinetic data are lacking for most of the drugs in the dihydropyridine class of CCB (with the exception of amlodipine in dogs); however, there is a significant amount of pharmacokinetic data in humans (see **Table 1**).[16–22] In general, the absorption, bioavailability, volume of distribution, and terminal elimination half-life of the dihydropyridines vary between drugs. Amlodipine has the highest bioavailability and volume of distribution.[16,17] All of the dihydropyridines are highly protein bound, extensively metabolized by the liver, and eliminated primarily through the kidneys.[16–22] The onset of action and time to peak plasma concentrations depend on the formulation, with immediate-release preparations being the shortest and controlled-onset extended-release preparations being the longest.[16–22]

CLINICAL SIGNS OF TOXICOSIS

The minimum oral toxic dose of each CCB has not been established in humans or animals. Signs of toxicity have been noted at therapeutic doses of verapamil, diltiazem, amlodipine, and nifedipine in some dog and cat cases (**Table 2**).[7,23] The diltiazem oral

Table 2
Therapeutic doses of selected calcium channel blockers commonly used in veterinary medicine

	Verapamil	Diltiazem	Amlodipine
Dog	IV: 0.05 mg/kg to a maximum cumulative dose of 0.15 mg/kg PO: 0.5–5.0 mg/kg q 8 h	IV: 0.05–0.35 mg/kg to a maximum cumulative dose of 0.75 mg/kg PO: 0.5–2.0 mg/kg	PO: 0.05–0.4 mg/kg q 12 h
Cat	IV: 0.025 mg/kg to a maximum cumulative dose of 0.15–0.2 mg/kg PO: 0.5–1.0 mg/kg q 8 h	IV: 0.125–0.35 mg/kg to a maximum cumulative dose of 0.75 mg/kg PO: 0.5–1.5 mg/kg q 8 h up to 10 mg/kg daily	PO: 0.625–1.25 mg daily
Human (Pediatric)	PO: 3–5 mg/kg daily in 3 divided doses	PO: 1.5–2 mg/kg daily in 3–4 divided doses to a maximum cumulative dose of 3.5 mg/kg daily	PO: 0.1 mg/kg q 12–24 h to a maximum of 0.6 mg/kg/d or 20 mg/d

Abbreviations: PO, by mouth; q, every.
Data from Refs.[10,14,17,23]

dose resulting in death of 50% of exposed patients (LD_{50}) in dogs has been reported as somewhere beyond 50 mg/kg but has not been reliably established.[23] Although the various classes of CCBs have distinct differences in their specificities for either the vascular smooth muscle or heart at therapeutic doses, in overdoses the tissue specificity may be lost.[3,4,24–26] Typically, the clinical signs seen are the result of an exaggeration of the normal pharmacologic activity of CCBs.[3,4,24–26] Clinical signs include sinus bradycardia and/or bradyarrhythmias (all degrees of heart block, QT interval prolongation, or junctional rhythms) caused by slowed cardiac conduction and hypotension caused by vasodilation and reduced cardiac inotropy.[7,24–27] Sinus tachycardia, likely caused by carotid sinus reflex stimulation, is possible as well.[24–27] Additional clinical signs associated with all CCBs include digestive upset; hypothermia (presumably caused by hypotension); central nervous system depression caused by hypotension and/or bradycardia; noncardiogenic pulmonary edema; hyperglycemia caused by inhibition of insulin release; hypokalemia; hyponatremia; metabolic acidosis caused by tissue hypoperfusion and increased lactate production; and, rarely, stimulatory signs such as seizures, agitation, or tremors (**Table 3**).[1,7,24–26,28] The exact mechanism of pulmonary edema is unknown. It may be secondary to aggressive fluid therapy combined with increased pulmonary capillary permeability, drug-induced changes to alveolar membrane permeability, or selective precapillary vasodilation from CCBs.[29,30]

DIAGNOSIS

The diagnosis of CCB toxicity in veterinary patients is largely based on clinical signs consistent with CCB toxicity and the history of a possible exposure. Serum drug levels for CCBs are not routinely evaluated on presentation because the tests are not widely available and drug levels for specific agents do not necessarily correspond with the degree of clinical signs seen.[1,30] Signs of toxicity can occur at therapeutic drug levels in humans.[1,28] When analytical tests for CCBs are available, they could be used to confirm an exposure.[1]

The clinical presentation of patients with hypotension and bradycardia or tachycardia can be consistent with other causes as well. Differential diagnoses may include toxicity from digoxin, cardiac glycoside–containing plants, β-adrenergic antagonists, α_2-adrenergic agonists, organophosphates, type 1a antiarrhythmic agents such as procainamide or quinidine, bufadienolides, and nontoxic causes such as myocardial infarction or other cardiac diseases.[31]

TREATMENT

Treatment of CCB toxicity focuses on reducing the absorption of the drug, providing good supportive care based on the clinical signs seen, and augmenting myocardial function. There is no specific antidote for treatment of CCB toxicity because of the number of mechanisms contributing to clinical signs; however, there are several therapies available that can counteract some of the toxic effects of CCBs.

Decontamination

For asymptomatic patients with a recent exposure of less than 2 hours, gastric decontamination is recommended.[25] This decontamination may be accomplished by inducing emesis, gastric lavage, and/or administration of activated charcoal (Toxiban; UAA Gel). In symptomatic patients, gastric decontamination should only be attempted once the patient's condition is stable. Inducing emesis is contraindicated for symptomatic patients; however, gastric lavage or activated charcoal administered via a

Table 3
Clinical signs of select calcium channel blocker toxicities in dogs

	Amlodipine	Nifedipine	Diltiazem	Verapamil
Frequent (25%–50% of Symptomatic Cases)	Tachycardia, hypotension	Tachycardia, lethargy	Bradycardia, hypotension, lethargy, vomiting	Lethargy
Possible (5%–25% of Symptomatic Cases)	Lethargy, respiratory signs (including pulmonary edema), vomiting, bradycardia, depression, hyperglycemia, cardiac arrhythmias[a]	Hypotension, vomiting, hyperthermia, hypertension, ataxia, respiratory signs (including pulmonary edema)	Cardiac arrhythmias,[b] respiratory signs (including pulmonary edema), ataxia, hypothermia, death, tachycardia	Tachycardia, vomiting, hypotension, cardiac arrhythmias,[c] bradycardia, respiratory signs (including pulmonary edema), hypertension, hypokalemia
Rare (<5% of Symptomatic Cases)	Azotemia, hypokalemia, hyponatremia, hyperkalemia, acidosis, tremors/fasciculation, seizures	Bradycardia, AV block, hyponatremia, hypernatremia	Azotemia, hyperglycemia, hypokalemia, hypophosphatemia, seizures, tremors, acidosis, hypoglycemia, hypertension, hypocalcemia, hypoproteinemia, hyponatremia, hypercalcemia, hypernatremia	Tremors, ataxia, hypernatremia, hyperphosphatemia

Total of 186 symptomatic amlodipine cases, 29 symptomatic nifedipine cases, 244 symptomatic diltiazem cases, and 31 symptomatic verapamil cases. Data were only used from patients having a single exposure that was either observed or there was evidence of exposure, with clinical signs assessed as having a high or medium likelihood of being related to the exposure. Clinical signs are listed in order of descending frequency.

[a] Cardiac arrhythmias included premature ventricular contractions, AV block, ventricular tachycardia, and unspecified arrhythmias.
[b] Cardiac arrhythmias included AV block, bigeminy, atrial standstill, atrial fibrillation, atrial premature contractions, premature ventricular contractions, and unspecified arrhythmias.
[c] Cardiac arrhythmias included second-degree AV block and premature ventricular contractions.
Data from ANTOX: ASPCA Animal Poison Control Center's toxicology database. Urbana (IL):2001–2018.

stomach tube could be considered, particularly with large ingestions or ingestion of sustained-release preparations.[24]

Emesis can be accomplished in asymptomatic patients using a few different methods. For dogs, apomorphine (Apokyn) or hydrogen peroxide 3% can be used as emetics.[23,32] The apomorphine dose recommended in dogs is 0.03 to 0.04 mg/kg intravenously (IV), intramuscularly (IM) or in the subconjunctival sac.[23,32] If given in the subconjunctival sac, the sac can be flushed with saline once emesis has occurred.[31] In dogs, hydrogen peroxide 3% can also be given as an alternative to apomorphine and is used at a dose of 1 to 2 mL/kg by mouth up to a maximum of 50 mL per patient.[32] In cats, xylazine (1.1 mg/kg IM or subcutaneously [SQ]) or dexmedetomidine (3.5 µg/kg IV or 7 µg/kg IM) causes emesis through stimulation of the α_2-adrenergic receptors in the emetic center.[33] Common adverse effects associated with xylazine include sedation, hypotension, bradycardia, and respiratory depression, although these effects can be reversed with atipamezole (0.2 mg/kg IV) or yohimbine (0.1 mg/kg IV).[23,32] For patients in whom emesis is contraindicated, gastric lavage performed under anesthesia may be considered.[32]

Activated charcoal can also be used for gastrointestinal decontamination. It is effective for both immediate-release and extended-release preparations of CCBs.[34] In a human study evaluating the effectiveness of activated charcoal for verapamil exposures, activated charcoal was effective in reducing the absorption of immediate-release verapamil when administered immediately following ingestion but not 2 hours after ingestion.[33] Activated charcoal was effective in reducing absorption of sustained-release verapamil 4 hours after ingestion (the longest time evaluated in the study).[33] Activated charcoal is used in dogs and cats at a dose of 1 to 3 g/kg by mouth with a cathartic such as sorbitol.[23,32] Activated charcoal can be repeated every 4 to 6 hours for 2 to 4 doses if a high dose of a sustained-release preparation is ingested.[23,32] Adverse effects associated with activated charcoal include aspiration pneumonia and hypernatremia.[23] If the patient is symptomatic, airway protection is critical and the risk versus the benefits of activated charcoal should be considered. For the ingestion of sustained-release preparations, a warm-water enema at a rate of 2.5 to 5 mL/kg could also be considered to facilitate evacuation of the intestinal contents.

Extracorporeal decontamination with hemodialysis is not expected to be of benefit in CCB toxicity. CCBs are highly protein bound, which minimizes the benefit of hemodialysis.[1] Continuous venovenous hemodiafiltration with charcoal hemoperfusion has rarely been used in people following amlodipine overdose, with variable effectiveness.[35]

Monitoring

When there has been a possible exposure to a CCB, close monitoring of the cardiovascular system, respiratory system, nervous system, electrolytes, and blood chemistries should be implemented for 12 to 24 hours or longer following exposure.[24] The blood pressure, heart rate, and cardiac rhythm should be monitored frequently. An electrocardiogram (ECG) should be used to monitor the cardiac rhythm. Respiratory system monitoring can involve auscultation, pulse oximetry, or arterial blood gas. The nervous system should also be monitored for depression or seizures. The serum glucose level, acid-base status, and electrolyte levels should be monitored for the development of hyperglycemia, lactic acidosis, hypokalemia, hypophosphatemia, hypomagnesemia, and hyponatremia.

As noted previously, plasma CCB levels can be performed to determine whether an exposure has occurred; however, monitoring CCB levels is not expected to be beneficial.[1,23,24,28]

Supportive Care

In symptomatic patients, stabilization and supportive care should be provided. Fluid therapy using a balanced isotonic crystalloid fluid should be administered for cardiovascular support and to help maintain hydration.[23–25] Aggressive fluid therapy should be used with care to minimize fluid overload and the development of pulmonary edema.[24,25,29,30] An antiemetic such as maropitant (Cerenia) (1 mg/kg SQ every 24 hours), metoclopramide (Reglan) (0.1–0.5 mg/kg SQ or IM or 0.01–0.02 mg/kg/h IV as a constant-rate infusion [CRI]), ondansetron (Zofran) (0.1–1 mg/kg IV every 12–24 hours), or dolasetron (Anzimet) (0.5–1 mg/kg IV every 24 hours) may be used to manage any vomiting.[23] If seizures develop, diazepam (Valium; Diastat) (0.5–1 mg/kg IV) or a barbiturate such as pentobarbital (Nembutal) (3–15 mg/kg IV) or phenobarbital (Tubex; Carpujects; Luminal Sodium) (2–20 mg/kg IV) may be used.[23] Potassium should be supplemented in the fluids when the serum potassium level is less than 2.5 mEq/L. If pulmonary edema develops, oxygen support should be provided.

CCBs are natriuretic. Dihydropyridines can increase sodium excretion 4-fold; they act directly on the renal tubules increasing sodium excretion and decreasing sodium reabsorption. Other mechanisms include a direct inhibitory effect on vasopressin-induced stimulation of water and sodium transport. In patients given amlodipine, the increase in sodium excretion may take a few days to develop. The serum sodium should be monitored and corrected if hyponatremia develops secondary to amlodpine exposure.

Specific Therapies

Specific CCB toxicity therapies can be divided into first-line therapies and additional therapies to consider if the first-line therapies fail. Common first-line therapies include administration of calcium, insulin-glucose, vasopressors, and atropine.[36,37] Atropine sulfate (0.02 mg/kg IV) can be used for persistent bradycardia.[23] Repeat atropine if and as needed. Other therapies that can be considered if the patient remains refractory to first-line treatment include glucagon, intravenous lipid emulsion, inamrinone, and temporary pacemaker placement.[36,37]

CALCIUM

After attempting cardiovascular stabilization, calcium is commonly administered for persistent hypotension and/or bradycardia.[1,24,25] The increased extracellular calcium available to cells may increase the intracellular calcium influx.[1,24,25] Increased calcium may also increase calcium release from the sarcoplasmic reticulum, enhancing contractility.[1,24,25] Calcium gluconate or calcium chloride may be used, although calcium chloride provides a higher concentration of calcium ion per milliliter compared with calcium gluconate (13.6 mEq vs 4.5 mEq in 10 mL of a 10% solution).[25] Calcium gluconate 10% can be used at a dose of 0.5 to 1.5 mL/kg IV slowly over 5 minutes while monitoring the ECG closely or as a CRI of 0.05 mL/kg/h.[23] Calcium chloride 10% is used at a dose of 0.1 to 0.5 mL/kg IV slowly over 5 minutes or as a CRI of 0.01 mL/kg/h.[23] If bradycardia develops or worsens during use, discontinue the calcium supplementation.[23] Adverse effects include hypercalcemia and local tissue irritation or necrosis if given extravascularly.[23]

INSULIN-GLUCOSE

High-dose insulin accompanied by dextrose to maintain euglycemia (High-dose insulin euglcyemic therapy [HIE]) has been determined to have a direct positive inotropic effect and is currently recommended in human cases of CCB intoxication with evidence of myocardial dysfunction as a first-line therapy.[36,37] In cardiac myocytes stressed from hypoperfusion, there is a shift from free fatty acid to glucose use as the energy substrate.[1,25,38–41] Hypoinsulinemia resulting from CCB effects on pancreatic β cells and insulin resistance leading to reduced glucose delivery to cardiac tissue combined with an increase in glucose use by the myocardium can have negative cardiac inotropic effects.[1,24,25,38,40,41] HIE enhances glucose uptake by the myocytes to increase energy substrate utilization.[1,25,39–43] HIE also suppresses phosphodiesterase III activity, thus increasing cyclic AMP (cAMP) levels, resulting in increased intracellular calcium influx.[1,41] In addition, HIE also enhances the intracellular potassium influx, resulting in hypokalemia, which can prolong phase 2 depolarization, increasing the intracellular calcium influx.[1] The end result is increased cardiac inotropy.[1,25,28,39–41] HIE also decreases capillary vascular resistance through increased nitric oxide synthase activity, leading to a reduction in acidosis.[41]

HIE can be used, but the ideal dose in companion animals has not been established. In a study of verapamil toxicity in anesthetized dogs, regular insulin was used at a dose of 4 U/min with 20% dextrose.[38,39] In a case report of HIE used for treatment of diltiazem toxicosis in a dog, 1 U/kg/h IV as a CRI (initial dose) was implemented 10 hours after exposure, and, combined with intravenous lipid emulsion (ILE), a response was seen within 1 hour. It was continued for 7 hours at this dose, then weaned down and finally discontinued over an additional 10 hours.[42] In human medicine, the dose typically used is the intravenous administration of a 1 U/kg bolus followed by 0.5 to 2 U/kg/h IV as a CRI along with 10% dextrose administration.[28,36,37,41] The dose may be titrated up to 10 U/kg/h IV as a CRI if the patient remains refractory to treatment.[36,37] The blood glucose should be monitored every 5–30 minutes.[41,42] Effects were seen after 30 to 45 minutes, and the most benefit was seen earlier in the course of CCB toxicity; if treatment with HIE is delayed, the benefits are reduced.[28,36,37,40] While using HIE, the serum glucose and potassium levels should be monitored closely to minimize the risk for hypoglycemia, hyperglycemia, and hypokalemia.[1,25,28,40,41] When administering 10% dextrose, a central catheter should be used to minimize the risk for phlebitis.[25]

VASOPRESSORS

Refractory hypotension or bradycardia may respond to sympathomimetic drugs, although no one agent has been proved to be consistently effective.[25] Norepinephrine (Levophed) is the first-choice vasopressor in humans (0.05–0.1 μg/kg/min IV).[23] Dopamine hydrochloride (Inotropin) (10–20 μg/kg/min IV), dobutamine hydrochloride (Dobutrex) (2–20 μg/kg/min IV), isoproterenol (Isuprel) (0.04–0.08 μg/kg/min IV), epinephrine (Adrenalin) (0.05–0.4 μg/kg/min IV), or phenylephrine hydrochloride (Neo-Synephrine) (0.5–3 μg/kg/min IV) may alternatively be used.[1,23,25]

GLUCAGON

Glucagon is a cardiac inotrope and chronotrope.[1,25] In addition to stimulating hepatic glycogenolysis, thus increasing blood glucose levels, it also acts on cardiac G protein–coupled receptors, stimulating an increase in intracellular cAMP and thus increasing the myocardial calcium influx.[1,25] The increased intracellular calcium level results in increased contractility and enhances impulse generation.[1,25] Glucagon may benefit patients with either hypotension or bradycardia, although it is expensive and may not be readily available. In case reports describing its use for verapamil toxicity in dogs, it was only transiently effective.[27,38] It can be used at an initial dose of 50 ng/kg body weight as an intravenous bolus followed by a CRI of 10 to 15 ng/kg/min up to 40 ng/kg/min[23]

INAMRINONE

As a phosphodiesterase III inhibitor, inamrinone prevents degradation of cAMP in vascular and cardiac muscle, resulting in increased intracellular cAMP levels.[1,24,28] Increased cAMP level leads to an increase in the myocardial calcium influx, resulting in improved contractility and increased impulse generation.[1,24,28] It can cause peripheral vasodilation, thus worsening hypotension if present.[28] It can be used at an initial dose of 1 to 3 mg/kg intravenous bolus followed by 10 to 100 μg/kg/min IV as a CRI.[23]

LIPID EMULSION

Treatment with an ILE, commonly used in total parenteral nutrition, has been investigated as an adjunctive therapy for various toxicities, particularly toxicity caused by local anesthetics, verapamil, or diltiazem, and has been proposed as a therapy for toxicity caused by other substances with high lipid solubility.[44] Although the exact mechanism by which ILE therapy works in toxicity is unknown, a few mechanisms have been suggested. One theory suggests that ILE sequesters lipophilic drug in an expanded plasma lipid phase, reducing the available free drug and promoting clearance of the compound through metabolism of drug-containing chylomicrons (the so-called lipid-sink theory).[44,45] Another theory for ILE benefit when used in treatment of cardiotoxic drugs suggests that the increased availability of free fatty acids provided by ILE may prevent the myocardium from switching to glucose as its preferred energy substrate.[44,46] In addition, the long-chain fatty acids in ILE may also activate myocyte calcium channels, resulting in increased calcium influx.[28,44] ILE may also increase nitric oxide and β-ketoacids, which stimulate insulin release.[28]

As with HIE, the ideal dose of ILE in companion animals has not been established. The most commonly suggested dose of ILE has been 1.5 mL/kg intravenous slow bolus of intralipid 20% followed by 0.25 mL/kg/min for 1 hour.[44,47] This therapy may be repeated in 3 to 4 hours if the serum is not lipemic. Adverse reactions to ILE therapy may include hyperlipidemia, fat overload syndrome (fat embolism, hepatomegaly, thrombocytopenia, hemolysis, increased clotting times, or neurologic deficits), and pancreatitis.[44]

MISCELLANEOUS AGENTS

Severe heart block may require the placement of a temporary cardiac pacemaker.[27] This therapy can improve cardiac output by increasing the heart rate; however, it does not have effects on the peripheral arterial vascular tone or cardiac contractility.[27] Another treatment using 4-aminopyridine (Ampyra) has been described in experimental studies.[48,49] 4-Aminopyridine is a potassium channel blocker; blockade of potassium channels leads to an increased intracellular calcium influx. At high doses it can also increase muscle contractility.[49] In an experimental cat study using anesthetized and manually ventilated cats, 4-aminopyridine was used effectively to treat verapamil toxicity at a dose of 0.5 mg/kg IV twice, 5 minutes apart.[48] This drug can have significant side effects in animals, including seizure activity, and the dose effective for CCB toxicity has not been definitively established.[24,25,49] At this time, 4-aminopyridine should be considered an experimental treatment and could be considered if all other treatments have failed.

SUMMARY

The prognosis of patients exposed to a CCB depends on the amount ingested, promptness of decontamination, severity of clinical signs, and response to treatment. CCB exposure can be life threatening, with the onset of signs potentially delayed by many hours depending on the individual medication and formulation (extended-release formulations vs regular formulations). The predominant signs of toxicosis include hypotension, cardiac rhythm changes, and hyperglycemia. Treatment can involve decontamination and cardiovascular stabilization with a variety of modalities. The most effective treatment regimen has not been established in companion animals.

REFERENCES

1. Brent J. Calcium channel-blocking agents. In: Brent J, Wallace KL, Burkhart KK, et al, editors. Critical care toxicology: diagnosis and management of the critically poisoned patient. Philadelphia: Elsevier Mosby; 2005. p. 413–26.
2. Johnson JT. Conversion of atrial fibrillation in two dogs using verapamil and supportive therapy. J Am Anim Hosp Assoc 1985;21:429–34.
3. Cooke KL, Snyder PS. Calcium channel blockers in veterinary medicine. J Vet Intern Med 1998;12:123–31.
4. Pion PD, Brown WA. Calcium channel blocking agents. Compend Contin Educ Vet 1995;17:691–706.
5. Mibefradil. In: IBM Micromedex® DRUGDEX® (electronic version). Greenwood Village (CO): Truven Health Analytics. Available at: http://www.micromedex solutions.com/. Accessed May 1, 2018.
6. Bepridil. In: IBM Micromedex® DRUGDEX® (electronic version). Greenwood Village (CO): Truven Health Analytics. Available at: http://www.micromedex solutions.com/. Accessed May 1, 2018.
7. ANTOX: ASPCA Animal Poison Control Center's toxicology database. Urbana (IL): 2001-2018.
8. Triggle DJ. L-type calcium channels. Curr Pharm Des 2006;12:443–57.
9. Kittleson MD. Drugs used to treat cardiac arrhythmias. In: Kittleson MD, Kienle RD, editors. Small animal cardiovascular medicine. St Louis (MO): Mosby; 1998. p. 517–8.
10. Verapamil. In: IBM Micromedex® DRUGDEX® (electronic version). Greenwood Village (CO): Truven Health Analytics. Available at: http://www.micromedex solutions.com/. Accessed May 1, 2018.
11. Diltiazem. In: IBM Micromedex (R) DRUGDEX (R) (electronic version). Greenwood Village (CO): Truven Health Analytics. Available at: http://www. micromedexsolutions.com/. Accessed August 6, 2018.
12. Kittleson MD. Drugs used in the management of heart failure and cardiac arrhythmias. In: Maddison JE, Page SW, Church D, editors. Small animal clinical pharmacology. London: WB Saunders; 2002. p. 371–2, 407–9.
13. Johnson LM, Atkins CE, Keene BW, et al. Pharmacokinetic and pharmacodynamic properties of conventional and CD-formulated diltiazem in cats. J Vet Intern Med 1996;10:316–20.
14. Diltiazem. In: IBM Micromedex® DRUGDEX® (electronic version). Greenwood Village (CO): Truven Health Analytics. Available at: http://www.micromedex solutions.com/. Accessed May 1, 2018.
15. Yabana H, Nagao T, Sato M. Cardiovascular effects of the metabolites of diltiazem in dogs. J Cardiovasc Pharmacol 1985;7:152–7.
16. Stopher DA, Beresford AP, Macrae PV, et al. The metabolism and pharmacokinetics of amlodipine in humans and animals. J Cardiovasc Pharmacol 1988; 12(Suppl 7):S55–9.

17. Amlodipine. In: IBM Micromedex® DRUGDEX® (electronic version). Greenwood Village (CO): Truven Health Analytics. Available at: http://www.micromedex solutions.com/. Accessed May 1, 2018.

18. Felodipine. In: IBM Micromedex® DRUGDEX® (electronic version). Greenwood Village (CO): Truven Health Analytics. Available at: http://www.micromedex solutions.com/. Accessed May 1, 2018.

19. Nifedipine. In: IBM Micromedex® DRUGDEX® (electronic version). Greenwood Village (CO): Truven Health Analytics. Available at: http://www.micromedex solutions.com/. Accessed May 1, 2018.

20. Nicardipine. In: IBM Micromedex® DRUGDEX® (electronic version). Greenwood Village (CO): Truven Health Analytics. Available at: http://www.micromedex solutions.com/. Accessed May 1, 2018.

21. Nisoldipine. In: IBM Micromedex® DRUGDEX® (electronic version). Greenwood Village (CO): Truven Health Analytics. Available at: http://www.micromedex solutions.com/. Accessed May 1, 2018.

22. Isradipine. In: IBM Micromedex® DRUGDEX® (electronic version). Greenwood Village (CO): Truven Health Analytics. Available at: http://www.micromedex solutions.com/. Accessed May 1, 2018.

23. Plumb D. Plumb's veterinary drugs. Tulsa (OK): Educational Concepts; 2018. dba Brief Media. Available at: http://www.plumbsveterinarydrugs.com. Accessed May 1, 2018.

24. Holder T. Calcium channel blocker toxicosis. Vet Med 2000;95:912–5.

25. Costello M, Syring RS. Calcium channel blocker toxicity. J Vet Emerg Crit Care (San Antonio) 2008;18:54–60.

26. Shepherd G. Treatment of poisoning caused by β-adrenergic and calcium-channel blockers. Am J Health Syst Pharm 2006;63:1828–35.

27. Syring RS, Costello MF. Temporary transvenous pacing in a dog with diltiazem intoxication. J Vet Emerg Crit Care 2008;18:75–80.

28. Arroyo AM, Kao LW. Calcium channel blocker toxicity. Pediatr Emerg Care 2009; 25:532–8.

29. Humbert VHJ, Munn NJ, Hawkins RF. Noncardiogenic pulmonary edema complicating massive diltiazem overdose. Chest 1991;99:258–9.

30. Brass BJ, Winchester-Penny S, Lipper BL. Massive verapamil overdose complicated by noncardiogenic pulmonary edema. Am J Emerg Med 1996;14:459–61.

31. Hayes C. Calcium channel blocker drug toxicosis. In: Côté E, editor. Clinical veterinary advisor: dogs and cats. 2nd edition. St Louis (MO): Elsevier Mosby; 2011. p. 170–2.

32. Poppenga R. Treatment. In: Plumlee KH, editor. Clinical veterinary toxicology. St Louis (MO): Mosby; 2004. p. 13–21.

33. Thawley VJ, Drobatz KJ. Assessment of dexmedetomidine and other agents for emesis induction in cats: 43 cases (2009-2014). J Am Vet Med Assoc 2015; 247:1415–8.

34. Laine K, Kivisto KT, Neuvonen PJ. Effect of delayed administration of activated charcoal on the absorption of conventional and slow-release verapamil. Clin Toxicol 1997;37:263–8.

35. Nasa P, Singh A, Juneja D, et al. Continuous venovenous hemodiafiltration along with charcoal hemoperfusion for the management of life-threatening lercanidipine and amlodipine overdose. Saudi J Kidney Dis Transpl 2014;25: 1255–8.

36. Rietjens SJ, de Lange DW, Donker DW, et al. Practical recommendations for calcium channel antagonist poisoning. Neth J Med 2016;74:60–7.

37. St-Onge M, Anseeuw K, Cantrell FL, et al. Experts consensus recommendations for the management of calcium channel blocker poisoning in adults. Crit Care Med 2017;45:e306–15.

38. Kline JA, Tomaszewski CA, Schroeder JD, et al. Insulin is a superior antidote for cardiovascular toxicity induced by verapamil in the anesthetized canine. J Pharmacol Exp Ther 1993;267:744–50.

39. Kline JA, Leonova E, Raymond RM. Beneficial myocardial metabolic effects of insulin during verapamil toxicity in the anesthetized canine. Crit Care Med 1995;23: 1251–63.

40. Lheureux PER, Zahir S, Gris M, et al. Bench to bedside review: hyperinsulinaemia/euglycaemia therapy in the management of overdose of calcium-channel blockers. Crit Care 2006;10:212.

41. Engebretsen KM, Kaczmarek KM, Morgan J, et al. High-dose insulin therapy in beta-blocker and calcium channel blocker poisoning. Clin Toxicol 2011;49: 277–83.

42. Maton BL, Simmonds EE, Lee JA, et al. The use of high-dose insulin therapy and intravenous lipid emulsion to treat severe, refractory diltiazem toxicosis in a dog. J Vet Emerg Crit Care 2013;23:321–7.

43. Yuan TH, Kerns WP, Tomaszewski CA, et al. Insulin-glucose as adjunctive therapy for severe calcium channel antagonist poisoning. Clin Toxicol 1999;37:463–74.

44. Fernandez AL, Lee JA, Rahilly L, et al. The use of intravenous lipid emulsion as an antidote in veterinary toxicology. J Vet Emerg Crit Care 2011;21:309–20.

45. Weinberg GL, VadeBoncouer T, Ramaraju GA, et al. Lipid emulsion infusion rescues dogs from bupivicaine-induced cardiac toxicity. Reg Anesth Pain Med 2003;28:198–202.

46. Bania TC, Chu J, Perez E, et al. Hemodynamic effects of intravenous fat emulsion in an animal model of severe verapamil toxicity resuscitated with atropine, calcium, and saline. Acad Emerg Med 2007;14:105–11.

47. Crandell DE, Weinberg GL. Moxidectin toxicosis in a puppy successfully treated with intravenous lipids. J Vet Emerg Crit Care 2009;19:181–6.

48. Agoston S, Maestrone E, van Hezik EJ, et al. Effective treatment of verapamil intoxication with 4-aminopyridine in the cat. J Clin Invest 1984;73:1291–6.

49. Kline JA. Calcium channel antagonists. In: Ford MD, Delaney KA, Ling LJ, et al, editors. Clinical toxicology. Philadelphia: WB Saunders; 2001. p. 370–7.

Management of Attention-Deficit Disorder and Attention-Deficit/Hyperactivity Disorder Drug Intoxication in Dogs and Cats: An Update

Laura Stern, DVM*, Mary Schell, DVM

KEYWORDS

- ADHD • ADD • Drug intoxication • Dog • Cat • Amphetamines • Atomoxetine

KEY POINTS

- Amphetamines and the nonamphetamine atomoxetine are commonly used in the treatment of attention-deficit disorder/attention-deficit/hyperactivity disorder in humans.
- Because these medications are often found in homes, dog and cat exposure to these medications is a common intoxication.
- Amphetamine intoxication can cause life-threatening central nervous system and cardiovascular stimulation, even when small amounts are ingested.
- This medication is quickly and well absorbed orally, and the onset of clinical signs is generally 30 minutes to 2 hours with immediate release products.
- Treatment is aimed at preventing absorption, controlling the stimulatory signs, and protecting the kidneys; prognosis is generally good, and treatment is very rewarding with control of the stimulatory signs.

Attention-deficit disorder/attention-deficit/hyperactivity disorder (ADD/ADHD) is defined as "a neurodevelopmental behavioral disorder resulting in a pattern of inattention and/or hyperactivity that causes impairment in social, emotional, cognitive, behavioral, and academic functioning,"[1] and it is treated with a variety of stimulants, in both immediate-release and extended-release formulations. The purpose of using the stimulant drugs is to improve brain levels of serotonin and norepinephrine.

This article is an update of the previously published article in the March 2012 issue of *Veterinary Clinics of North America: Small Animal Practice*.
The authors have nothing to disclose.
ASPCA Animal Poison Control Center, 1717 South Philo Road, Suite 36, Urbana, IL 61802, USA
* Corresponding author.
E-mail address: laura.stern@aspca.org

Specific drugs prescribed for the management of ADHD include both amphet-amine class stimulants and nonstimulants, such as atomoxetine (Strattera) (**Table 1**).[1] When these drugs are ingested by dogs and cats, although the drugs differ in rate of absorption and time to onset of clinical signs, those signs are very similar and can be managed similarly. Key to the treatment of dogs and cats is to manage signs as they develop and not delay treatment while the ingested agent is identified.

Second-line therapy may include the use of antidepressant class medications, such as imipramine, bupropion, or nortriptyline, for patients who do not respond adequately to the first-line stimulants or who have coexisting mood disorders. This article does not address these nonstimulant agents beyond noting that they may be included in the general grouping of "ADHD drugs" in the case of ingestion by a household pet.[1]

AMPHETAMINE SALTS AND OTHER SIMILAR AGENTS
Use in Veterinary Medicine

Amphetamines were used in veterinary medicine to increase the respiratory rate and depth in animals undergoing anesthesia with barbiturates, due to its stimulatory ef-fects on the medulla oblongata.[2] Methylphenidate has also been used for the treat-ment of narcolepsy in dogs, although it has been only partially effective when used as the sole treatment.[3] Amphetamine use was placed under strict control by the 1970 Controlled Substances Act. Amphetamines are no longer available for veterinary use in the United States.

Mechanism of Toxicity

Amphetamines cause release of catecholamines, resulting in the stimulation of the ce-rebrospinal axis, especially the brainstem, cerebral cortex, medullary respiratory cen-ter, and reticular activating system.[2,4] Amphetamines cause marked increased in the release of norepinephrine, dopamine, and serotonin from presynaptic terminals.[5,6] Monoamine oxidase is also inhibited, which is one of the metabolic pathways of catecholamine metabolism.[6] This increase in catecholamine release and inhibition of reuptake cause both α and β stimulation. This catecholamine effect results in vaso-constriction with sequelae of hypertension, tachycardia, cardiac dysrhythmias, and central nervous system (CNS) stimulatory signs. Cardiac output is generally not appre-ciably affected, due to reflex bradycardia.[7] Methylphenidate is a CNS stimulant that is structurally related to amphetamines.[8] Methylphenidate is "thought to block the reup-take of norepinephrine and dopamine into the presynaptic neuron and increase the release of these monoamines into the extraneuronal space."[9]

Pharmacokinetics, Toxicity, and Metabolism

The median lethal dose (LD_{50}) for orally administered amphetamine sulfate in dogs is 20 to 27 mg/kg.[10] Generally, the LD_{50} for most amphetamines is between 10 and 23 mg/kg.[11] The LD_{50} for methylphenidate has not been established. Experimentally, healthy beagle dogs survived dosage regimens of greater than 20 mg/kg/d for 90 days.[12]

Following rapid absorption from the gastrointestinal tract, amphetamines enter the cerebrospinal fluid at up to 80% of plasma concentrations.[13] Amphetamines are pri-marily excreted in the urine without any biotransformation. However, in vivo research shows that amphetamines do undergo oxidative deamination and aromatic hydroxyl-ation in the liver of dogs.[14] Deaminated metabolites are oxidized to benzoic acid and excreted in the urine as the glycine conjugate of hippuric acid. Amphetamines are

Table 1
Amphetamine class attention-deficit/hyperactivity disorder drugs

Trade Name	Generic Name	Available Formulations
Adderall	Amphetamine	5-, 7.5-, 10-, 12.5-, 15-, 20-, and 30-mg tablet
Adderall XR	Amphetamine (extended release)	5-, 10-, 15-, 20-, 25-, and 30-mg capsule
Concerta	Methylphenidate (long acting)	18-, 27-, 36-, and 54-mg tablets
Daytrana	Methylphenidate patch	10, 15, 20, and 30 mg/9-h patch
Desoxyn	Methamphetamine hydrochloride	2.5-, 5-, 10-, and 15-mg tablets; 5-, 10-, and 15-mg SR tablets
Dexedrine	Dextroamphetamine	5-, 10-, and 15-mg Spansule XR
Dextrostat	Dextroamphetamine	5- and 10-mg tablets
Focalin	Dexmethylphenidate	2.5-, 5-, and 10-mg tablets
Focalin XR	Dexmethylphenidate (extended release)	5-, 10-, 15-, 20-, 30-, and 40-mg XR capsules
Metadate ER	Methylphenidate (extended release)	20-mg extended-release tablet
Metadate CD	Methylphenidate (extended release)	10-, 20-, 30-, 40-, 50-, and 60-mg XR capsules
Methylin	Methylphenidate (oral solution and chewable tablets)	2.5-, 5-, and 10-mg chewable tablets; 5-, 10-, and 20-mg tablets; 5- and 10-mg/tsp solution; 10- and 20-mg XR tablets
Ritalin	Methylphenidate	5-, 10-, and 20-mg tablets
Ritalin SR	Methylphenidate	20-mg SR tablet
Ritalin LA	Methylphenidate (long acting)	10-, 20-, 30-, and 40-mg XR capsules
Strattera	Atomoxetine	10-, 18-, 25-, 40-, 60-, 80-, and 100-mg capsules
Vyvanse	Lisdexamfetamine dimesylate	20-, 30-, 40-, 50-, 60-, and 70-mg capsules

Abbreviations: SR, sustained release; XR, extended release.

weak bases, and urinary excretion is pH dependent.[13] Because the metabolism varies widely between species that were studied, these data cannot be extended to cats.

Clinical Signs

Clinical signs commonly seen with amphetamine intoxication are cardiovascular (CV) signs, including significant hypertension (often in conjunction with reflex bradycardia), tachycardia, and tachyarrhythmias; CNS stimulatory signs are common, including hyperactivity, agitation, mydriasis, circling, head bobbing, apprehension, and tremors. Seizures can occur but are rare. Lethargy, depression, and coma have been reported later in the course of intoxication. Gastrointestinal upset can also be seen, as well as anorexia. Animals may be mildly to severely hyperthermic secondary to stimulatory signs. Disseminated intravascular coagulopathy (DIC) can be seen as sequelae to the hyperthermia.

Diagnosis

Diagnosis is supported by history of exposure or recovery of pills or capsules in the vomitus. One study group took a human on-site urine multidrug test and evaluated it for the use in dogs; it was found to be sensitive and specific for the detection of amphetamines. It has not been validated for use in cats.[15] Thin layer chromatography is commonly used, and immunologic assays can also be used for urine and plasma. Gas chromatography–mass spectrometry can also be used for detecting amphetamines in urine or plasma samples, especially in legal cases.[10] Necropsy findings in experimental dogs showed subendocardial and epicardial hemorrhage and myocardial necrosis.[10]

Differential Diagnoses

Differential diagnoses include pseudoephedrine, cocaine, methamphetamine, phenylpropanolamine, methylxanthines (caffeine, theobromine, theophylline), ma huang, 5-hydroxytryptophan (5-HTP), and other serotonergic medication intoxications.

ASPCA Animal Poison Control Center's Experience

A review of the ASPCA Animal Poison Control Center's (APCC) toxicology database from 2010 to June 2018 found amphetamine salt and methylphenidate toxicity cases involving 4189 dogs and 844 cats.[16] These cases involved exposure to one agent (an amphetamine or methylphenidate) only and were assessed as medium or high suspect cases (history of exposure and clinical signs were consistent with amphetamine or methylphenidate toxicosis). These cases were not confirmed via analytical methods.

Of the canine cases, full recovery was noted in 128 cases, 13 dogs died, 3 dogs were euthanized, and final outcome was unknown in 4045 cases. The most commonly reported clinical signs (reported in 4% or more of the cases) were hyperactivity or agitation in 2930 (71%) of 4120, hyperthermia 1312 (32%) of 4120, tachycardia 1215 (30%) of 4120, mydriasis 873 (21%) of 4120, panting 750 (18%) of 4120, restlessness 601 (14%) of 4120, pacing 466 (11%) of 4120, head bobbing 380 (9%) of 4120, circling 380 (9%) of 4120, hypertension 371 (9%) of 4120, anxiety 344 (8%) of 4120, behavior change 319 (8%) of 4120, hypersalivation 317 (8%) of 4120, vocalization 292 (7%) of 4120, hyperesthesia 289 (7%) of 4120, disorientation 257 (6%) of 4120, vomiting 252 (6%) of 4120, staring 257 (6%) of 4120, and bradycardia 178 (4%) of 4120.

With the 844 feline cases, 25 made a full recovery, 2 died, and final outcome for 817 cases were not available. The most commonly reported clinical signs (reported in 5% or more of the cases) were mydriasis in 423 (50%) of 844, tachycardia 343 (41%) of 844, agitation 236 (28%) of 844, hyperthermia 161 (19%) of 844, tachypnea 133 (16%) of 844, vocalization 128 (15%) of 844, panting 125 (15%) of 844, disorientation 115 (14%) of 844, behavior change 112 (13%) of 844, pacing 96 (11%) of 844, head bobbing 86 (10%) of 844, staring 86 (10%) of 844, hyperesthesia 78 (9%) of 844, circling 75 (9%) of 844, vomiting 75 (9%) of 844, restlessness 72 (9%) of 844, hypersalivation 60 (7%) of 844, hypertension 54 (6%) of 844, mouth breathing 44 (5%) of 844, anxiety 44 (5%) of 844.

Clinical signs with amphetamine salt medications started at 0.09 mg/kg with hyperactivity, agitation, and restlessness. Tachycardia, hyperthermia, mydriasis, tachypnea, head bobbing, pacing, disorientation, vocalizing, tachypnea, anxiety, hypersalivation, staring, and hiding were seen starting at dosages from 0.2 mg/kg. Hyperesthesia was seen starting at dosages of 0.5 mg/kg; circling was seen at dosages starting at 0.6 mg/kg; tremors were seen starting at 0.7 mg/kg, and seizures were seen starting at 1.3 mg/kg.

Clinical signs with methylphenidate started at slightly higher doses than with amphetamines. Tachycardia and hyperthermia were seen starting at 0.3 mg/kg, hyperactivity and hyperthermia at 0.6 mg/kg, vocalizing at 0.8 mg/kg, and hypertension at 0.85 mg/kg.

A case report involving a dog ingesting 19 mg/kg amphetamine (Adderall) in the literature showed increased alanine aminotransferase (ALT), alkaline phosphatase (ALP), and metarubricytosis. The dog was also mildly hypoglycemic. The metarubricytosis was attributed to pyrexia with ensuing damage to the bone marrow sinusoidal epithelium and vascular endothelium. The increased ALT may have occurred due to direct thermal damage to hepatocytes or secondary to hypoperfusion. The increased ALP was attributed to release of endogenous corticosteroids.[17] Blood work abnormalities resolved without treatment. No such bone marrow abnormalities were found in the APCC database.

Treatment Recommendations

There is no specific antidote for amphetamine toxicosis. When a pet is suspected to have ingested a stimulant medication, the immediate response depends on whether there are clinical signs on presentation for evaluation, the potential dose, and the formulation.

The goal of treatment is to prevent absorption of the medication, control the stimulatory signs, treat hyperthermia, treat cardiovascular effects, and protect the kidneys.

Emesis can be induced with apomorphine or hydrogen peroxide, if the exposure to a prompt release product was very recent (<30 minutes). Animals ingesting an extended-release product may benefit from emesis for up to 2 hours after exposure, if clinical signs are not yet being shown. Animals that are showing stimulatory signs, such as hyperactivity, pacing, or tremoring, are at risk for aspiration, and emesis should not be induced. Activated charcoal can be given. With extended-release products, a second half-dose can be given 8 hours after the first dose if stimulatory signs are still observed, but the pet should be monitored for signs of hypernatremia. With very high doses, gastric lavage can be performed under anesthesia with a cuffed endotracheal tube in place, if emesis cannot be safely induced. Activated charcoal can then be instilled via the orogastric tube before anesthesia is discontinued.

Phenothiazines should be considered the mainstay of controlling stimulatory signs with amphetamine intoxication. Phenothiazine tranquilizers are effective because of their effects on dopamine. They inhibit its release, block postsynaptic binding, and increase the turnover of dopamine in the CNS. In addition, they also help to block the α-adrenergic activity induced by amphetamines.[18] Acepromazine can initially be given at 0.05 mg/kg intravenously (IV) and titrated to effect for stimulatory signs. The dose can be gradually increased to 0.1 to 1.0 mg/kg if clinical signs do not resolve with lower doses. Blood pressure should be monitored at higher doses to ensure that hypotension does not occur. Chlorpromazine can be used as an alternative treatment and is given at 0.5 mg/kg IV initially, and it may also be titrated up as needed to control stimulatory signs. Large doses of phenothiazines may be needed to control the clinical signs. Chlorpromazine has also been shown to have antiarrhythmic effects because it protects the heart from β_1 simulation due to an excess of epinephrine and norepinephrine, which can help alleviate tachycardia and tachyarrhythmias. Phenothiazines can also cause hypotensive and hypothermic effects, both of which are helpful in the treatment of amphetamine intoxication, due to the potential for hypertension and hyperthermia.[19]

Another important part of amphetamine toxicosis involves treatment of cardiac arrhythmias, although they often resolve with the treatment of the CNS stimulatory signs.[10] If the pet has been treated with phenothiazines and is resting quietly but still showing significant tachycardia, propranolol at 0.02 to 0.06 mg/kg slowly IV can be used. The total dosage is based on the clinical response of the tachycardia; monitoring an electrocardiogram (ECG) may be needed while giving propranolol, so it can be titrated to the target heart rate. Do not use this in hypertensive animals, because administration of propranolol can further worsen the hypertension. Treatment of tachycardia with propranolol has not been shown to improve survival in amphetamine intoxication cases.[11] Esmolol, which is a specific β_1-blocking agent, can be used if propranolol is not helping to resolve the tachycardia (25–200 μg/kg/min constant rate infusion).

IV fluids should be instituted to help maintain normal hydration status, enhance renal excretion of the medication, and help protect the kidneys, should myoglobinuria occur. If giving fluids above the maintenance rate to a hypertensive animal, the lungs should be monitored for pulmonary edema.

Animals should be kept in a dark and quiet area of the hospital to decrease stimulation, especially in hyperesthetic animals. Thermoregulation in the form of fans and cool towels should help to cool hyperthermic animals. Control of stimulatory signs will usually also help prevent the worsening of hyperthermia.

The use of diazepam is generally avoided in patients showing stimulatory signs because its use can increase the chances of paradoxic hyperactivity and dysphoria.[10] If seizures are seen, they should be controlled with barbiturates. Phenobarbital can be dosed at 3 to 4 mg/kg IV. Gas anesthesia, levetiracetam, or propofol can be used for seizures that are refractory to barbiturates. Diazepam, although not generally used with patients showing stimulatory signs, can also be used with seizing patients. Antiepileptics will stop the physical signs of the seizures until levels of the amphetamines in the brain drop and the seizures are controlled in the brain. Tremors can be controlled with methocarbamol 50 to 220 mg/kg IV, given slowly to effect. The rate of infusion should not exceed 2 mL/min.

Urine acidification may be helpful, because amphetamine elimination in the urine is enhanced at a pH between 4.5 and 5.5. This pH level can be achieved with ammonium chloride administration at 100 to 200 mg/kg/d orally divided 4 times daily or ascorbic acid 20 to 30 mg/kg orally, subcutaneously, intramuscularly (IM), or IV. Urinary acidification should not be attempted if the urine is already in the target pH range, the pet is acidotic, acid-base status cannot be monitored, or if rhabdomyolysis or evidence of acute renal failure is present.[11]

IV lipid emulsion (ILE) infusion is not indicated for cases of amphetamine toxicoses, due to a lack of efficacy. Clinical signs may worsen with the administration of ILE, because the efficacy of some therapeutic medications may decrease, if they are affected by ILE.

Monitoring of the Patient

Pet should have blood pressure and heart rate monitored closely. An ECG should be instituted in all pets with noted tachycardia or reflex bradycardia. Pets should be monitored for hyperactivity and CNS stimulation signs.

Urinalysis can be performed to watch for myoglobinuria. Pets with poorly controlled signs or pets that were significantly hyperthermic may need to have complete blood count and coagulation profile monitored to detect DIC.

The onset of clinical signs is generally 30 minutes to 2 hours. Pets may require hospitalization, monitoring, and treatment for up to 72 hours depending on the dosage and whether the medication is a prompt- or extended-release product. Patients are generally ready to be released when 8 hours has passed since any treatments were indicated.

PROGNOSIS

Prognosis is generally good, as long as CNS stimulation and CV signs can be controlled. Seizures and seizurelike activity and cardiac failure pose the highest risk to the pet. Pets with underlying cardiac disease may be at increased risk of developing life-threatening arrhythmias and may be more susceptible to severe signs.[10] Cause of death in amphetamine toxicity is generally attributed to DIC secondary to hyperthermia and respiratory failure.[20] No long-term effects are expected in animals making a full recovery.

ATOMOXETINE

Very little information has been published about the toxicity, mechanism of action, or treatment of atomoxetine in dogs and cats; therefore, information is generally limited to clinical experience in the treatment of atomoxetine intoxication and human data. Atomoxetine is a selective norepinephrine reuptake inhibitor that is used to treat ADHD. The exact mechanism by which produces its therapeutic effects in ADHD is unknown.[21]

Pharmacokinetics and Metabolism

Atomoxetine was well absorbed from the gastrointestinal tracts of dogs. Atomoxetine is highly protein bound at 97% in dogs. The bioavailability in the dog was about 74%. The bioavailability appears to have great variability between species and cannot be extrapolated to the cat. Atomoxetine is highly metabolized in the liver of dogs by N-demethylation, aromatic ring hydroxylation, benzylic ring hydroxylation, glucuronidation, and sulfonation. Atomoxetine and its metabolites were excreted 48% in the urine and 42% in the feces of dogs. The fecal excretion appears to be due to biliary elimination and not due to unabsorbed drug. In fact, very little atomoxetine was eliminated intact.[20]

Mechanism of Action

Atomoxetine is a methyl phenoxy-benzene propanamine derivative with antidepressant activity. Atomoxetine purportedly enhances noradrenergic function via selective inhibition of the presynaptic norepinephrine transporter. The mechanism of action by which produces its therapeutic effects in ADHD is unknown.[16]

ASPCA Animal Poison Control Center's Experience

A review of the APCC toxicology database from 2010 to June 2018 found atomoxetine toxicity cases involving 53 dogs and 14 cats.[16] These cases involved exposure to one agent (atomoxetine) only and were assessed as medium or high suspect cases (history of exposure and clinical signs were consistent with atomoxetine toxicosis). In the 53 canine cases, follow-up was not available on any of the cases. Mild gastrointestinal signs were seen starting at 0.4 mg/kg, but stimulatory signs, such as hyperactivity, tachycardia, and disorientation, were not seen until 2.2 mg/kg. The most commonly reported clinical signs (reported in 5% or more of the cases) were mydriasis in 12 (23%) of 53 cases, hyperactivity in 10 (19%) of 53, vomiting in 10 (19%) of 53, tachycardia in 10 (19%) of 53, hypersalivation in 9 (17%) of 53, lethargy in 6 (11%) of 53, agitation in 5 (9%) of 53, ataxia in 5 (9%) of 53, hyperthermia in 4 (8%) of 53, behavior change in 4 (8%) of 53, diarrhea in 3 (6%) of 53, head bobbing in 3 (6%) of 53, polydipsia in 3 (6%) of 53, and trembling in 3 (6%) of 53.

In the 21 feline cases, follow-up was not available in any of the cases. Mild, gastrointestinal signs were reported at 0.7 mg/kg, with stimulatory signs (disorientation, tachycardia) starting at 2.2 mg/kg. The most commonly reported clinical signs (reported in 6% or more of the cases) were hypersalivation in 14 (67%) of 21, mydriasis in 8 (38%) of 21, tachycardia in 4 (19%) of 21, disorientation in 2 (10%) of 21, hiding in 2 (10%) of 21, tremors in 2 (10%) of 21, and vomiting in 2 (10%) of 21. With the feline and canine cases, vomiting was seen at 0.4 mg/kg, lethargy and hypersalivation were seen starting at 0.73 mg/kg, ataxia was seen starting at 1.7 mg/kg, mydriasis at 1.4 mg/kg, tachycardia, hyperactivity, hypertension, and disorientation at 2.2 mg/kg, hypertension at 2.0 mg/kg, hyperactivity and agitation at 3.5 mg/kg, vomiting at 4.0 mg/kg, head bobbing at 8.8 mg/kg, and tremors at 19.6 mg/kg.

Diagnosis

Diagnosis is based on history and recovery of pills or capsules in the vomitus. There is no on-site test for this medication. Serum levels may be available at a human hospital.

Differential Diagnoses

Differential diagnoses include methylxanthines (caffeine, theobromine, theophylline), cocaine, methamphetamine, 5-HTP, and other serotonergic medication intoxications.

Monitoring

The onset of clinical signs is generally 30 minutes to 2 hours. The duration of signs is between 12 and 24 hours. Pets should have heart rate, blood pressure, and CNS status monitored. Electrolytes and hydration status should be monitored in pets with significant vomiting.

Treatment

Treatment is based largely on providing good supportive care to patients exhibiting clinical signs, because there are little published data about the treatment of atomoxetine toxicity in dogs and cats.

Emesis can be induced in asymptomatic animals (as discussed in the section on amphetamine treatment). Activated charcoal can be given following emesis, but the animals should be monitored for hypernatremia. If a high dosage has been ingested, gastric lavage can be performed with the animal under anesthesia with a cuffed endotracheal tube in place, if emesis cannot be safely induced. Activated charcoal can then be instilled via the orogastric tube before anesthesia is discontinued.

Vomiting can be managed symptomatically with antiemetic medications. IV fluids should be given to help support the pet's CV system and to help prevent dehydration secondary to gastrointestinal upset.

Diazepam at 0.1 to 0.5 mg/kg IV to effect or methocarbamol 50 to 220 mg/kg IV to effect can be used to treat tremors. Nitroprusside 0.5 to 10 µg/kg/min in D5W titrated to effect can be used to treat hypertension. Diphenhydramine 2 mg/kg IM can be used for atomoxetine-induced dystonia (involuntary muscle spasms and contractions).

Affected animals should be kept in a dark and quiet area in order to decrease stimulation, if the animal is hyperesthetic. Thermoregulation in the form of fans and cool towels should help to cool hyperthermic animals. Control of stimulatory signs will also help prevent the worsening of hyperthermia.

Prognosis

Prognosis should be considered good, and animals generally respond well to treatment. Animals with underlying liver disease, hypertension, tachycardia, or other CV or cerebrovascular disease may be more sensitive to this medication. No long-term effects are expected.

SUMMARY

In summary, amphetamines or similar stimulants and the nonamphetamine atomoxetine are commonly used in the treatment of ADD/ADHD in humans. Because these medications are often found in homes, dog and cat exposure to these medications is a fairly common intoxication. Amphetamine intoxication can cause life-threatening CNS and CV stimulation, even when small amounts are ingested. This medication is quickly and well absorbed orally, and the onset of clinical signs is generally 30 minutes to 2 hours with immediate release products. Treatment is aimed at preventing absorption, controlling the stimulatory signs, and protecting the kidneys. Prognosis is generally good, and treatment is very rewarding with control of the stimulatory signs.

Atomoxetine also has a fast onset of action with development of clinical signs within 30 minutes to 2 hours. Stimulatory signs, such as hyperactivity and tachycardia, are often seen with atomoxetine toxicosis. Treatment is aimed at providing symptomatic and supportive care to patients showing clinical signs. Prognosis is generally good with animals receiving prompt and appropriate treatment.

REFERENCES

1. DRUGDEX System [intranet database]. Version 5.1. Greenwood Village (CO): Thomson Reuters (Healthcare) Inc. Accessed January 2, 2012.
2. Adams HR. Adrenergic agonists and antagonists. In: Riviere JE, Papch MG, editors. Veterinary pharmacology and therapeutics. Ames (IO): Wiley-Blackwell; 2009. p. 141–2.
3. Mitler MM, Soave O, Dement WC. Narcolepsy in seven dogs. J Am Vet Med Assoc 1976;168:1036–8.
4. Beasley VR, Dorman DC, Fikes JD, et al, editors. A systems affected approach to veterinary toxicology. Urbana (IL): University of Illinois; 1999. p. 133–4.
5. Volmer P. Human drugs of abuse. In: Bonaguara JD, Twedt DC, editors. Kirk's current veterinary therapy XIV. St Louis (MO): Elsevier; 2009. p. 144–5.
6. Diniz PP, Sousa MG, Gerardi DG, et al. Amphetamine poisoning in a dog: case report, literature review and veterinary medicine perspectives. Vet Hum Toxicol 2003;45:315–7.
7. Amphetamines. Drugdex system [intranet database]. Version 5.1. Greenwood Village (CO): Thomson Reuters (Healthcare) Inc. Accessed January 2, 2012.
8. Genovese DW, Gwaltney-Brant SM. Methylphenidate toxicosis in dogs: 128 cases (2001-2008). J Am Vet Med Assoc 2010;12:1438–43.
9. Methylphenidate. In: POISINDEX® System (electronic version). Greenwood Village (CO): Thomson Reuters (Healthcare) Inc; 2011. Available at: http://www.thomsonhc.com. Accessed January 12, 2012.
10. Bischoff K. Toxicity of drugs of abuse. In: Gupta R, editor. Veterinary toxicology: basic and clinical principles. Amsterdam: Elsevier; 2007. p. 401–3.
11. Wismer T. Amphetamines. In: Osweiler GD, Howvda LR, Brutlag AG, et al, editors. Clinical companion: small animal toxicology. Ames (IO): Wiley-Blackwell; 2011. p. 125–30.
12. Teo SK, Stirling DI, Thomas SD, et al. A 90 day oral gavage toxicity study of d-methylphenidate and d,l methylphenidate in beagle dogs. Int J Toxicol 2003; 22:215–26.
13. Kisseberth WC, Trammel HL. Toxicology of selected pesticides, drugs, and chemicalsIllicit and abused drugs. Vet Clin North Am Small Anim Pract 1990; 20(2):405–18.

14. Green CE, LeValley SE, Tyson CA. Comparison of amphetamine metabolism using isolated hepatocytes from five species including human. J Pharmacol Exp Ther 1986;237:931–6.

15. Teitler J. Evaluation of a human on-site urine multidrug test for emergency use with dogs. J Am Anim Hosp Assoc 2009;45:59–66.

16. ANTOX: ASPCA Animal Poison Control Center's toxicology database. Urbana (IL): 2003–2011, in press.

17. Wilcox A, Russell KE. Hematologic changes associate with Adderall toxicity in a dog. Vet Clin Pathol 2008;37:184–9.

18. Mensching D, Volmer PA. Neurotoxicity. In: Gupta R, editor. Veterinary toxicology: basic and clinical principles. Amsterdam: Elsevier; 2007. p. 135.

19. Gross ME, Booth NH. Tranquilizers. In: Adams HR, editor. Veterinary pharmacology and therapeutics. Ames (IO): Iowa State University Press; 1995.

20. Atomoxetine. In: POISINDEX® System (electronic version). Greenwood Village (CO): Thomson Reuters (Healthcare) Inc; 2010. Available at: http://www.thomsonhc.com. Accessed January 12, 2012.

21. Mattuiz EL, Ponsler GD, Barbuch RJ, et al. Disposition and metabolic fate of atomoxetine hydrochloide: pharmacokinetics, metabolism, and excretion in the fischer 344 rat and beagle dog. J Pharmacol Exp Ther 2003;31:88–97.

Toxicology of Frequently Encountered Nonsteroidal Anti-inflammatory Drugs in Dogs and Cats: An Update

Mary Kay McLean, DVM, MS[a], Safdar A. Khan, DVM, MS, PhD[b],*

KEYWORDS

- Toxicology • Nonsteroidal anti-inflammatory drugs • Incidents • Dogs • Cats
- Treatment

KEY POINTS

- Nonsteroidal anti-inflammatory drugs (NSAIDs) are extensively used in both human and veterinary medicine for their antipyretic, anti-inflammatory, and analgesic properties.
- Each year, thousands of dogs and cats are intentionally and accidentally exposed/overdosed to NSAIDs.
- In dogs and cats, NSAIDs are approved for osteoarthritis and postoperative pain. Along with their benefits, NSAIDs also have some undesirable effects that can be seen both with therapeutic use and in overdose situations.

GENERAL USES AND CLASSIFICATION

Nonsteroidal anti-inflammatory drugs (NSAIDs) are used to treat a variety of conditions, including headaches and migraines, rheumatoid arthritis, osteoarthritis, inflammatory arthropathies, acute gout, dysmenorrhea, metastatic bone pain, postoperative pain, mild-to-moderate pain caused by inflammation and tissue injury, pyrexia, ileus, and renal colic. In dogs and cats, NSAIDs are approved for osteoarthritis and postoperative pain. Along with their benefits, NSAIDs also have some undesirable effects that can be seen both with therapeutic use and in overdose situations.

This article originally appeared in *Veterinary Clinics of North America: Small Animal Practice*, Volume 42, Issue 2, March 2012.

The authors have nothing to disclose. The views and opinions expressed in this article are those of authors and do not necessarily reflect policy or position of the editors or their employer or the publisher.

[a] US Army, Veterinary Treatment Facility, Building 265, 10th Division Road, Fort Benning, GA 31905, USA; [b] Global Pharmacovigilance, Zoetis Animal Health, 333 Portage Road, Kalamazoo, MI 49007, USA

* Corresponding author.

E-mail address: Safdar.khan@zoetis.com

The first NSAID discovered in 1897 was acetylsalicylic acid, or aspirin. In 1961, ibuprofen was discovered after scientists had been searching for an option that had less risk for adverse gastrointestinal (GI) effects compared with aspirin. Ibuprofen became available on an over-the-counter basis in the United States in 1984. In a continued attempt to discover an NSAID with even less risk for adverse effects, the first selective cyclooxygenase (COX)-2 inhibitor was approved by the US Food and Drug Administration (FDA) in 1999, and the first prostaglandin E2 (PGE2) EP4 receptor antagonist was approved by the FDA for use in dogs in 2016. Most NSAIDs are substituted organic acids classified into 3 main groups: carboxylic acids, enolic acids, and COX-2 inhibitors. The carboxylic acids can be further divided into salicylic acids, acetic acids, propionic acid, and fenamic acid. The enolic acid group can be further divided into pyazolones and oxicams. NSAIDs are placed in each of these groups based on their mechanism of action or chemical structure if the mechanism of action is not, or was not, known at the time of classification. Grapiprant is a non-COX inhibiting NSAID in the piprant class. Some veterinary approved NSAIDs (approved by the FDA) for use in dogs include carprofen, deracoxib, etodolac, firocoxib, grapiprant, meloxicam, robenacoxib, and tepoxalin. NSAIDs approved for use in cats include meloxicam and robenacoxib.

INCIDENT DATA

The widespread availability of NSAIDs has resulted in a marked increase in the number of overdose cases in people. From 1985 to 1988, 55,800 cases of ibuprofen exposure were reported to the American Association of Poison Control Centers (AAPCC). In 1994 alone, the total number of NSAID exposures was 50,154, of which 35,703 cases were related to ibuprofen exposure. Despite their widespread use, the adverse effects associated with NSAID use are relatively few. One report suggests the incidence of adverse drug reactions associated with NSAID use is 24.4 cases per 1 million prescriptions. The fatal adverse reactions are estimated at 1.1 fatal reaction per 1 million prescriptions.[1] According to more recent information compiled by the AAPCC from 2003 to 2007, approximately 4% of all human incidents reported to AAPCC involved exposure to an NSAID. This translates to about 90,000 to 100,000 calls annually. The fatality review board of the AAPCC, in its annual report during 2006 and 2007, assigned 5 fatalities and 107 life-threatening manifestations to NSAID exposures.[2]

Although there are several case reports that discuss toxicity reactions resulting from exposure to different NSAIDs in dogs and cats, the total incidence of adverse effects resulting from NSAID ingestion in dogs and cats is not known. Data from the American Society for the Prevention of Cruelty to Animals (ASPCA) Animal Poison Control Center (APCC) electronic medical record database involving exposure to different NSAIDs (human and veterinary approved NSAID) were reviewed from 2010 to 2017. This review included information retrieved from the APCC public database. During this time period, the APCC received 60,177 reports of animals exposed to different types of NSAIDs. These cases accounted for approximately 4.2% of the total cases called into the APCC. The dog was the most commonly reported species (55,084 dogs), followed by the cat (4227 cats). The other animals exposed to NSAIDs included birds, horses, ferrets, and pigs. The most common NSAID involved was ibuprofen (21,518 incidents), followed by carprofen (14,441 incidents), aspirin (7844 incidents), naproxen (6533 incidents), meloxicam (2787 incidents), deracoxib (2288 incidents), diclofenac (1191 incidents), firocoxib (1186 incidents), celecoxib (802 incidents), indomethacin (350 incidents), piroxicam (326 incidents), grapiprant (315 incidents), nabumetone (167 incidents), and robenacoxib (101 incidents). Of the 3 classes of NSAIDs, exposures to carboxylic acid-derivative was most commonly reported, with ibuprofen being the most commonly reported ingredient, followed by carprofen and aspirin.

GENERAL INFORMATION REGARDING ABSORPTION, DISTRIBUTION, METABOLISM, AND EXCRETION

Most NSAIDs are absorbed rapidly and almost completely following oral administration. Peak plasma concentration is usually achieved within 2 to 4 hours after oral administration. Absorption occurs mainly in the stomach and upper small intestine and is influenced by pH. Because NSAIDs are weak acids, they are un-ionized in the highly acidic gastric environment. In this state, NSAIDs are lipid soluble and easily diffuse into gastric cells, where the pH is higher, and the drug dissociates. In this manner, NSAIDs become ion trapped within the gastric cells. These high local concentrations contribute to the GI adverse effects of NSAIDs.[3]

Concurrent administration of aluminum or magnesium antacids or presence of food may delay absorption of NSAIDs. Although presence of antacids may delay absorption, the total amount of drug absorbed is unaffected. A larger fraction of the NSAID dose is absorbed in the small intestine under these circumstances. Rectal administration of NSAIDs does not provide any advantage, because absorption is erratic and incomplete.[3]

All NSAIDs are highly protein bound (98%–99%), mainly to albumin; only the unbound drug is biologically active. NSAIDs are metabolized in the liver and metabolites are mainly excreted in the urine. The major mechanism of conjugation is with glucuronic acid, which in some cases is preceded by oxidation and hydroxylation.[1] In general, less than 10% of a dose is excreted unchanged by the kidneys; however, larger amounts of indomethacin, flurbiprofen, tolmectin, and piroxicam are eliminated by this route.[1,3,4] The high degree of protein binding restricts these drugs to the plasma compartment, accounting for small volumes of distribution. Most NSAIDs bind only to albumin. The concentration of free drug rapidly increases after the albumin binding sites are saturated, leading to rapid efficacy of most NSAIDs. The kidney rapidly excretes the unbound drug, so that accumulation is prevented. Because the NSAIDs are strongly protein bound, they can be displaced from binding sites or can displace other protein-bound drugs (eg, corticosteroids), potentiating the effects of these drugs.[3]

Elimination half-lives of NSAIDs vary considerably, ranging from 1 to 1.5 hours for tolmectin, ketoprofen, and diclofenac and 25 to 50 hours for oxaprozin and piroxicam.[1,3,4] In neonates and patients with renal or hepatic disease, half-lives of NSAIDs are usually increased. Many NSAIDs such as naproxen, sulindac, indomethacin, diclofenac, flufenamic acid, ibuprofen, phenylbutazone, and piroxicam undergo significant enterohepatic recirculation.[3] Naproxen in dogs is known to have much longer half-life (74 hours) compared with other NSAIDs.

GENERAL MECHANISMS OF ACTIONS

Salicylates inhibit the enzyme COX that enables the synthesis of prostaglandins (PGs), which mediate inflammation and fever. All members of the salicylate class have similar properties, because the parent compound is first metabolized to salicylic acid. Salicylic acid is then further metabolized to the primary metabolite salicyluric acid by glycine, and then to the more minor metabolites phenolic glucuronide, acylglucuronide, and gentisic acid by glucuronidation and oxidation. Salicylic acid is also eliminated unchanged in the urine. Alkaline urine allows for a greater percentage to be eliminated unchanged than acidic urine.

The 2 forms or isoenzymes of COX are COX-1 and COX-2.[5,6] COX-1 appears to be present naturally in the body and is involved in important physiologic functions such as autoregulation of renal blood flow. It is mainly found in the stomach, kidney, endothelium, and platelets. COX-2, which is an inducible form of COX, is believed to be responsible for production of inflammatory mediators.[5] COX-2 is mainly produced by monocytes, fibroblasts, synoviocytes, and chondrocytes in association with inflammation. It has been suggested that inhibition of COX-2 helps decrease inflammation and that inhibition of COX-1 may lead to adverse effects associated with the use of NSAIDs such as GI ulceration and kidney damage.[5] Thus, the NSAIDs that act mainly against COX-1 are more likely to result in GI tract injury compared with NSAIDs that act mostly against COX-2.

Other NSAIDs, including carboxylic acids, enolic acids, and COX-2 selective inhibitors, all share the ability to inhibit PG synthesis by inhibiting COX just like salicylates. Lipoxygenase (LOX) also aids in the synthesis of PG, and most NSAIDs are unable to directly affect the LOX enzyme.

PROSTAGLANDINS

PGs are unsaturated fatty acid compounds derived from 20-carbon essential fatty acids found in tissue membranes, primarily phospholipids.[3,7] PGs are synthesized from the dietary essential fatty acids linoleic acid and linolenic acid. The most important precursor to PG synthesis is arachidonic acid (AA). PG synthesis is started within the cell by cleavage of AA from the membrane phospholipids through the action of cellular phospholipase. Synthesis is stimulated because of membrane damage from any mechanisms such as trauma, infection, fever, or platelet aggregation. The phospholipase causes phospholipids in the membrane to release AA into the cytoplasm. AA is then available for use in the COX or LOX pathways.[7] The COX pathway leads to production of PG (PGH_2, PGI_2, PGE_2, $PGF_{2\alpha}$), prostacyclin, and thromboxane (TX)A_2, and the LOX cascade results in the production of leukotrienes (**Fig. 1**).[5] Collectively, PGs, TXs, and leukotrienes are known as eicosanoids. TXs are primarily

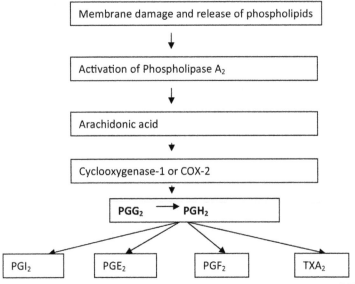

Fig. 1. Pathway involved in the production of prostaglandins. (*Data from* Refs.[5,6,8,11])

produced by platelets and are potent vasoconstrictors and inducers of platelet aggregation.[5] PGs are known as local hormones, as they have an effect on target cells in the immediate vicinity of their site of synthesis. PGs are produced in small quantities, have a short half-life (seconds to minutes), are not stored in appreciable quantities, and are present throughout the body.

PGs are involved in several activities including inflammation, protection of the GI mucosa against injury, and regulation of renal blood flow.[6] Decreased acid production, increased gastric mucus production, increased gastric mucosal cytoprotection, and enhancement of renal blood flow during times of reduced renal perfusion are some of the beneficial effects of PGs.[8] PGI_2 is the main PG produced in the renal cortex, whereas PGE_2 is the primary PG produced in the renal medulla.[5] PGE_2 and prostacyclin are potent vasodilators and hyperalgesics. They presumably contribute to erythema, swelling, and pain during inflammation.[6]

GI tract abnormalities and renal toxicity are the most common adverse effects associated with NSAID use.[5,9] It has long been recognized that some NSAIDs are associated with a greater risk of GI toxicosis than others. The reason for this has been partly explained recently with the identification of different forms of COX. The 2 forms or isoenzymes of COX are COX-1 and COX-2.[5,6] COX-1 appears to be present naturally in the body and is involved in important physiologic functions such as autoregulation of renal blood flow. It is mainly found in the stomach, kidney, endothelium, and platelets. COX-2, which is an inducible form of COX, is believed to be responsible for production of inflammatory mediators.[5] COX-2 is mainly produced by monocytes, fibroblasts, synoviocytes, and chondrocytes in association with inflammation. It has been suggested that inhibition of COX-2 helps decrease inflammation, and inhibition of COX-1 may lead to adverse effects associated with the use of NSAIDs such as GI ulceration and kidney damage.[5] Thus, the NSAIDs that act mainly against COX-1 are more likely to result in GI tract injury compared with NSAIDs that act mostly against COX-2.

Role of Prostaglandins in Gastropathies Associated with Nonsteroidal Anti-inflammatory Use

There are several defense mechanisms that play a role in preventing gastric ulceration resulting from normal insults to the GI tract. It is believed that endogenous PGs play an integral part in these defense mechanisms. The most superficial barrier to gastric ulceration is a protective mucous gel layer that provides a defense against gastric acid. This layer contains a bicarbonate-rich fluid secreted by the gastric epithelium. Bicarbonate mixes with the gel to produce a gradient that forms an effective barrier to acid penetration. The gel also contains phospholipids that make it hydrophobic and prevent back diffusion of acid from the gastric lumen to the epithelial cells. The second defense mechanism is due to the ability of surface epithelial cells to rapidly migrate and divide to repair small defects. Moreover, the vasculature of the stomach is designed so that bicarbonate can be rapidly transported from parietal cells to the surface epithelium to replenish used bicarbonate. Adequate mucosal blood flow allows the epithelium to tolerate a wide array of insults, whereas reduced mucosal blood flow may result in severe mucosal injury.[6,9]

It is generally believed that NSAIDs can induce gastric damage through local and systemic effects. Local effects are associated with the physical properties of NSAIDs. Most NSAIDs are slightly acidic and may become concentrated in the gastric mucosa through a process known as ion trapping. This can lead to direct cellular injury. Aspirin is especially known to cause these local toxic effects. Systemic effects are thought to be associated with the inhibition of endogenous PG production. Decreased PG production can result in decreased mucin quality and bicarbonate content of the mucous gel layer, making the mucosa more vulnerable to acid-induced injury. NSAIDs are also thought to decrease mucosal proliferation, although it has been suggested recently that alterations in gastric cellular proliferation may not play a significant role in the development of NSAID-induced gastropathy. NSAIDs may also cause areas of reduced blood flow within the mucosa by inhibiting endogenous prostanoids that have a vasodilatory effect.[6,8,9] Adherence of neutrophils to vascular endothelium contributes to gastric mucosal injury as a result of activation of neutrophils and release of oxygen-derived free radicals and other enzymes.[6] The NSAID-induced gastropathy may be reduced in dogs by administering exogenous PGs. Misoprostol, a synthetic PGE_1 analogue, has been shown to reduce aspirin-induced gastropathy in clinical studies in dogs.[10]

Role of Prostaglandins in Renal Toxicosis Associated with Nonsteroidal Anti-inflammatory Drug Use

PGE_2 and PGI_2 function as vasodilatory agents to regulate renal blood flow. During a period of decreased renal perfusion, PGE_2 and PGI_2 cause afferent arteriolar dilation, which in turn helps maintain renal blood flow, counteracting the effect of systemic vasoconstrictors such as vasopressin, angiotensin, and norepinephrine.[5,11] Clinically, important adverse renal effects of NSAIDs are primarily the result of decreased PG production. Usually, short-term use of NSAIDs by healthy individuals has little effect on renal hemodynamics and function. During periods of hemodynamic compromise such as dehydration, hemorrhage, anesthesia, heart failure, or liver or kidney disease, circulating vasoconstrictors are released to maintain vascular resistance and blood pressure at the expense of organ blood flow. Under these conditions, the kidney becomes increasingly dependent on the vasodilatory effects of PG to maintain renal blood flow and glomerular filtration rate. The use of NSAIDs during hemodynamic compromise may result in ischemic injury of the kidneys, which may progress to acute renal failure.[5,6] NSAID-induced nephropathy is characterized by papillary necrosis and interstitial nephritis. This condition has been associated with the use of several different types of NSAIDs.

GENERAL TREATMENT RECOMMENDATIONS FOR ACUTE NONSTEROIDAL ANTI-INFLAMMATORY DRUG OVERDOSE

The goals of treatment of acute NSAID overdose in dogs and cats consist of aggressive decontamination, supportive care, GI protection, and monitoring of renal functions. In clinically normal patients, within a few hours of exposure with no clinical signs of toxicosis present, emesis should be induced with 3% hydrogen peroxide or apomorphine in dogs. In cats, emesis can be tried with xylazine or dexmedetomidine with varying degrees of success. Gastric lavage or enterogastric lavage should be considered in animals in which emesis cannot be induced because of the presence of neurologic signs such as coma, ataxia, or seizures. Induction of emesis should be followed with administration of activated charcoal (1–3 g/kg by mouth; use labeled dose for commercial products). Because many NSAIDs are known to undergo enterohepatic recirculation, multiple doses (2–6 doses) of activated charcoal every 6 to 8 hours may be needed. Patients receiving activated charcoal need to be watched for signs of hypernatremia (eg, ataxia, tremors, or seizures) and aspiration.[12,13] GI irritation and ulceration can be treated with GI protectants such as H2 blockers (eg, cimetidine, famotidine, or ranitidine) or proton pump inhibitors (eg, omeprazole, esomeprazole, or pantoprazole) and sucralfate. Misoprostol, a synthetic PG analogue, has been successfully used to prevent GI ulcers when used concurrently with some NSAIDs; however, its usefulness in acute NSAID overdose is not known. Treatment with GI protectants may be needed for 7 to 10 days or more depending on the dose of the NSAID and severity of the clinical signs present. Vomiting can be controlled with antiemetics like maropitant (1 mg/kg subcutaneously) or metoclopramide (0.2–0.5 mg/kg intramuscularly or subcutaneously). Broad-spectrum antibiotics and surgical repair may be needed for perforated ulcers and associated peritonitis.

Animals ingesting nephrotoxic doses of NSAIDs often require intravenous fluids at twice the maintenance rate for 48 to 96 hours depending on the dose and the type of NSAID involved. The use of dopamine (2.5 μg/kg/min) may increase renal perfusion and minimize the degree of renal impairment. The use of sodium bicarbonate (1–3 mEq/kg) in salicylate poisoning may increase excretion of parent compound and its metabolites in alkaline urine. With nephrotoxic dose ingestion, monitoring of renal functions (eg, blood urea nitrogen [BUN], serum creatinine, phosphorous, and electrolytes) on presentation and then daily for 3 to 5 days and serial urinalysis analysis with monitoring of specific gravity are often needed. Large NSAID overdoses can also result in an increase in liver enzymes along with signs of renal damage. For such patients, monitor liver-specific enzymes (eg, alanine aminotransferase, aspartate aminotransferase, alkaline phosphatases, and gamma-glutamyl transferase) for few days. SAMe (S-adenosylmethionine) may be helpful for patients showing signs of increased liver enzymes.

Control seizures with diazepam or barbiturates as needed. Repeated doses (2–3 doses within 5–10 minutes) of naloxone (0.01–0.02 mg/kg intravenously) can be tried in comatose and severely depressed dogs, such as those that have had large doses of ibuprofen (>400 mg/kg). Provide respiratory support and treat hypothermia and acidosis as needed. Treat any other associated clinical signs supportively.

SPECIFIC TOXICITY INFORMATION REGARDING FREQUENTLY REPORTED NONSTEROIDAL ANTI-INFLAMMATORY DRUGS IN DOGS AND CATS
Ibuprofen

Ibuprofen [2-(4-isobutylphenyl) propionic acid] is an NSAID with anti-inflammatory, antipyretic, and analgesic properties in animals and people. Ibuprofen has similar pharmacologic actions to other NSAIDs such as aspirin, phenylbutazone, and indomethacin.[14]

Ibuprofen is commonly used to treat acute and chronic rheumatoid arthritis and osteoarthritis, as well as headaches and fever and various joint, musculoskeletal, and gynecologic disorders.[12] It is available over the counter in 50-, 100-, and 200-mg tablets and 100 mg/5 mL suspension. Prescription strengths are available at 400, 600, and 800 mg. Ibuprofen is also available in combination with decongestant products.[14,15]

Before the availability of veterinary approved NSAID, ibuprofen was recommended in dogs at a dose of 5 mg/kg.[12,16,17] However, ibuprofen may cause gastric ulcers and perforations in dogs at this dose and is generally not recommended for prolonged use anymore.[16,17] GI irritation, GI hemorrhages, and renal damage are the most commonly reported toxic effects of ibuprofen ingestion in dogs.[12,14,15,18–20] In addition, central nervous system (CNS) depression, hypotension, ataxia, cardiac effects, and seizures can be seen. Ibuprofen has a narrow margin of safety in dogs.[17] Dogs dosed with ibuprofen orally at 8 mg/kg/d or 16 mg/kg/d for 30 days showed gastric ulceration or erosions along with clinical signs of GI disturbances.[21] According to 1 report, acute single ingestion of ibuprofen in dogs at 100 to 125 mg/kg can lead to clinical signs of vomiting, diarrhea, nausea, abdominal pain, and anorexia.[18] Renal failure can be seen with 175 to 300 mg/kg. CNS effects (seizure, ataxia, depression, and coma) along with renal and GI signs can be seen when dosage is greater than 400 mg/kg. Greater than 600 mg/kg is considered a lethal dose in the dog.[13,18,22]

Cats are susceptible to ibuprofen toxicosis at approximately half the doses required to cause toxicosis in dogs, although no experimental data are available to confirm this observation.[18] Cats are especially sensitive to NSAID toxicosis, because they have a limited glucuronyl-conjugating capacity.[23,24] Clinical signs of ibuprofen toxicosis in ferrets are more severe than those expected at similar doses in dogs. Typical toxic effects of ibuprofen in ferrets include CNS, GI, and renal effects.[25,26]

Carprofen

Carprofen, (6-chloro-alpha-methy-9H-carbazole-2-acetic acid) is an NSAID approved for use in dogs for its analgesic, anti-inflammatory, and antipyretic properties. Carprofen has shown to selectively inhibit COX-2 versus COX-1 in vitro, inhibiting the production of osteoclast-activating factor (OAF), PGE1, and PGE2.

Carprofen is available in 25, 75, or 100 mg tablets and caplets or as an injectable solution (50 mg/mL). Carprofen is recommended at 4.4 mg/kg once daily or divided and given as 2.2 mg/kg twice daily orally. Carprofen can also administered subcutaneously in the injectable form at the same dosage administered 2 hours before the procedure.

When administered at high doses, carprofen loses its selectivity for COX-2, and toxicity can result from inhibition of the COX-1. As with other NSAIDS, adverse reactions may include decreased appetite, vomiting, diarrhea, dark or tarry stools, increased water consumptions, increased urination, pale or yellow gums, lethargy, incoordination, seizure, or behavior change. In 1 study, dogs administered 2.2 mg/kg twice daily showed no clinically significant adverse reactions. Even at therapeutic levels, some dogs have exhibited an idiosyncratic hepatocellular toxicosis.[27]

Carprofen has nearly 90% to 100% bioavailability when ingested orally, with a peak plasma concentration in 1 to 3 hours.[28] In dogs, the elimination half-life ranges from 8 to 18 hours and because 70% to 80% of carprofen is metabolized via glucuronidation, the elimination half-life in cats is longer (20 plus or minus 16.6 hours).[29]

In otherwise healthy dogs, significant GI signs have been seen in dogs ingesting more than 20 mg/kg, with diuresis being recommended at 40 mg/kg. In cats, more than mild GI signs have been seen with ingestions greater than 4 mg/kg.[30]

Aspirin

Aspirin (acetylsalicylic acid or ASA), the salicylate ester of acetic acid, is the prototype of salicylate drugs. It is a weak acid derived from phenol.[14,31] Aspirin is available as plain, film-coated, buffered, time-release, and enteric-coated tablets, suppositories, and capsules.[32] Oral bioavailability of aspirin may vary due to differences in drug formulation. Aspirin reduces PG and TX synthesis by inhibition of COX. Salicylates also uncouple mitochondrial oxidative phosphorylation and inhibit specific dehydrogenases.[14,31,33–35] Platelets are incapable of synthesizing new COX. This fact causes an effect on platelet aggregation.[14,33] Salicylates also inhibit the formation and release of kinins, stabilize lysosomes, and remove energy needed for inflammation by uncoupling oxidative phosphorylation.[32]

Aspirin is recommended at 10 to 20 mg/kg twice daily in dogs and 10 to 20 mg/kg every 48 hours in cats.[33] Aspirin has a relatively good margin of safety in most species. Aspirin toxicosis is usually characterized by depression, fever, hyperpnea, seizures, respiratory alkalosis, metabolic acidosis, coma, gastric irritation or ulceration, liver necrosis, or increased bleeding time.[31,32] Ataxia and seizures may occur because of aspirin intoxication, although the exact etiology is unknown.

Aspirin is a phenolic compound. Cats are deficient in glucuronyl transferase and have prolonged excretion of aspirin (half-life in cats is 37.5 hours). Half-life of salicylates can increase with dose. In 1 study, no clinical signs of toxicosis occurred when cats were dosed with 25 mg/kg of aspirin every 48 hours for up to 4 weeks. Doses of 5 grains (325 mg) twice a day were lethal to cats. Erosive gastritis has been seen after a single 5-grain dose in dogs.[31]

Dogs can tolerate aspirin better than can cats. Doses of 25 mg/kg 3 times daily of regular aspirin caused mucosal erosions in 50% of dogs in 2 days, while there was minimal damage seen in animals receiving buffered and enteric-coated aspirin.[32] Gastric ulcers were induced in 4 of 6 dogs at a dose of 35 mg/kg of aspirin given orally 3 times a day on day 30 of dosing.[6,10] Similarly, gastric ulcers were seen in 3 of 7 dogs following aspirin administration at 50 mg/kg orally twice after 5 to 6 weeks of dosing.[18] In dogs, toxicity has been noted at doses of 100 to 300 mg/kg/d taken orally for 1 to 4 weeks.[32] Acute ingestion at 450 to 500 mg/kg can cause signs of GI disturbances, hyperthermia, panting, seizure, or coma.[18] Alkalosis caused by stimulation of the respiratory center can occur in the early course of intoxication. Metabolic acidosis with an elevated anion gap usually develops later.[18]

Naproxen

Naproxen, a propionic acid derivative, is an NSAID available over the counter as an acid or the sodium salt. Structurally and pharmacologically, naproxen is like carprofen and ibuprofen. In people and dogs, it has been used for its anti-inflammatory, analgesic, and antipyretic properties. It is generally better tolerated than aspirin or indomethacin at therapeutic doses.[36,37] Because of its relatively long plasma half-life (12–15 hours) in people, it may be conveniently administered twice daily. The half-life of naproxen in dogs is very long, at 74 hours.[38]

Several cases of naproxen toxicity have been described in dogs. In 1 case report, naproxen was administered to a dog at 11.11 mg/kg orally for 3 days and resulted in melena, frequent vomiting, and abdominal pain. Abdominal radiographs revealed generalized gastric wall thickening. Further investigation with barium sulfate suspension (barium meal) confirmed the presence of a perforating duodenal ulcer. Because of the perforating nature of the ulcer, bacteria- and barium sulfate-induced peritonitis was also diagnosed. Surgical resection of the ulcer along with supportive care (eg, antibiotics, fluids, cimetidine, sucralfate, and B-complex) resulted in complete recovery. The authors concluded that because of the lack of efficacy and safety information of naproxen, this drug should not be used in dogs at doses comparable to those for people.[39]

Similarly, a 34 kg dog developed vomiting, progressive weakness, and stumbling following naproxen administration by the owner at 5.6 mg/kg/d for 7 days. Feces were tarry, and the dog had paled mucous membranes. On radiography, hepatomegaly and prostatomegaly were observed. Blood work showed regenerative anemia, neutrophilia with a left shift, high BUN (66 mg/dL) and creatinine (2.1 mg/dL), and lower total protein (4 g/dL), albumin (2.1 g/dL), potassium (3.1 mEq/L), and total CO_2 (15 mm/L). Treatment with fluids, antacids, and antihistamines, along with multivitamins resulted in recovery in 11 days.[38]

A 13-year-old Basenji dog was given naproxen 250 mg twice a day for 7 days by the owner for the treatment of rheumatoid arthritis. The dog showed signs of anorexia, weight loss, and lethargy over a period of 2 weeks. Physical examination showed pale mucous membranes, moderate abdominal pain, and melena. Blood work showed left shift regenerative anemia. Abdominal radiography revealed mild splenomegaly and prostatomegaly. Urinalysis also indicated the presence of increased granular and hyaline casts. The dog recovered with supportive care in 3 weeks.[36]

Toxicity of naproxen from a single oral dose of 35 mg/kg (250 mg tablet in a 7 kg dachshund) resulted in clinical signs of listlessness, vomiting, diarrhea, abdominal pain, and profound depression within the first 24 hours of administration, followed by profuse hematemesis and melena and low plasma proteins. The dog recovered with supportive care over the next 3 days.[37] The same author reported another case of naproxen toxicosis in which naproxen was administered twice, approximately 48 hours apart, to an aged Labrador at 14.2 mg/kg. Within 12 hours after the last dose, the dog developed severe hemorrhagic dysentery. Because of his age and the severity of illness, the dog was euthanized. On postmortem examination, the gastric mucosa was erythematous and hemorrhagic. Similar but more severe lesions were found in small intestinal and colonic mucosae.[37]

There are several other reports of naproxen toxicosis in the dog described in the literature.[40–45] In the author's experience, as is the case with most NSAIDs, cats appear particularly more sensitive to the toxic effects of naproxen than dogs.

Deracoxib

Deracoxib is a coxib, COX-2 inhibitor used in veterinary medicine to treat osteoarthritis in dogs. Deracoxib is available in chewable tablets that have beef flavoring to make them more palatable. Tablets are either 25, 75, or 100 mg. It is not approved or recommended for use in cats.[46] For control of pain and inflammation, the recommended dose is 1 to 2 mg/kg once daily or 3 to 4 mg/kg/d as needed for postoperative pain, not to exceed 7 days of therapy.[46]

Deracoxib is a coxib-class NSAID. In vitro studies have shown that deracoxib predominantly inhibits COX-2 and spares COX-1 at therapeutic dosages.[46,47] This, theoretically, would inhibit production of the PGs that contribute to pain and inflammation (COX-2) and spare those that maintain normal GI and renal function (COX-1).

After oral administration to dogs, bioavailability is greater than 90%; the time to peak serum concentration occurs at approximately 2 hours.[46] The presence of food in the gut can enhance bioavailability. Terminal elimination half-life in the dog depends on dose and is about 3 hours after dosages up to 8 mg/kg. The half-life at a dose of 20 mg/kg is approximately 19 hours.[46] Drug accumulation can occur with higher dosages, leading to increased toxic effects, as increased COX-1 inhibition can occur at higher concentrations.

After administering 1 mg of deracoxib in cats orally, peak levels (0.28 mcg/mL) occurred about 3.6 hours after administration. Elimination half-life was about 8 hours.

There are few data available regarding this drug's acute toxicity. A 14-day study in dogs demonstrated no clinically observable adverse effects in the dogs that received 10 mg/kg. Dogs that received 25, 50, or 100 mg/kg/d for 10 to 11 days survived but showed vomiting and melena; no hepatic or renal lesions were demonstrated in these dogs.[46]

Because nonlinear elimination occurs in dogs at dosages of 10 mg/kg and above, dogs acutely ingesting dosages above this amount should be observed for GI[48] erosion or ulceration and treated symptomatically for vomiting and GI bleeding. Aggressive decontamination and fluid therapy to prevent renal damage should be considered for dogs ingesting acute dosages greater than 20 mg/kg.

Meloxicam

Meloxicam has analgesic and fever-reducing effects. It is approved for human and veterinary use. Veterinary formulations are available as an oral suspension at

1.5 mg/mL and an injectable solution of 5 mg/mL. Meloxicam is principally used for treatment of osteoarthritis in dogs; however, single-dose injectable use is also approved for use in cats to control postoperative pain and inflammation associated with orthopedic surgery, ovariohysterectomy, and castration when administered prior to surgery. Dogs should receive 0.2 mg/kg initially orally, intravenously, or subcutaneously on the first day of treatment, with subsequent doses of 0.1 mg/kg orally once daily.[38] Cats should receive 0.3 mg/kg subcutaneously once.[38,48]

Like other NSAIDs, meloxicam exhibits analgesic, anti-inflammatory, and antipyretic activity probably through its inhibition of COX, of phospholipase A_2, and of PG synthesis. It is considered COX-2 preferential (not COX-2 specific), because at higher dosages, its COX-2 specificity is diminished.

In dogs, meloxicam is well absorbed after oral administration. Food does not appear to alter absorption. Peak blood levels occur in about 7 to 8 hours after administration.[38,48] Meloxicam is extensively metabolized in the liver, and most of the metabolites (and unchanged drug) are eliminated in the feces. A significant amount of enterohepatic recirculation occurs. The elimination half-life in dogs averages 24 hours (range, 12–36 hours). In cats, subcutaneous injection is nearly completely absorbed. Peak levels occur about 1.5 hours after injection. Meloxicam is relatively highly bound to feline plasma proteins (97%). After a single dose, total systemic clearance is approximately 130 mL/h/kg, and elimination half-life is approximately 15 hours.[38,48]

In a 6-month target animal safety study, meloxicam was administered orally at 1, 3, and 5 times ($\times$) the recommended dose with no significant clinical adverse reactions.[49] All animals in all dose groups (controls and $1\times$, $3\times$, and $5\times$ the recommended dose) exhibited some GI distress (diarrhea and vomiting). Treatment-related changes seen in hematology and chemistry included decreased red blood cell counts in 7 of 24 dogs (4 dogs at the $3\times$ dose and 3 dogs at the $5\times$ dose); decreased hematocrit in 18 of 24 dogs (including 3 control dogs); dose-related neutrophilia in 1 dog at the $1\times$ dose, 2 dogs at the $3\times$ dose, and 3 dogs at the $5\times$ dose; and evidence of regenerative anemia in 2 dogs at the $3\times$ dose and 1 dog at the $5\times$ dose. Also noted were increased BUN in 2 dogs at the $5\times$ dose and decreased albumin in 1 dog at the $5\times$ dose. Endoscopic changes consisted of reddening of the gastric mucosal surface covering less than 25% of the surface area. This was seen in 3 dogs at the recommended dose, 3 dogs at the $3\times$ dose, and 2 dogs at the $5\times$ dose. Two control dogs exhibited reddening in conjunction with ulceration of the mucosa covering less than 25% of the surface area. Gross GI necropsy results observed included mild discoloration of the stomach or duodenum in 1 dog at the $3\times$ dose and 1 dog at the $5\times$ dose. Multifocal pinpoint red foci were observed in the gastric fundic mucosa in 1 dog at the recommended dose and in 1 dog at the $5\times$ dose. No macroscopic or microscopic renal changes were observed in any dogs receiving meloxicam in this 6-month study. Microscopic GI findings were limited to 1 dog at the recommended dose and 2 dogs at the $3\times$ dose. Mild inflammatory mucosal infiltrate was observed in the duodenum of 1 dog at the recommended dose. Mild congestion of the fundic mucosa and mild myositis of the outer mural musculature of the stomach were observed in 2 dogs receiving the $3\times$ dose.

There have been anecdotal reports of acute renal failure and death associated with the use of meloxicam in cats.

Diclofenac

Diclofenac is a phenylacetic acid–derivative NSAID. It structurally related to meclofenamate sodium and mefenamic acid, but unlike these anthranilic acid (2-aminobenzoic acid) derivatives, diclofenac is a 2-aminobenzeneacetic acid derivative. Diclofenac is commercially available as diclofenac sodium delayed-release and extended-release tablets and as diclofenac potassium conventional tablets. Diclofenac is also available as a fixed combination of diclofenac sodium in an enteric-coated core with an outer shell of misoprostol. The primary uses of diclofenac in human medicine are for inflammatory diseases, pain, and dysmenorrhea. The usual initial dosage of diclofenac sodium in adults is 75 mg twice daily or 50 mg 3 times daily, but this can be increased to 200 mg daily if needed. Dosages of diclofenac greater than 225 mg/d are not recommended by the manufacturer because of the increased risk of adverse effects. The usual adult dosage of diclofenac potassium is 100 to 200 mg daily.[50]

Diclofenac sodium and diclofenac potassium are rapidly and almost completely absorbed from the GI tract in people but undergo extensive first-pass metabolism in the liver. Only about 50% to 60% of a dose of diclofenac reaches the systemic circulation as unchanged drug. After oral administration, peak plasma concentrations of diclofenac generally occur within 1 hour for diclofenac potassium conventional tablets and 2 to 3 hours for delayed-release diclofenac sodium tablets. Food decreases the rate of absorption of diclofenac tablets, resulting in delayed and decreased peak plasma concentrations. Significant accumulation of diclofenac during repeated dosing reportedly does not occur, although the degree of accumulation of metabolites is unknown. Following intravenous administration of diclofenac in rats, it is widely distributed, with highest concentrations achieved in bile, liver, blood, heart, lungs, and kidneys, and lower concentrations in adrenals, thyroid glands, salivary glands, pancreas, spleen, muscles, brain, and spinal cord. Like other NSAIDs, diclofenac is also distributed into synovial fluid. Diclofenac is 99% to 99.8% reversibly protein bound, mainly to albumin. Along with its metabolites, diclofenac has been shown to cross the placenta in mice and rats. The exact metabolic fate of diclofenac is unknown, but it is rapidly and extensively metabolized in the liver via hydroxylation and then conjugation with glucuronic acid, taurine amide, sulfuric acid, and other biogenic ligands. Diclofenac is excreted in urine (50%–70%) and feces (30%–35%), with only minimal amounts eliminated as unchanged drug (<1%). Although there is some evidence that diclofenac undergoes enterohepatic recirculation, this appears to be minimal in people. Following oral administration of delayed-release diclofenac sodium tablets, the elimination half-life is approximately 1.2 to 2 hours but may by prolonged in individuals with severe renal impairment.[50]

After a single injection of 1 mg/kg of diclofenac sodium in the dog, 35% to 40% is excreted in the urine.[51] In the dog, the major metabolite of diclofenac found in urine is the taurine conjugate of unchanged diclofenac. In the urine of rats, baboons, and people, conjugates of the hydroxylated metabolites predominate.[52] The dog does not oxidize diclofenac. An unstable ester glucuronide of diclofenac found in dog bile has also been found in rat bile. It is presumed to hydrolyze in the duodenum, releasing diclofenac that then undergoes enterohepatic recirculation.[51]

The oral LD_{50} of diclofenac sodium is 55 to 240 mg/kg in rats, 500 mg/kg in dogs, and 3200 mg/kg in monkeys. Another source reported the LD_{50} in dogs to be 59 mg/kg.[53] Hydroxylated metabolites exhibited less toxic potential than did the unchanged drug in LD_{50} studies in rats.[50]

Grapiprant

Grapiprant is a first-in-class piprant; a non-COX-inhibiting, prostaglandin receptor antagonist (PRA) sold under the trade name Galliprant. Grapiprant specifically blocks the EP4 receptor that is the primary mediator of canine OA pain and inflammation.[54] Grapiprant is available in 20, 60, and 100 mg tablets, and the recommended dose is 2 mg/kg by mouth once daily.

There are few data available regarding this drug's acute toxicity. In a 9-month toxicity study, Grapiprant was suspended in a methylcellulose solution and administered by oral gavage at 1, 6, and 50 mg/kg/d to 28 dogs.[54] All groups developed vomiting and soft stools.[54] Decreases in serum albumin and total protein were seen with increasing doses of Grapiprant.[54]

Robenacoxib

Robenacoxib is a non-narcotic, nonsteroidal, NSAID of the coxib class approved for use in dogs and cats to control postoperative pain and inflammation. Robenacoxib is available as 6 mg tablets for cats, 10, 20, and 40 mg tablets for dogs, and as a 20 mg/mL injectable solution. The recommended dose for dogs is 2 mg/kg orally once daily for a maximum of 3 days, and 1 mg/kg orally once daily for a maximum of 3 days in cats. Subcutaneous dosing in dogs and cats is 2 mg/kg once daily for up to 3 days.

In vitro, whole-blood assays in cats have shown that robenacoxib demonstrates selective COX-2 inhibition.[55] Like other NSAIDs in this class, it is possible that at high doses, robenacoxib loses its specificity for COX-2. Absorption occurs in 0.5 hours, and the elimination half-life in exudate is 27 hours versus 2.5 hours for blood.[55] Elimination in dogs and cats is primarily through the biliary route.[55,56]

There are few data available regarding this drug's acute toxicity. A 21-day study in cats demonstrated that robenacoxib may be tolerated at doses up to 24 mg/kg/d for 21 days.[55] In a controlled field study, 6 mg tablets of robenacoxib were administered postoperatively to 167 cats, and a placebo was administered to 87 cats.[55] Adverse reactions included incision site bleeding (4%), incision site infection (3.5%), inappetence (2%), lethargy (2%), vomiting (3%), hematuria (1.7%), diarrhea (1.7%), hair loss (1.2%), respiratory problems, cardiac arrest (0.5%), and incoordination (0.5%).[55] In a 6-month oral dosing study in dogs receiving 10 mg/kg doses once daily, treatment-related adverse events included 1 dog with increased buccal mucosal bleeding times, and 1 dog with red mucosal discoloration of the duodenum.[56]

REFERENCES

1. Donovan JW. Nonsteroidal anti-inflammatory drugs and colchicine. In: Haddad LM, Shannon MW, Winchester JF, editors. Clinical management of poisoning and drug overdose. 3rd edition. Philadelphia: WB Saunders; 1998. p. 687–99.
2. Holubek W. Nonsteroidal anti-inflammatory drugs. In: Nelson LS, Hoffman RS, Lewin NA, editors. Goldfrank's toxicologic emergencies. 9th edition. New York: McGraw-Hill; 2011. p. 528–36.
3. Bryson PD. Nonsteroidal anti-inflammatory agents. In: Simmons HF, editor. Comprehensive review in toxicology for emergency clinicians. 3rd edition. Washington, DC: Taylor and Francis; 1996. p. 565–75.
4. Ellenhorn MJ. Nonsteroidal anti-inflammatory drugs. In: Ellenhorn MJ, Schonwald S, Ordog G, et al, editors. Ellenhorn's medical toxicology: diagnosis and treatment of human poisoning. 2nd edition. Baltimore (MD): Williams & Wilkins; 1997. p. 196–206.
5. Forrester SD, Troy GC. Renal effects of nonsteroidal antiinflammatory drugs. Compend Contin Educ Pract Vet 1999;21(10):910–9.
6. Johnston SA, Fox SM. Mechanisms of action of anti-inflammatory medications used for the treatment of osteoarthritis. J Am Vet Med Assoc 1997;210:1486–92.
7. Lees P, May SA, McKeller QA. Pharmacology and therapeutics of non-steroidal anti-inflammatory drugs in the dog and cat: I. General pharmacology. J Small Anim Pract 1991;32:183–93.

8. MacAllister CG. Nonsteroidal anti-inflammatory drugs: their mechanism of action and clinical uses in horses. Vet Med 1994;89:237–40.

9. Wolfe MM. NSAIDs and the gastrointestinal mucosa. Hosp Pract 1996;15:37–48.

10. Bowersox TS, Lipowitz AJ, Hardy RM, et al. The use of a synthetic prostaglandin E_1 analog as a gastric protectant against aspirin-induced hemorrhage in the dog. J Am Anim Hosp Assoc 1996;32:401–7.

11. Rubin SI. Nonsteroidal anti-inflammatory drugs, prostaglandins, and the kidney. J Am Vet Med Assoc 1986;188:1065–8.

12. Kore AM. Toxicology of nonsteroidal anti-inflammatory drugs. Vet Clin North Am Small Anim Pract 1990;20:419–30.

13. Dunayer E. Ibuprofen toxicosis in dogs, cats, and ferrets. Vet Med 2004;99: 580–5.

14. McEvoy GK. AHFS Drag Information. Bethesda (MD): American Society of Health-System Pharmacists; 2000. p. 1815.

15. Rumack BH. Ibuprofen (toxicologic managements). Poisindex System, vol. 100. Englewood (CO): Micromedex; 2000.

16. Roush JK. Diseases of joints and ligaments. In: Morgan RV, editor. The handbook of small animal practice. 3rd edition. New York: Churchill Livingstone; 1997. p. 813–29.

17. Osweiler G, Carson TL. Household drugs. In: Morgan RV, editor. The handbook of small animal practice. 3rd edition. New York: Churchill Livingstone; 1997. p. 1279–83.

18. Villar D, Buck WB. Ibuprofen, aspirin, and acetaminophen toxicosis and treatment in dogs and cats. Vet Hum Toxicol 1998;40:156–62.

19. Smith KJ, Taylor DH. Another case of gastric perforation associated with administration of ibuprofen in a dog. J Am Vet Med Assoc 1993;202:706.

20. Spyridakis LK, Bacia JJ, Barsanti JA, et al. Ibuprofen toxicosis in a dog. J Am Vet Med Assoc 1986;188:918–9.

21. Adams SS, Bough RG, Cliffe EE, et al. Absorption, distribution and toxicity of ibuprofen. Toxicol Appl Pharmacol 1969;15:310–30.

22. Richardson JA. Management of acetaminophen and ibuprofen toxicoses in dogs and cats. J Vet Emerg Crit Care 2000;10:285–91.

23. Rumbeiha WK. Nephrotoxins. In: Bonagura JD, editor. Kirk's current veterinary therapy XIII Small animal practice. Philadelphia: W.B. Saunders Co; 2000. p. 212–7.

24. Owens-Clark J, Dorman DC. Toxicity from newer over the counter drugs. In: Bonagura JD, editor. Kirk's current veterinary therapy XIII Small animal practice. Philadelphia: W.B. Saunders Co; 2000. p. 227–31.

25. Richardson JA, Balabuszko RA. Ibuprofen ingestion in ferrets: 43 cases (January 1996–March 2000). J Vet Emerg Crit Care 2001;11:53–9.

26. Cathers TE. Acute ibuprofen toxicosis in a ferret. J Am Vet Med Assoc 2000;216: 1426–8.

27. MacPhail CM, Lappin MR, Meyer DJ, et al. Hepatocellular toxicosis associated with administration of carprofen in 21 dogs. J Am Vet Med Assoc 1998; 212(12):1895–901.

28. Schmitt M, Guentert TW. Biopharmaceutical evaluation of carprofen following single intravenous, oral, and rectal doses in dogs. Biopharm Drug Dispos 1990; 11(7):585–94.

29. Parton K, Balmer TV, Boyle J, et al. The pharmacokinetics and effects of intravenously administered carprofen and salicylate on gastrointestinal mucosa and

selected biochemical measurements in healthy cats. J Vet Pharmacol Ther 2000; 23(2):73–9.

30. Volmer PA, Mensching D. Toxicology brief: managing acute carprofen toxicosis in dogs and cats. Vet Med 2009;104:326.

31. Rumack BH, editor. Aspirin (toxicologic managements). Poisindex System, vol. 100. Englewood (CO): Micromedex; 2000.

32. Booth DM. The analgesic-antipyretic-antiinflammatory drugs. In: Richard AH, editor. Veterinary and pharmacology and therapeutics. 7th edition. Ames (IA): Iowa State University Press; 1995. p. 432–9.

33. Plumb DC. Veterinary drug handbook. 3rd edition. Ames (IA): Iowa State University Press; 1999. p. 56–8, 221, 434, 462, 518–9, 562, 583.

34. Brogden RN, Heel RC, Speight TM, et al. Naproxen up to date: a review of its pharmacological properties and therapeutic efficacy and use in rheumatic diseases and pain states. Drugs 1979;18:241–77.

35. Brogden RN, Pinder RM, Sawer PR, et al. Naproxen: a review of its pharmacological properties and therapeutic efficacy and use. Drugs 1975;9:326–63.

36. Roudebush P, Morse GE. Naproxen toxicosis in a dog. J Am Vet Med Assoc 1981;179:805–16.

37. Steel RJS. Suspected naproxen toxicity in dogs. Aust Vet J 1981;57:100–1.

38. Gilmour MA, Walshaw R. Naproxen-induced toxicosis in a dog. J Am Vet Med Assoc 1987;191:1431–2.

39. Gfeller RW, Sandors AD. Naproxen-associated duodenal ulcer complicated by perforation and bacteria- and barium sulfate-induced peritonitis in a dog. J Am Vet Med Assoc 1991;198:644–6.

40. Hallesy D, Shott L, Hill R. Comparative toxicology of naproxen. Scand J Rheumatol Suppl 1973;2:20–8.

41. Dye TL. Naproxen toxicosis in a puppy. Vet Hum Toxicol 1997;39:157–9.

42. Daehler MH. Transmural pyloric perforation associated with naproxen administration in a dog. J Am Vet Med Assoc 1986;189:694–5.

43. Dean SP, Reid JFS. Use of naproxen [letter]. Vet Rec 1985;116:479.

44. Smith RE. Naproxen toxicosis [letter]. J Am Vet Med Assoc 1982;180:107.

45. Shiltz RA. Naproxen in dogs and cats [letter]. J Am Vet Med Assoc 1982;180: 1397.

46. Deramaxx (Deracoxib) package insert Greensboro (NC): Novartis Animal Health. US Inc; 2011. NADA # 141-203, approved by FDA. Available at: http://valleyvet.naccvp.com/index.php?m=product_view_basic&u=country&p=msds&id=113 1012. Accessed January 10, 2012.

47. Anti-inflammatory agents. In: Kahn Cynthia M, editor. The Merck veterinary manual. 10th edition. NJ: Merck & Co; 2010. p. 2313–28.

48. Plumb DC. Veterinary drug handbook. 5th edition. Ames (IA): Blackwell Publishing; 2005. p. 222.

49. Boehringer Ingelheim Vetmedica, Inc. Freedom of information summary new animal drug application Metacam (meloxicam) 0.5 mg/mL and 1.5 mg/mL oral suspension. 2003. NADA 141–219. Available at: http://www.fda.gov/downloads/animalveterinary/products/approvedanimaldrugproducts/foiadrugsummaries/ucm118026.pdf. Accessed January 10, 2012.

50. McEvoy GK. AHFS Drag Information. Bethesda (MD): American Society of Health-System Pharmacists; 2000. p. 1800.

51. Stierlin H, Faigle JW. Biotransformation of diclofenac sodium (Voltaren in animals and man: II. Quantitative determination of the unchanged drug and principal phenolic metabolites, in urine and bile. Xenobiotica 1979;9:611–21.

52. Stierlin H, Faigle JW, Sallmann A, et al. Biotransformation of diclofenac sodium (Voltaren) in animals and in man: I. Isolation and identification of principal metabolites. Xenobiotica 1979;9:601–10.

53. RTECS:Registry of Toxic Effects of Chemical Substances. National Institute for Occupational Safety and Health. Cincinnati, OH (CD-ROM. 2002). MICROMEDEX, Greenwood Village, CO.

54. Galliprant (grapiprant) package insert. Leawook (KS): Aratana Therapeutics, Inc; 2016. NADA #141-455, approved by FDA. Available at: https://assets.ctfassets. net/0kto1cmw1iq5/5PEbZTfRluMA00u4MaQYUU/8df5bee10c6fa00d378f86de02 59c429/galliprantpi.pdf. Accessed May 1, 2018.

55. Onsior (robenacoxib) for cats package insert Elanco Animal Health, 2015. NADA #141-320, approved by FDA. Available at: https://assets.ctfassets.net/ kvimhx6nhg7h/3lqYXVToVqWsgEiikumWs8/b641f1f0c40e3fe26a2c35fdc5170e69/ Onsior_Tablets_for_Cats_PI_Oct_2016.pdf. Accessed May 1, 2018.

56. Onsior (robenacoxib) for dogs package insert Elanco Animal Health, 2015. NADA #141-463, approved by FDA. Available at: https://assets.ctfassets.net/ kvimhx6nhg7h/3LU0AgHxcAGGeQGc6Mky26/c87b61be5f9c171953733ffeb703 7f89/Onsior_Tablets_for_Dogs_PI_Oct_2016.pdf. Accessed May 1, 2018.

Xylitol Toxicosis in Dogs
An Update

Lisa A. Murphy, VMD[a],*, Eric K. Dunayer, VMD[b,c]

KEYWORDS

- Xylitol • Hypoglycemia • Liver failure • Coagulopathy

KEY POINTS

- Xylitol ingestions in dogs may result in severe hypoglycemia and/or acute hepatic necrosis and associated coagulopathies.
- Aggressive treatment may be needed, but the prognosis is generally expected to be good for dogs developing uncomplicated hypoglycemia.
- Because of increased availability of xylitol-containing products in the market and in the dog's environment, it is likely that there will continue to be increased exposures and toxicity in dogs.

The 5-carbon sugar alcohol xylitol is used as a sweetener in many products including gums, candies, and baked goods. In recent years, the use of xylitol has increased because of the popularity of low-carbohydrate diets and low–glycemic index foods.[1] Xylitol also prevents oral bacteria from producing acids that damage the surfaces of teeth, leading to its inclusion in toothpaste and other oral care products.[1,2] Although xylitol is considered safe in people, canine ingestions have resulted in severe and life-threatening signs, likely associated with increased insulin secretion leading to hypoglycemia and acute hepatic damage/failure. Death caused by severe hypoglycemia if untreated is possible, and acute liver failure may develop 1 to 3 days after xylitol ingestion.

SOURCES

Initially xylitol was used as a sugar substitute during World War II in Scandinavian countries, when sucrose availability was low. During that time, xylitol was derived from birch and other hardwoods.[3] More recently, the sweetener has been used as a sugar

This article originally appeared in Veterinary Clinics of North America: Small Animal Practice, Volume 42, Issue 2, March 2012.
The authors have nothing to disclose.
[a] Department of Pathobiology, University of Pennsylvania School of Veterinary Medicine, PADLS New Bolton Center Toxicology Laboratory, 382 West Street Road, Kennett Square, PA 19348, USA; [b] Department of Veterinary Clinical Sciences, St. Matthew's University School of Veterinary Medicine, Grand Cayman, Cayman Islands; [c] ASPCA Animal Poison Control Center, 1717 South Philo Road, Suite 36, Urbana, IL 61802, USA
* Corresponding author.
E-mail address: murphylp@vet.upenn.edu

substitute for human diabetics. It has a similar sweetness to sucrose but has fewer calories (4 calories/g vs 2.4 calories/g, respectively).[4] It has also been eagerly embraced by dental care professionals and the general public because of its anticariogenic properties.[5] Its presence in gum, mints, and candies including gumballs, lollypops, and taffy has been fairly well known for years; however, recently, several additional, lesser-known products have also been made with xylitol. Veterinarians and pet owners should be aware that this sugar substitute may be found in several common household products, both edible and nonedible, and even in some prescription drugs.

Based on a 2018 search of the American Society for the Prevention of Cruelty to Animals (ASPCA) Animal Poison Control Center's (APCC) product database, xylitol was present in over 1900 products including several vitamins (ie, iron, vitamin D, calcium chews, multivitamin tablets, gummy vitamins) and nutritional supplements (coenzyme Q10, 5-hydroxytryptophan, caffeine, omega 3 fish oils, melatonin). Xylitol can also be found in chocolate, baked goods, puddings, syrup, fruit preserves, jellies, peanut butter, ice cream, nutritional/diet bars, and drink powders. It is also available in its pure form as a sugar substitute under several different brand names. Xylitol is also used as an ingredient in toothpaste, tooth wipes and towelettes for babies, oral lozenges, moisturizing mouth sprays and gels, and mouthwash because of its ability to prevent cavity formation. It can additionally be found in exfoliating facial wipes, personal lubricants, deodorants, sunscreens, and night creams.

Xylitol is used in medicinal products, most notably both brand-name and generic nicotine gums. It is also found in oral drug suspensions, cold remedies, some sublingual tablets, and nasal sprays including aripiprazole disintegrating tablets, Bach flower remedies (BFRs), and gabapentin oral solution.

If an exposure to any of the previously mentioned substances has occurred, the ingestion of xylitol should be considered. Xylitol may be listed on product labels using a number of possible synonyms, including Eutrit, Kannit, Klinit, Newtol, xylite, Torch, or Xyliton.[6]

Xylitol is also an ingredient in drinking water additives for dogs and cats. Exposures have been reported to the APCC; however, no evidence of associated xylitol toxicity has been documented to date (ASPCA APCC, unpublished data, Eric Dunayer, VMD, 2018). A study involving dogs that received 5 times the recommended xylitol drinking water dose failed to demonstrate any toxic effects.[7]

TOXICOKINETICS

Xylitol is quickly absorbed from the canine gastrointestinal tract, with peak plasma levels occurring within 30 minutes of ingestion.[8] Approximately 80% of xylitol metabolism occurs in the liver, where it is rapidly oxidized to D-xylulose, then metabolized to glucose, glycogen, and lactate via the pentose-phosphate pathway.[9]

Xylitol ingestion in dogs results in a dose-related insulin release that is greater than the response to an equal dose of glucose.[10,11] Peak serum insulin concentrations have been observed to be sixfold greater following ingestion of xylitol compared with glucose[8] and so may lead to severe hypoglycemia. Xylitol does not cause similar insulin release or blood glucose changes in people, rats, and horses, although increased insulin releases have been documented in cows, goats, and rabbits.[12] Dogs experimentally orally dosed with 1 or 4 g of xylitol per kilogram of body weight showed sharp increases in plasma insulin concentrations within 20 minutes, peaking at 40 minutes.[13] Another study indicates that xylitol directly stimulates secretion of insulin by pancreatic islet β cells.[8]

A recently published paper in 2018 looked at the effects of xylitol in cats. Six cats were given xylitol at 100, 500, and 1000 mg/kg in separate trials. None of the cats developed hypoglycemia at any of the doses, and blood glucose remained within the reference range, although the cats in the 1000 mg/kg group showed significant increase in blood glucose levels. Liver enzymes, renal functions, and electrolytes were monitored for 72 hours after exposure. There were no significant changes seen in any of these values in the cats.[14]

Xylitol ingestion has appeared to be fatal to at least one species of nectar-feeding birds, Cape sugarbirds (Proerops cafer). After feeding on a solution of 21.8% xylitol in water, the birds developed signs of ataxia, lethargy, and inability to fly within 15 to 30 minutes. Approximately 29 birds died, and 15 birds appeared to eventually recover. Necropsies did not reveal a definitive cause of death, and it was presumed to be hypoglycemia caused by xylitol toxicosis.[15]

The mechanism of action for liver damage in dogs is not fully understood; however, it is thought to be related to either ATP depletion during the metabolism of xylitol, leading to hepatic necrosis, or the production of hepatocyte-damaging reactive oxygen species.[14] Histopathologic changes observed in 3 dogs with known xylitol toxicosis included severe acute periacinar and midzonal hepatic necrosis with periportal vacuolar degeneration, diffuse hepatic necrosis, and moderate-to-marked subacute centrilobular hepatocyte loss and atrophy with lobular collapse and disorganization.[16]

TOXICITY

Oral xylitol has a wide margin of safety in most species. The estimated oral LD_{50} of xylitol in rabbits is 4 to 6 g per kilogram of body weight.[17] People consuming more than 130 g of xylitol per day may develop diarrhea but no other abnormalities.[18] Anecdotal reports indicate ferrets have shown evidence of hypoglycemia following ingestion, but this has not been confirmed. In fact, the 3 cases of xylitol exposure received by the APCC in ferrets did not show evidence of hypoglycemia or other adverse effects as reported in dogs.

Based on canine xylitol ingestions reported to the APCC, only mild clinical signs of hypoglycemia are expected with the ingestions of less than 100 mg of xylitol per kilogram of body weight (100 mg/kg), although typically exposures greater than 50 mg/kg may at least warrant decontamination and blood glucose monitoring. Ingestions involving more than 500 mg/kg of xylitol in dogs can be associated with hepatic failure.[3]

CLINICAL SIGNS AND LABORATORY CHANGES

A 2001 to 2018 search of canine xylitol ingestions in the APCC database was performed. The search was limited to cases where the xylitol concentration of the product involved was known, and no other potentially toxic exposures were known to have occurred. Although ingestions involving mints and 100% xylitol-containing products appear to often develop clinical signs quickly (usually within 30 minutes, possibly because of quick disintegration and release of xylitol from these products), the current database search supports previously reported observations that dogs ingesting xylitol-containing gums may not develop clinical signs of hypoglycemia until 12 hours later.[3] These variations in the onset of clinical signs may be related to the formulation of the specific product involved and the amount of mastication (chewing) that may have occurred during consumption. When dogs ingest xylitol-containing gums, they usually do not chew/masticate it. This may be the main reason for a delayed release and absorption of xylitol, leading to delay in onset time of hypoglycemia. Increased mastication of chewing gum would cause an increased likelihood of developing clinical signs relatively quickly due to an increased release of the product's total available xylitol.[19]

Clinical signs most commonly noted in dogs in the APCC database include vomiting, lethargy, and weakness. Vomiting was most commonly reported with gum ingestions (especially those containing xylitol in the outer coating), mints, and 100% xylitol products, typically within 30 minutes and up to several hours after exposure. In many of these cases, the dogs partially self-decontaminated themselves, and the xylitol-containing product could be seen in the vomitus.

In cases where lethargy and weakness were reported by the owners, dogs were generally also hypoglycemic on presentation to the veterinary clinic. However, not all animals exhibited hypoglycemia on presentation for veterinary care and sometimes appeared clinically normal on initial examination. Dogs that were presented either nonresponsive or with seizure activity were often hypoglycemic, although in some cases, blood glucose levels performed postictally showed levels within the normal limits. Of the cases reviewed, ingestions involving less than 100 mg of xylitol per kilogram of body weight usually resulted in mild signs. Hyperglycemia has sometimes been reported following xylitol ingestion, which may be the result of the Somogyi phenomenon (rebound hyperglycemia) that occurs with insulin overdose.[3]

Some dogs in the APCC database developed mild-to-moderate hypokalemia or an initial hypophosphatemia, typically within 12 hours of the initial exposure, and appeared to respond well to supplementation. Hyperphosphatemia associated with subsequent hepatic damage in dogs is considered a poor prognostic indicator.

The time at which liver enzyme elevations were first detected generally varied from 4 to 24 hours, but in some cases, alanine aminotransferase became elevated in less than 4 hours after exposure. This early development of mild liver enzyme elevations is consistent with a recent research study performed in China.[13] Dogs in the APCC database that developed hypoglycemia did not always develop evidence of liver damage. Additionally, there were several cases of dogs that developed liver enzyme elevations but not hypoglycemia. Many dogs with elevated liver enzymes did eventually recover, even in some cases in which coagulopathies (prolonged prothrombin and activated partial thromboplastin times) were noted (APCC, unpublished data, 2018).

TREATMENT AND MONITORING

On arrival to the veterinary clinic, a baseline blood glucose level should be measured. Emesis should be induced if the dog has not vomited prior to presentation (either by induction or self-decontamination) and no contraindications are present by the patient's history or physical examination findings. Apomorphine can be administered either by injection (0.03 mg/kg intravenously or 0.04 mg/kg intramuscularly) or by subconjunctival administration (a crushed quarter of a 6-mg tablet).[20] If excessive sedation occurs, naloxone can be used as a reversal agent, but the depression associated with apomorphine is generally mild. Following apomorphine administration to the conjunctiva, a thorough ocular flushing should occur once vomiting has been initiated in order to avoid excessive ocular irritation and retching. As an alternative to apomorphine for the induction of emesis, 3% active hydrogen peroxide can be orally administered at a dosage of 1 to 2.2 mL/kg (generally not exceeding 45 mL as a total dose). If vomiting does not occur after the first dose, it can be repeated once.[21] Additional doses could result in gastric irritation and protracted vomiting. Vomitus should be thoroughly evaluated for the presence of the ingested xylitol product(s) to determine if decontamination was successful.

Emesis is not recommended in patients that have ingested 100% xylitol products more than 30 minutes prior to presentation. Because of the rapid absorption of this form of xylitol, an insulin peak plasma effect can occur within 40 minutes, meaning that clinical signs of hypoglycemia (ataxia, disorientation, and seizures) may develop rapidly before or during decontamination.[13] If significant clinical signs and weakness associated with xylitol toxicosis develop during emesis, aspiration may occur.

Activated charcoal is not typically recommended, because xylitol is so readily absorbed from the gastrointestinal tract. Also, in vitro studies suggest that activated charcoal binds poorly to xylitol.[22]

Initial blood work on presentation should include monitoring of electrolytes (including potassium), blood glucose, a baseline liver profile, a baseline complete blood count, and a serum phosphorus level. The electrolytes can be repeated in 8 to 12 hours after exposure in several affected animals, and hypokalemia should be corrected as needed. Blood glucose should be evaluated every 2 hours for the first 12 hours and checked more frequently in severely affected patients. Monitoring of blood glucose levels for more than 12 hours may be necessary if hypoglycemia develops and persists. Baseline liver enzymes should be reevaluated 12, 24, and 48 hours later. If liver enzymes become elevated, the patient's coagulation parameters (to monitor for coagulopathies) should be monitored,[3] and the complete blood cell count should be examined for evidence of mild-to-moderate thrombocytopenia.[16] Serum phosphorus should be evaluated once daily.

An intravenous catheter should be placed in dogs exposed to doses suspected to result in hypoglycemia. If hypoglycemia is identified, an intravenous dextrose bolus should be administered, followed by parenteral fluids containing 2.5% to 5% dextrose.[3] The dextrose may prevent hypoglycemia in mild intoxications and may be hepatoprotective in patients at risk for hepatic necrosis. S-Adenosyl-L-methionine (SAMe) or Denosyl (20 mg/kg/d) and Marin (per label instructions) or milk thistle (50 mg/kg/d) may also be used,[20] although the efficacy of these hepatoprotectants for xylitol toxicosis has not been established. There may also be some benefit for using 5% N-acetylcysteine (140 mg/kg by mouth initially, then 70 mg/kg by mouth every 6–8 hours for 7 additional treatments).[20] The hepatoprotective efficacy of N-acetylcysteine for xylitol toxicosis has not been determined. If evidence of hepatic damage develops and the patient's coagulation profile becomes abnormal, vitamin K_1 therapy should be initiated, and plasma transfusions may be considered.

Dogs should be hospitalized for a minimum of 12 to 24 hours after ingestion because of the risk of delayed-onset of hypoglycemia, particularly with chewing gum exposures.[3] If symptoms develop, the patient should receive veterinary care and frequent feedings until the blood glucose level has been stabilized. The addition of dietary fiber to the diet may be useful for facilitating the elimination of concurrently consumed wrapper materials and packaging.

Prognosis is generally good with early decontamination and effective management of hypoglycemia, even in cases in which mild liver enzyme elevations have developed. The prognosis becomes more guarded for dogs that develop repeated bouts of profound hypoglycemia (often with central nervous system signs), or significant prolonged liver enzyme elevations, with or without coagulopathy, suggestive of hepatic necrosis. Patients that develop hyperphosphatemia tend to have a poor prognosis for survival; however, even some of these severely affected dogs have successfully recovered.

SUMMARY

Xylitol ingestions in dogs may result in severe hypoglycemia followed by acute hepatic failure and associated coagulopathies. Aggressive treatment may be needed, but the prognosis is generally expected to be good for dogs developing uncomplicated hypoglycemia. Because of increased availability of xylitol-containing products in the market and in the dog's environment, it is likely that there will continue to be increased exposures and toxicity in dogs.

REFERENCES

1. Gare F. The sweet miracle of xylitol. North Bergen (NJ): Basic Health Publications; 2003.
2. Cronin JR. Xylitol: a sweet for healthy teeth and more. Altern Complement Ther 2003;9:139–41.
3. Dunayer EK. New findings on the effects of xylitol ingestion in dogs. Vet Med 2006;12:791–6.
4. Dills WL. Sugar alcohols as bulk sweeteners. Annu Rev Nutr 1989;9:161–86.
5. Todd JM, Powell LP. Xylitol intoxication associated with fulminant hepatic failure in a dog. J Vet Emerg Crit Care 2007;17:286–9.
6. Budavari S, editor. The Merck index: an encyclopedia of chemicals, drugs, and biologicals. Rahway (NJ): Merck; 1989. p. 9996.
7. Anthony JP, Weber LP, Alkemade S. Blood glucose and liver function in dogs administered a xylitol drinking water additive at zero, one and five times dosage rates. Veterinary Science Development 2011;1:7–9.
8. Kuzuya T, Kanazawa Y, Kosaka K. Stimulation of insulin secretion by xylitol in dogs. Endocrinology 1969;84:200–7.
9. Froesch ER, Jakob A. The metabolism of xylitol. In: Sipple HL, McNutt KW, editors. Sugars in nutrition. New York: Academic Press; 1974. p. 241–58.
10. Kuzuya T, Kanazawa Y, Kosaka K. Plasma insulin response to intravenously administered xylitol in dogs. Metabolism 1966;15:1149–52.
11. Hirata Y, Fujisawa M, Sato H, et al. Blood glucose and plasma insulin responses to xylitol administered intravenously in dogs. Biochem Biophys Res Commun 1966;24:471–5.
12. Kuzuya T, Kanazawa Y, Hayashi M, et al. Species difference in plasma insulin responses to intravenous xylitol in man and several mammals. Endocrinol Jpn 1971;18:309–20.
13. Xia Z, He Y, Yu J. Experimental acute toxicity of xylitol in dogs. J Vet Pharmacol Ther 2009;32:465–9.
14. Jerzsele Á, Karancsi Z, Pászti-Gere E, et al. Effects of p.o. administered xylitol in cats. J Vet Pharmacol Ther 2018;41(3):409–14.
15. Gardner BR, Mitchell EP. Acute, fatal, presumptive xylitol toxicosis in Cape sugarbirds (Promerop cafer). J Avian Med Surg 2017;31(4):356–8.
16. Dunayer EK, Gwaltney-Brant SM. Acute hepatic failure and coagulopathy associated with xylitol ingestion in eight dogs. J Am Vet Med Assoc 2006;229:1113–7.
17. Wang YM, King SM, Patterson JH, et al. Mechanism of xylitol toxicity in the rabbit. Metabolism 1973;22:885–94.
18. Brin M, Miller ON. The safety of oral xylitol. In: Sipple HL, McNutt KW, editors. Sugars in nutrition. New York: Academic Press; 1974. p. 591–606.
19. Kvist CL, Andersson SB, Berglund J, et al. Equipment for drug release testing of medicated chewing gums. J Pharm Biomed Anal 2000;22:405–11.
20. Plumb DC. Veterinary drug handbook. 6th edition. Stockholm (WI), Ames (IA): PharmaVet, Blackwell; 2005. p. 14–5, 91–2, 1086–7, 1101–2.
21. Poppenga R. Treatment. In: Plumlee KH, editor. Clinical veterinary toxicology. St Louis (MO): Mosby; 2004. p. 15.
22. Cope RB. A screening study of xylitol binding in vitro to activated charcoal. Vet Hum Toxicol 2004;46:336–7.

Toxicology of Avermectins and Milbemycins (Macrocyclic Lactones) and the Role of P-Glycoprotein in Dogs and Cats

Valentina M. Merola, DVM, MS, MPH[a],*, Paul A. Eubig, DVM, MS, PhD[b]

KEYWORDS

- Macrocyclic lactones • Ivermectin • Dogs • Cats • P-glycoprotein

KEY POINTS

- Overdoses of macrocyclic lactones in dogs and cats can result in such signs as tremors, seizures, coma, and blindness.
- Dogs with the ABCB1-1Δ gene defect are predisposed to macrocyclic lactone toxicosis at lower dosages than dogs without the defect.
- Intravenous lipid emulsion therapy has been suggested for treatment of macrocyclic lactone toxicosis but evidence of efficacy is limited.
- Initial decontamination and supportive care remain the mainstays of therapy for macrocyclic lactone toxicosis.

The macrocyclic lactones (MLs) are parasiticides able to kill a wide variety of arthropods and nematodes. They have a high margin of safety for labeled indications, and ivermectin has become the best-selling antiparasitic in the world.[1] Dogs of certain breeds and mixtures of those breeds have a defect in the *ABCB1* gene (formerly *MDR1* gene) that results in a lack of functional permeability glycoprotein (P-gp), which leads to accumulation of the MLs in the central nervous system (CNS) and a higher risk of adverse effects when exposed. With toxicosis, such CNS signs as ataxia, lethargy, coma, tremors, seizures, mydriasis, and blindness predominate. In general, the MLs have a long half-life and therefore exposure results in a long duration of illness

The authors have nothing to disclose.
[a] 78th Medical Group, United States Air Force, Robins AFB, Building 700, 655 Seventh Street, Warner Robins, GA 31098, USA; [b] College of Veterinary Medicine, Department of Physiology & Pharmacology, University of Georgia, 501 DW Brooks Drive, Room# 2215, Athens, GA 30602, USA
* Corresponding author.
E-mail address: valentina.m.merola.mil@mail.mil

when overdoses occur. Recent case reports detail the use of intravenous lipid emulsion (ILE) therapy in the treatment of ML toxicosis, but evidence of efficacy for this treatment modality is limited. Given that there is no specific antidote for ML toxicosis, the most important aspects of treatment are timely decontamination and good supportive care.

CHEMISTRY OF MACROCYCLIC LACTONES

The MLs (macrolides) include two groups: avermectins and milbemycins. The avermectins include abamectin, ivermectin, eprinomectin, doramectin, and selamectin. The milbemycins consist of moxidectin, milbemycin, and nemadectin. These structurally similar compounds are derived from natural compounds produced by soil-dwelling fungi from the genus *Streptomyces*.[1] The natural compound avermectin is composed of eight closely related compounds: four A- and B-components (A_1, A_2, B_1, B_2), each of which further contains two homologous a- and b-components (eg, B_{1a} and B_{1b}).[1] Abamectin and ivermectin are both composed of avermectin B_1 components, differing only in the absence of a double bond in ivermectin.[1] Further modification of B_1 produces eprinomectin.[1] Doramectin and selamectin are closely related and contain A_1 and B_1 components, respectively.[2] Moxidectin is produced from the *Streptomyces* fermentation product nemadectin.[2] Milbemycin oxime (milbemycin) is composed of 5-oxime derivatives of milbemycins A_4 and A_3.[1]

MECHANISMS OF TOXICITY AND THE ROLE OF P-GLYCOPROTEIN

Avermectins and milbemycins have minor differences in some substituents, but they share the same general structure that confers on them the ability to bind to chloride channel receptors.[1] One main mechanism by which the MLs exert their effect is by binding ligand-gated chloride channels.[2,3] Binding of glutamate-gated chloride channels, which are specific to invertebrates, causes influx of chloride ions into the parasite neurons leading to hyperpolarization, paralysis, and death.[2]

In mammals, MLs bind to γ–aminobutyric acid type A–gated chloride channels (GABA$_A$ receptors).[4] GABA is the primary inhibitory neurotransmitter in the brain, and postsynaptic binding of GABA to its receptors serves to modulate firing of excitatory neurons, such as glutamatergic neurons. MLs are believed to bind GABA$_A$ receptors at sites different than those where GABA, benzodiazepines, barbiturates, or picrotoxin separately bind.[5] Because GABA$_A$ receptors are only present in the CNS, binding of MLs is prevented by the blood-brain barrier (BBB), as discussed later. However, in overdoses, enough ML permeates the BBB that binding to GABA$_A$ receptors, and to glycine- and voltage-gated chloride channels, occurs.[3,6] Subsequent chloride influx causes hyperpolarization and decreased firing of the excitatory neurons that express these chloride receptors and channels, leading to clinical signs. Of interest, avermectins actually may reduce GABA effects at lower concentrations, resulting in such signs as tremoring (excitatory signs), and then start to enhance GABA effects as concentrations at the receptor increase, causing a progression of signs to ataxia and CNS depression (inhibitory effects).[3] So avermectins may have stimulatory CNS effects (tremors) at lower concentrations but inhibitory effects (ataxia, depression) at higher concentrations.

P-gp is a transmembrane efflux protein that influences the pharmacokinetics of many of its substrates, including MLs, by actively transporting absorbed substrates back across a variety of cell membranes in the body.[7] P-gp, which is a member of the ATP-binding cassette (ABC) superfamily of transporters, is found in all mammalian species[8] and is well distributed throughout the tissues of dogs[9] and cats.[10] It is characteristically located along the apical border of cell types that serve a barrier function (eg, enterocytes, bile canalicular cells, renal tubular cells, and endothelial cells), so P-gp is viewed as having a protective function because it limits entry of substrates into internal compartments.[11]

P-gp is important in limiting the entry of MLs and other xenobiotics into the CNS.[12] The BBB regulates entry of endogenous substances and xenobiotics from the circulation into the brain. Tight junctions between endothelial cells prevent paracellular diffusion of substances into the CNS. Also, endothelial cells in the brain are specialized in that they lack pinocytotic vacuoles and fenestrations in their plasma membranes, thus making the BBB selectively permeable.[13] Substances that enter the brain must either diffuse through the endothelial cells or be actively transported into the endothelial cells by uptake transporters.[14] As substances enter the endothelial cells in the brain, they are potentially subject to being extruded back across the apical membrane by P-gp and other efflux proteins,[13,14] as shown in **Fig. 1.** Further components of the BBB include the basal lamina on the abluminal side of the endothelial cells and the foot processes of the glial astrocytes.[13]

The *ABCB1* gene (formerly called *MDR1*) codes for P-gp in vertebrates[8] and has been sequenced in dogs.[15] In some dog breeds there is a genetic defect in P-gp: a four-base pair deletion in the *ABCB1* gene (*ABCB1-1Δ*) results in production of an extremely truncated, nonfunctional P-gp.[15] Having the *ABCB1-1Δ* mutation can result in accumulation of P-gp substrates in the brain that would normally be removed by P-gp,[12] so the BBB is compromised and becomes permeable to P-gp substrates, including MLs. In dogs with this defect, treatment with doses of MLs above those used for heartworm prevention may result in accumulation of the drug in the CNS, resulting in neurologic effects. Adverse neurologic effects can also occur in animals without the gene defect when overdoses of MLs are administered, in which case

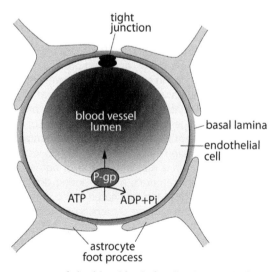

Fig. 1. P-gp is a component of the blood-brain barrier. P-gp actively transports substrates entering CNS endothelial cells back into the systemic circulation, thus preventing entry of substrates, such as ivermectin, into the parenchyma of the brain. (*Data from* Refs.[50,60,89–91]; and *Adapted from* Linnet K, Ejsing TB. A review on the impact of P-glycoprotein on the penetration of drugs into the brain. Focus on psychotropic drugs. Eur Neuropsychopharmacol 2008;18:159; with permission.)

saturation of the transport capacity of P-gp likely occurs. Dogs may be homozygous or heterozygous for the defect, with homozygous dogs being at greater risk of developing toxicosis from ML exposure.[7]

EXPOSURE SOURCES, FORMULATIONS, AND THERAPEUTIC AND TOXIC DOSAGES

Because the MLs are commonly used as parasiticides in many species, they are available in a wide array of formulations.[1] Some of the most common small animal veterinary products include tablets with ivermectin, moxidectin, or milbemycin and topical products with selamectin that are used for heartworm prevention. Ivermectin, moxidectin, milbemycin, and doramectin are also used off-label for various indications including as a heartworm microfilaricide and for treating demodectic and sarcoptic mange and other ectoparasites and endoparasites.[16] Dogs and cats may also be exposed to large animal products either accidentally or by intentional administration. Many formulations intended for large animals are concentrated so it is easy for accidental overdoses to occur.

Signs of intoxication with MLs generally are related to the CNS. Neurologic depression, ataxia, mydriasis, blindness, tremors, and hypersalivation all may be seen and, as signs progress, an animal may become comatose. Seizures may also occur. The blindness is typically temporary and has been associated with retinal edema and electroretinogram abnormalities in the case of ivermectin.[17,18] The signs seen are similar in dogs and cats for all the MLs. Depending on the dose and the breed involved and because of the long half-life of these agents, toxicosis may persist for days to weeks.

Formulations, labeled and off-label therapeutic dosage ranges, and documented "safe" versus toxic dosages for specific MLs are discussed next. When possible, distinctions are made between dosages that affect dogs with or without the *ABCB1-1Δ* gene defect. **Table 1** provides a summary of the information in this section.

Ivermectin

Ivermectin is available in numerous forms for large animal applications including injectable liquid, oral bolus, pour-on, paste, and feed premix. It is available as chewable tablets for heartworm prevention in small animals. Ivermectin is also produced as a 3-mg tablet (Stromectrol) for humans indicated for treatment of gastrointestinal (GI) strongyloidiasis in the United States and for onchocerciasis and strongyloidiasis in other countries. Many of the large animal formulations are of high concentration, from 1% to 1.87% (10–18.7 mg/mL), so it is easy for accidental overdose to occur either from miscalculation of a dosage when using these products off-label, from accidental exposure to the remnants in a discarded tube of equine dewormer, or from blobs of dewormer that fall from a horse's mouth during deworming. Exposure to concentrated (eg, ivermectin 1.87%) MLs eliminated in the dung of treated large animals is also a potential source of exposure (American Society for the Prevention of Cruelty to Animals [ASPCA] Animal Poison Control Center [APCC], Urbana, IL, unpublished information, 2011). In one study, ivermectin concentrations in horse dung were monitored after horses were treated with a manufacturer's recommended therapeutic dosage.[19] Peak ivermectin levels of 2.4 mg/kg of dung were measured 2.5 days after exposure. To place this concentration in perspective, a 27.3 kg (60 lb) collie homozygous for *ABCB1-1Δ* would need to ingest 1.1 kg (2.4 lb) of dung to attain a dosage of 0.1 mg/kg of ivermectin, which is mildly toxic in sensitive collies.[20] In contrast, tablets for heartworm prevention range from 0.068 to 0.272 mg of ivermectin per tablet so toxicosis is rare even when small animals ingest several of these pills.

Table 1
Therapeutic, nontoxic, and toxic dosages of macrocyclic lactones in normal and sensitive dogs and in cats

Agent	Formulations	Therapeutic Dosages (Labeled and Off-Label, mg/kg)	Acute, Subacute, or Chronic Dosages Published as Safe (mg/kg)	Toxic Dosages ML Sensitive Dogs (mg/kg)	Acute Toxic Dosage Normal Dog/Cat (mg/kg)	References
Ivermectin	Tablets, oral liquid, oral paste, feed premix, injectable, topical, otic	0.006–0.6 PO D 0.024 PO C 0.2–0.4 SC D, C	0.5 PO daily × 12 wk[a] D 0.06 PO Collies 0.2–1.33[a] PO or SC C 0.72 PO C	0.1–0.4[b] PO 0.2–0.25[b] SC	0.2–2.5 PO D 0.3 SC C	16,23,26 27,28,33 71,92,94,99
Selamectin	Topical	6 topical D, C	6 PO D, C[c] 40 topical Collies 72–114 topical D 236–367 topical C	5 PO[d]	None found	16,95,100
Moxidectin	Tablets, oral drench, injectable, topical	0.003 PO D 0.17 sustained-release SC D 2.5 topical D 1 topical C	1.15 PO daily × 1 y D 0.09 PO Collies 0.85 SC D, Collies	1 PO[e]	1.9–2.8 PO D 1 PO C[f]	2,16,29 96,97,101 102,103
Doramectin	Injectable, pour-on	0.6 SC D, C	0.5–1 PO daily × 91 d D 0.2 SC C	0.2[a]–0.7 SC	None found	16,38,39 93,98
Milbemycin	Tablets	0.5–2 PO D 2 PO C	10 PO Collies 10 PO C	5–10[g] PO 0.8 PO × 2 d 1.5 PO × 13 d	None found	16,34,35 99

Abbreviations: C, cat; collies, ivermectin-sensitive collies; D, dog; PO, orally; SC, subcutaneously.
[a] It should be noted that some animals are also reported to have problems at this dosage.
[b] Many of the collies in these reports were not tested for the ABCB1-1Δ gene defect.
[c] Cats exhibited drooling and intermittent vomiting with oral dosing.
[d] One collie was ataxic after this dosage in the safety studies, but others tolerated up to 15 mg/kg PO.
[e] Administered as a product containing 2.5% moxidectin and 10% imidacloprid.
[f] Generally only mild signs seen.
[g] Collies at these dosages were not tested for the ABCB1-1Δ gene defect.

Ivermectin is used for heartworm prevention at dosages of 0.006 to 0.012 mg/kg in dogs and 0.024 mg/kg in cats. It is also used off-label in dogs as a microfilaricide at 0.05 to 0.2 mg/kg and to treat ectoparasites at 0.3 to 0.6 mg/kg.[16]

Clinical signs have been reported in breeds with a history of ivermectin sensitivity at dosages ranging from 0.08 to 0.34 mg/kg.[21–23] However, none of these dogs were tested for the *ABCB1* gene deletion. In breeds considered to be normal in their response to ivermectin, mild clinical signs have been documented at dosages starting from 0.2 mg/kg,[23] with more severe signs developing at dosages of 1 to 2.5 mg/kg or greater.[23,24] Some of the dogs reported to show signs at low ivermectin dosages in one retrospective study[23] were German shepherds. A small percentage of this breed does carry the *ABCB1* gene defect,[25] which might partly explain the presence of signs in "normal" dogs at low dosages. It is important to emphasize that problems are not expected with standard heartworm preventative dosages even in *ABCB1-1Δ* dogs. Ivermectin-sensitive collies were treated with 10 times the heartworm preventative dosage (0.06 mg/kg) without signs developing.[26] However, when ivermectin is used at higher dosages as a microfilaricide or for demodicosis, problems can easily occur in patients with the *ABCB1* gene deletion, and sometimes even in dogs with normal *ABCB1* genotype. Clinical signs have developed following oral dosages of 0.1 mg/kg in ivermectin-sensitive collies.[20] In overdoses, the most frequent clinical signs reported in dogs were lethargy, ataxia, hypersalivation, tremors, mydriasis, blindness, and bradycardia.[23,27] Coma, seizures, and death have been seen in severely affected animals. Similar signs have been seen in cats[28] (ASPCA APCC, unpublished information, 2011), although miosis rather than mydriasis was noted in one case report.[28]

Moxidectin

Moxidectin is available in many forms including injectable, pour-on, and oral drench for ruminants and horses. It is available as a topical preparation, a subcutaneous (SC) injection, and a monthly tablet for heartworm prevention in small animals. As with ivermectin, moxidectin products intended for use in horses and ruminants are of high concentration (0.5%–2% or 5–20 mg/mL), so small animals may be exposed to high doses from small amounts of these products. Also similar to ivermectin, horse dung could be another potential source of moxidectin exposure for dogs, with peak moxidectin concentrations of 2.6 mg/kg of horse dung measured 2.5 days after horses were treated with a manufacturer's recommended therapeutic dosage.[19]

Moxidectin is used in dogs for heartworm prevention orally at 0.003 mg/kg monthly and in sustained-release SC injection at 0.17 mg/kg every 6 months. It is also used topically in dogs at 2.5 mg/kg and in cats at 1 mg/kg monthly for heartworm prevention.[16]

At oral dosages of 1.9 to 2.8 mg/kg, adverse effects have been documented in dogs with normal P-gp genotype.[29] Signs in dogs exposed to equine moxidectin dewormers include ataxia, tremors, seizures, hyperthermia, tachycardia, blindness, hypersalivation, bradycardia, coma, and respiratory depression.[29–32]

Selamectin

Selamectin is available as a topical formulation for dogs and cats that is labeled for prevention of heartworm and for killing fleas and ear mites at a minimum dosage of 6 mg/kg, with concentrations of 60 and 120 mg/mL. It is also used at the same dosages to treat sarcoptic mange and tick infestation in dogs and hookworms and ascarids in cats.[16] Because it is not available as a more concentrated form, overdose is less likely. The most common clinical signs following selamectin exposure include vomiting, drooling, retching, licking of lips, lethargy, agitation, anorexia, and ataxia (ASPCA APCC, unpublished information, 2011). Many of these signs likely result from inadvertent oral exposure or administration.

Abamectin (Avermectin B₁)

Abamectin is generally used in products used to control ants, cockroaches, mites, and other insects. Sometimes abamectin products are labeled as containing avermectin B_1. These are usually found in the form of plastic traps ("baits") for ants and cockroaches, insect spikes, granules, or liquids intended to be sprayed for outdoor and indoor use. The liquids range in concentration from 0.15% to 2%. Generally, the ant/cockroach traps contain between 0.01% and 0.05% of abamectin. A typical ant "bait" weighs about 1.6 to 2 g, giving a range of 0.16 to 1 mg of abamectin per trap; thus, it is rare to see significant signs with exposure. Subchronic studies in several species (dogs, rats, rabbits, and mice) suggest that abamectin and ivermectin have a similar degree of toxicity and that abamectin is marginally more toxic than ivermectin.[33] Dogs are primarily exposed to these insecticide products because some contain attractants, such as peanut butter, which are intended to lure insects but are also appealing to dogs. The clinical signs most commonly reported to the APCC following abamectin exposure are vomiting, ataxia, hypersalivation, lethargy, mydriasis, and diarrhea (ASPCA APCC, unpublished information, 2011). Many of the clinical signs are also likely related to the inert ingredients that can cause mild GI upset.

Milbemycin

Milbemycin is available as an oral chewable tablet (2.3–27 mg) for heartworm prevention in dogs and cats and a 0.1% otic solution for treating ear mites.[16] It is not available in a more concentrated dosage form, so overdoses are rare.

The therapeutic dosages of milbemycin for heartworm prevention are 0.5 mg/kg in dogs and 2 mg/kg in cats. Mild clinical signs of ataxia, hypersalivation, mydriasis, and lethargy have been documented in ivermectin-sensitive dogs dosed at 5 to 10 mg/kg.[34] In a separate report, two *ABCB1*-defective dogs developed mild signs (ataxia) after being dosed repeatedly with milbemycin for demodicosis; one dog received 0.8 mg/kg 2 days in a row and the other dog received 1.5 mg/kg daily for 13 days before developing signs.[35] Mild clinical signs have been reported to develop in normal dogs at 10 to 20 mg/kg and in cats and in dogs with suspected *ABCB1* gene deletions at greater than 5 to 10 mg/kg (ASPCA APCC, unpublished information, 2011). The most common clinical signs reported include ataxia, tremors, lethargy, vomiting, mydriasis, disorientation, and hypersalivation.

Doramectin, Eprinomectin, and Nemadectin

Doramectin is available as an injectable formulation (10 mg/mL) for ruminants and pigs and a pour-on for cattle (5 mg/mL).[2] Doramectin has been used off-label to treat demodicosis in dogs and cats at 0.6 mg/kg SC once weekly.[16] Eprinomectin is available as a pour-on for cattle (5 mg/mL).[2] Eprinomectin has been used experimentally to treat *Toxocara canis* at 0.1 mg/kg in dogs,[36] whereas nemadectin has been used at 0.2 to 0.6 mg/kg in dogs to treat GI helminths.[37] Side effects were not seen in either study. Further information about eprinomectin and nemadectin use in small animals could not be located.

Exposure of small animals to these products occurs less frequently than to some of the more common MLs, but these products are of high concentration so it is plausible that accidental exposure could result in toxicosis. Two case reports regarding dogs exposed to doramectin give an idea of what clinical signs are seen. One report involved a collie given 0.2 mg/kg of doramectin SC,[38] and the other involved two white Swiss shepherds exposed to 0.7 mg/kg doramectin SC.[39] The dogs in the latter report were confirmed to have the *ABCB1* gene defect, whereas the collie was assumed to have the gene defect. Clinical signs included blindness, restlessness, CNS depression, recumbency, hypersalivation, tremors, tachypnea, ataxia, head pressing, disorientation, lack of menace response, and bradycardia. Clinical signs from eprinomectin or nemadectin overdose in animals with normal P-gp are expected to be similar, but it is uncertain at what dosage signs would emerge.

TOXICOKINETICS OF MACROCYCLIC LACTONES AND THE ROLE OF P-GLYCOPROTEIN

In general, the MLs have fast oral absorption but a much more gradual absorption rate after SC injection.[40] They also are all highly fat soluble, have a large volume of distribution, and accumulate in fat tissue resulting in a long elimination half-life.[1,41] The authors were unable to locate specific information about metabolism and amounts of drug or metabolites eliminated in bile and urine in the dog or cat. Data from species where this information is known indicate that generally large percentages of MLs are eliminated in the bile with the degree of metabolism varying among the different compounds.[1] Studies in large animal species[1] and humans[42] suggest that enterohepatic circulation, by which xenobiotics are eliminated in the bile and then reabsorbed from the gut, occurs with MLs. However, differences in product formulation can alter pharmacokinetic parameters significantly even for the same agent.[40,43]

In dogs, it takes about 4 hours for orally administered ivermectin to reach maximum plasma levels (t_{max} = 4 hours).[44,45] SC absorption is slower, with t_{max} being 32 to 36 hours in dogs[44,46] and about 28 hours in cats.[41] The elimination half-life after oral administration of ivermectin to dogs is 3.3 days,[44,45] whereas after SC administration, the half-life is 3.2 days in dogs[44] and 3.4 days in cats.[41] One study evaluated the differences in pharmacokinetic parameters after SC injection of the same dosage of seven different ivermectin preparations in dogs.[46] The maximum plasma concentrations ranged from 26.5 to 49.6 ng/mL and the area under the curve ranged from 2523 to 4956 ng • h/mL. The area under the curve, which reflects bioavailability, is a measure of the amount of free drug that reaches systemic circulation.[46] These significant differences illustrate the influence of formulation on pharmacokinetic parameters.

Moxidectin is absorbed faster than ivermectin following oral administration, with a t_{max} of 2 to 3 hours in dogs.[45,47] Moxidectin is highly bioavailable after oral dosing: about 90% of the drug is absorbed in dogs.[48] Reported elimination half-lives in dogs vary from 13.9 to 25.9 days.[45,47,48] This variability is associated with body condition. More obese dogs had a higher volume of distribution,[47,48] resulting in indirectly prolonged elimination caused by distribution of the lipophilic drug into their larger fat compartment.

Selamectin is used in dogs and cats topically. With dermal exposure, peak blood levels are reached in 72 hours in dogs and 15 hours in cats; if given orally, t_{max} is 8 hours in dogs and 7 hours in cats.[49] The elimination half-life in dogs is 11.1 days after dermal exposure and 1.9 days with oral exposure. In cats, the half-life is 8.25 days after dermal exposure and 1.1 days after oral exposure.[49] Selamectin is much more bioavailable in cats than in dogs after dermal applications: 72% bioavailability in cats versus 4.4% in dogs.[49] However, it is not known how much of this difference is caused by grooming behavior (and therefore oral absorption) in cats. Oral bioavailability of selamectin was 109% in cats and 62% in dogs,[49] which, especially in cats, suggests enterohepatic circulation of selamectin.

Doramectin reaches peak blood levels in 2 hours after oral dosing and 1.4 days after SC administration in dogs, whereas the half-life in dogs is 3 to 3.7 days.[44] Kinetic information in small animals could not be located for eprinomectin and nemadectin.

P-gp potentially limits drug absorption, by moving substrates out of enterocytes and back into the intestinal tract, and enhances drug elimination, by depositing substrates into the bile, intestine, and renal tubules.[7,50] Several factors can affect the ability of P-gp to alter the kinetics of MLs. One factor is the affinities of the MLs for P-gp, with MLs that have higher affinities being more readily transported at lower concentrations. Ivermectin, abamectin, doramectin, and eprinomectin all have higher affinities for P-gp compared with selamectin and moxidectin.[51] The concentration of MLs presented to transporters is another potentially important factor. P-gp substrates can often stimulate their own transport at lower concentrations while inhibiting transport at higher concentrations,[52] so as levels of an ML crossing the cellular apical border increase, P-gp may become less able to effectively transport it back across the plasma membrane.

Unfortunately, the ability of P-gp to alter the pharmacokinetics of MLs has not been closely examined. One way to evaluate for this is to compare kinetic parameters of MLs between dogs with and without the *ABCB1-1Δ* gene defect. Ivermectin plasma levels did not differ between normal and ivermectin-sensitive collies administered 0.1 mg/kg ivermectin orally,[53] but 0.1 mg/kg may be too small a dose for pharmacokinetic differences to be evident. It has been demonstrated that dogs with the *ABCB1* defect are impaired in the ability to eliminate P-gp substrates into the bile[54] but do not seem to have enhanced intestinal absorption of P-gp substrates.[55] However, MLs were not evaluated in the latter two studies.

SENSITIVE POPULATIONS
Dogs with the ABCB1-1Δ Gene Defect

The *ABCB1-1Δ* mutation is typically seen in herding-type breeds, primarily collies and Shetland sheepdogs and Australian shepherds; in addition, it has been detected in longhaired whippets, old English sheepdogs, silken windhounds, white Swiss shepherds, German shepherds, and some mixes of these breeds.[39,56]

Dogs are easily tested for the gene defect.[7] However, it is difficult to know whether the frequencies of the gene defect in populations of dogs that are tested are representative of the general population because there may be bias in submitting samples (eg, dogs may be more likely to be tested after an ML-related toxicosis develops or if they are related to dogs known to have the *ABCB1* defect). Mealey and Meurs[25] found that of 5368 client-owned dogs, the breeds with the highest frequency of the *ABCB1-1Δ* mutation were collies and Australian shepherds: of 1424 collies tested, 35% were homozygous and 42% were heterozygous, and of 1421 Australian shepherds tested, 10% were homozygous and 37% were heterozygous. In miniature Australian shepherds, silken windhounds, and longhaired whippets, between 30% and 60% of the dogs tested had one or both copies of the gene defect. In border collies, German shepherds, herding breed mixes, old English sheepdogs, Shetland sheepdogs, and other mixed breeds, less than 15% of dogs had one or both copies of the gene defect. They also tested 659 purebred dogs of other breeds with none having the gene defect. In a smaller study of dogs in Australia, higher rates of the gene defect in collies and Australian shepherds were seen compared with rates in the United States.[56] In both of these studies, it was rare (about 1% frequency) to find the *ABCB1* mutation in border collies. However, a recent report of an *ABCB1* mutation that differs from the *ABCB1-1Δ* mutation in an ivermectin-sensitive border collie[57] demonstrates that other gene defects can produce the ivermectin-sensitive phenotype. Thus, just because a dog does not have the *ABCB1-1Δ* genotype does not mean that it is absolutely certain that it will tolerate higher dosages of MLs.

Animals Treated with Other P-Glycoprotein Substrates

Chronic administration of MLs for demodicosis has resulted in toxicosis in dogs of breeds in which the *ABCB1-1Δ* mutation has not been documented[58] (ASPCA APCC, unpublished information, 2011), suggesting that factors other than genetics might play a role in the development of ML toxicosis. These dogs developed signs, such as ataxia, lethargy, and tremors, after administration of extralabel doses of ivermectin, moxidectin, or milbemycin for periods ranging from days to weeks. Bissonnette and colleagues[58] had 28 of these dogs genotyped and found that 27 were normal, whereas one was heterozygous for the *ABCB1-1Δ* gene mutation. Of these dogs, 10 were on other medications that also are P-gp substrates. Acquired P-gp dysfunction caused by drug interactions may make animals more susceptible to ML toxicosis.[7] It also may be possible that in these dogs there were other, as yet unidentified, mutations that may impair P-gp function.

Mechanisms by which other P-gp substrates can potentially cause elevated levels of MLs in the brain or plasma include competing with MLs for transport by P-gp and inhibiting P-gp function. These effects can be concentration dependent where a substrate can become an inhibitor as its concentrations at the transporter rise.[52] **Table 2** lists several medications that are known P-gp substrates or inhibitors. In many cases it is not known if an interaction between MLs and these drugs will occur, so this list should be taken as a guideline for when caution should be exercised when coadministering avermectins or milbemycins with the listed medications. However, combining a P-gp substrate with a P-gp inhibitor is more likely to be problematic than treating a patient with two P-gp substrates. Two commonly used veterinary drugs that are P-gp inhibitors (and substrates) and that interact unfavorably with MLs in dogs, as discussed next, illustrate this principle.

The antifungal drug ketoconazole can cause problems when administered concurrently with ivermectin. Hugnet and colleagues[59] reported that administration of ketoconazole to dogs over a period spanning from 5 days before through 5 days after ivermectin administration resulted in higher plasma concentrations and longer residence time of ivermectin than in dogs treated with ivermectin alone. Ketoconazole is an inhibitor of P-gp, which may result in decreased elimination of ivermectin from the CNS and decreased biliary excretion of ivermectin.

When ivermectin and the insecticide spinosad were coadministered, signs of ivermectin toxicosis sometimes developed at dosages not typically expected to cause problems.[60] One study determined that ivermectin pharmacokinetics were altered when ivermectin was given with spinosad: maximum plasma concentrations and area under the curve of ivermectin were increased, whereas clearance was decreased compared with dogs given ivermectin alone.[60] It was determined that spinosad is a substrate and inhibitor of human P-gp, prompting the authors to hypothesize that this inhibition is responsible for the increased risk of ivermectin toxicosis when spinosad is coadministered in dogs.[60] A different study assessed the effects of coadministration of spinosad and milbemycin in collies with the *ABCB1-1Δ* mutation.[61] Up to 10 times the heartworm preventative dose of milbemycin along with spinosad at either three or five times the labeled therapeutic dose did not result in signs of milbemycin toxicosis. It is interesting to speculate

Table 2
P-gp substrates and inhibitors

P-gp Substrates	P-gp Inhibitors
Antibiotics	
Erythromycin	Erythromycin
Tetracycline	Clarithromycin
Doxycycline	
Antifungals	
Ketoconazole	Ketoconazole
Itraconazole	Itraconazole
Antidepressants	
Paroxetine	Paroxetine
Venlafaxine	Fluoxetine
Amitriptyline	St. John's wort
Chemotherapeutics	
Vinblastine	
Vincristine	
Doxorubicin	
Actinomycin D	
Mitoxantrone	
Etoposide	
Docetaxel	
Cardiac drugs	
Digoxin	Amiodarone
Diltiazem	Quinidine
Verapamil	Verapamil
	Carvediol
	Nicardipine
Opioids	
Loperamide	Methadone
Morphine	Pentazocine
Steroid hormones	
Dexamethasone	
Triamcinolone	
Hydrocortisone	
Aldosterone	
Methylprednisolone	
Proton pump inhibitors	Omeprazole
	Esomeprazole
	Lansoprazole
	Pantoprazole
Miscellaneous agents	
Cyclosporine	Cyclosporine
Phenothiazines	Chlorpromazine
Spinosad	Spinosad
Cimetidine	
Fexofenadine	

Data from Refs.[50,60,89–91]

whether milbemycin has a poorer affinity for P-gp, as does moxidectin,[51] compared with ivermectin, which might explain the difference between the two studies. However, the authors cannot locate information regarding the affinity of milbemycin for P-gp in the literature.

Neonatal and Elderly Dogs and Cats

An important question is whether very young dogs and cats have an immature BBB that would make them more susceptible to ML toxicosis. However, studies that would directly address this question could not be located. Tight junctions between endothelial cells in the brain, which begin forming in conjunction with the development of blood vessels in the fetal brain, are vital for sealing the BBB.[62] Evidence suggests that tight junctions exist in the brain prenatally in dogs, with further modifications occurring between 6 days before birth and 3 days postpartum.[63] In the authors' opinion, adequate P-gp expression in the endothelial cells is the other important component necessary for the BBB to be able to prevent MLs from accumulating in the brain. Information on P-gp expression in fetal or neonatal dogs or cats could not be located in the literature. In other species, times when there are marked increases in P-gp expression range from, at the earliest, during fetal development in humans[64] to, at the latest, postnatal days 16 to 21 in mice.[65] Given that times for increased P-gp expression are not expected to vary greatly beyond the times seen in other mammalian species, it is best to avoid ML exposure in neonatal dogs and cats. However, the authors speculate that sensitivity to MLs diminishes by weaning, if not sooner, in dogs and cats.

Aging also significantly affects the BBB. Brain P-gp expression is significantly decreased in aged dogs, with a 72% decrease occurring in expression in dogs older than 8.3 years of age compared with dogs less than 3 years of age.[66] It is not known if this change is significant in reducing elimination of MLs from the CNS, but it does suggest that older patients could be more susceptible to ML toxicosis than adults.

Obese and Malnourished Animals

An animal's nutritional plane and body condition may also impact the likelihood of ML toxicosis developing and the duration of treatment needed when toxicosis occurs. In moxidectin pharmacokinetic studies, obese dogs, which have a larger volume of distribution, had a significantly longer elimination half-life for moxidectin.[47,48] It is not known if this difference is clinically significant, but it suggests that obese patients may require a longer duration of treatment after overdose because of the longer length of time needed for MLs to redistribute out of the fat compartment. Conversely, obesity could have a protective effect by basically providing more body volume for a given ML dose to distribute into, thus lowering plasma and tissue concentrations. So it is difficult to predict which effect might have more impact in ML toxicosis. A case report describing three rottweilers that ingested moxidectin noted that, of the three, the obese dog received the lowest dose but had the most severe signs.[29] Two of the three dogs in the study (including the obese dog) were negative for the *ABCB1-1Δ* gene defect, whereas the third dog's sample was not adequate for testing.

But what if a patient is has a low body condition score? *In vitro* binding studies in dogs have shown that ivermectin binds extensively to plasma albumin and lipoproteins.[43] In a malnourished or hypoalbuminemic patient, it is possible that a higher free drug concentration could develop resulting in more severe clinical signs. A recent report of ivermectin overdose in a colony of cats reported that cats with low body condition scores were more likely to develop clinical signs, and the signs were more severe, than in cats with higher body condition scores.[67] For now, the influence of body condition on ML toxicosis remains mostly speculative, but should be considered in clinical cases.

TREATMENT

There are no specific antidotes for ML toxicosis. Appropriate decontamination and good supportive care are the cornerstones of treatment. Some patients need to be hospitalized for several days, so it is important that animal owners are advised up front regarding this possibility. However, with commitment to treatment, it is possible for even severely affected animals to make a complete recovery.

Decontamination

Inducing emesis may be considered if oral exposure was recent and the animal is asymptomatic. There are no established criteria for when emesis should be induced or avoided with ML ingestion. Rather, several factors must be considered. Liquid or paste formulations of MLs are anticipated to empty from the stomach rather quickly compared with solid formulations,[68] although mixing with recently ingested food may slow the emptying of nonsolid formulations.[69] Also, inducing emesis not only delays the administration of activated charcoal, which is likely to be of greater benefit in reducing absorption of MLs than emesis, but also makes it more likely that subsequently administered activated charcoal is vomited. Additionally, care must be taken to avoid aspiration if neurologic signs have already developed,[70] so emesis should not be induced in patients who are already showing signs, such as tremors, seizures, or CNS depression. Ultimately, the decision to induce emesis is best determined on a case-by-case basis, but a rule-of-thumb is to induce emesis if ingestion was within the past 30 to 60 minutes. Emesis could also be considered beyond 1 hour postingestion in such circumstances as the consumption of a large meal before oral ML exposure.

An initial dose of activated charcoal is likely to be of benefit if given within the first 4 hours of ingestion, given what is known regarding the absorption rate of MLs. Administering repeated doses of activated charcoal as frequently as every 8 hours for 2 days has been advised for ivermectin toxicosis,[23,71] although the efficacy of activated charcoal in treating overdoses of MLs has not been established. Whether a substance undergoes enterohepatic circulation is a key factor in whether repeated doses of activated charcoal are beneficial in enhancing elimination.[69] Because there is evidence that MLs are enterohepatically circulated, it is reasonable to consider repeated doses of activated charcoal in small animal patients regardless of the route of exposure. However, this recommendation caries some caveats. As with emesis, the risk of aspiration is higher when administering charcoal in a symptomatic patient, especially a comatose patient, so this should not be attempted in a patient with an absent gag reflex. Intubation may offer some degree of airway protection during charcoal administration, but it does not completely remove risk of aspiration.[72] Other complications of activated charcoal administration to consider include hypernatremia and hypermagnesemia, likely caused by the loss of free water osmotically drawn into the GI lumen.[69] These electrolyte disturbances are considered infrequent in humans, with an incidence of 6% and 3.1%, respectively, in one study,[73] but the incidence of either has not been reported in small animal patients. An additional consideration is that dogs with the *ABCB1-1Δ* gene defect may have minimal biliary elimination of P-gp substrates because of nonfunctional P-gp.[54] Therefore, repeated doses of activated charcoal may not be of much benefit in these animals, although this has not been proven. Because the amounts of MLs eliminated in bile in canines have not been evaluated, this is an excellent avenue for further research that would help better answer questions about the role of repeated administration of activated charcoal in wild-type and P-gp-defective dogs. In summary, decisions on the frequency of administration of activated charcoal are also best decided on a case-by-case basis, with the authors urging caution and moderation. An initial dose of charcoal given within 4 hours of exposure is strongly advised, provided that marked CNS signs are not present. Subsequent doses administered every 8 hours may be of some benefit, more so in animals with a normal *ABCB1* genotype. Risks of hypernatremia and aspiration should always be kept in mind whenever activated charcoal is used.

Supportive and Symptomatic Care

Fluid therapy, good nursing care of the recumbent animal, and thermoregulation are essential for these patients.[74] If respiratory depression develops, patients may require oxygen, intubation, and positive pressure ventilation. Nutritional support may also be needed. If bradycardia develops, a preanesthetic dose of atropine or glycopyrrolate may be given.

Treatment of tremors or seizures resulting from ML toxicosis is a challenging topic, with the uncertainty of which drugs to use being the main question. In clinical case reports, administration of diazepam either seemed to be of no benefit[31] or resulted in improvement of CNS stimulation soon followed by worsening of CNS depression.[27,29,30] This led Hopper and colleagues[27] to suggest that diazepam be avoided in favor of other suitable drugs, such as barbiturates or propofol. Yet a progression of signs from tremors or seizures to severe CNS depression describes a typical clinical course as concentrations of MLs rise in the brain. It is likely that an onset of CNS depression would have occurred regardless of whether diazepam was given. Although benzodiazepines, such as diazepam, can potentiate GABAergic effects, so can barbiturates and propofol, which both bind GABA$_A$ receptors, albeit at different sites than benzodiazepines and MLs.[5] Moreover, an experimental study in rodents suggests that ivermectin worsens the CNS effects caused by barbiturates.[6] The present state of knowledge is that there are several different binding sites on GABA$_A$ receptors, each of which binds different types of xenobiotics. The different binding sites interact allosterically, with binding of a compound to one site influencing the likelihood of different compounds binding to other sites, all of which then influence opening of the channel in the receptor and subsequent chloride influx.[4,75] Assessment of allosteric relationships in the GABA$_A$ receptor is challenging,[5] and the relationships between MLs and drugs that bind GABA$_A$ receptors have not been well investigated. Until these allosteric relationships are better established, it is the authors' opinion that diazepam, barbiturates, levetiracetam, or propofol may be cautiously used to control tremors or seizures.

Specific Therapies

ILE has been suggested to be a treatment that may shorten the duration of clinical signs of ML toxicosis. Lipid therapy has been used to treat moxidectin intoxication in dogs and ivermectin intoxication in cats and dogs.[30,67,76] In a 16-week old Jack Russell terrier, ILE was used after ingestion of an unknown amount of moxidectin. The puppy recovered quickly compared with other cases of moxidectin toxicosis, but it is difficult to draw conclusions because the dose of moxidectin was unknown.[30] In two other dogs exposed to moxidectin, both developed significant signs and then recovered in less than 24 hours, suggesting that ILE may have hastened recovery, given that signs resolved quicker than anticipated.[76] Lipid therapy has also been successfully used in a border collie that ingested up to 6 mg/kg of ivermectin paste.[77] The authors demonstrated decreasing blood levels of ivermectin and a rapid improvement in clinical signs with use of lipid therapy in this case. The dog in this case report was found to not have the *ABCB1-1Δ* gene mutation, which may be why the therapy seemed effective: the ability of P-gp to clear ivermectin from the CNS and the circulation was intact in this patient. In a different report, three dogs from the same household were exposed to ivermectin, and the two that were most symptomatic and had the highest dose of ivermectin were given ILE.[76] These two dogs recovered quicker than their housemate who had a lower initial ivermectin dose but did not receive ILE. Unfortunately, none of the dogs were tested for the *ABCB1-1Δ* gene mutation. In a separate case report, lipid therapy was administered several hours after ivermectin exposure to three dogs homozygous for the P-gp gene defect, but failed to improve stupor or coma.[78] Speculatively, these dogs may have had higher CNS levels or been impaired in the elimination of ivermectin because of nonfunctional P-gp, resulting in the lack of efficacy of lipid therapy.

Lipid therapy may also be beneficial in treating blindness associated with ivermectin in dogs. In two separate cases, blindness resolved less than 1 hour after ILE administration to dogs that were avisual but had no other significant clinical signs postivermectin exposure.[79,80]

ILE have also been used in feline cases of ivermectin exposure. A cat breeder gave 20 cats 4 mg/kg ivermectin SC, and ILE was administered to all of the cats 2 hours postexposure.[67] Only 6 of the 20 cats developed signs of toxicity, so it may be reasonable to conclude that ILE was beneficial in some of these cats. However, subgroups of cats received different courses of ILE, and signs took 72 to 168 hours to resolve in the three most severely affected cats despite receiving multiple doses of ILE over several days,[67] complicating the interpretation of the report.

It is hypothesized that the lipids act as a "sink" and draw lipophilic xenobiotics into the plasma lipid phase, thus removing the harmful agent from the target tissues[30] and increasing the likelihood for more rapid elimination. Intralipid therapy also has other beneficial effects, particularly improvement in myocardial performance (see Fernandez and colleagues[81] for a review). Although moxidectin may be the best candidate for this ILE therapy because of its high lipid solubility, all of the MLs are lipophilic so lipid therapy is potentially beneficial in treating toxicity from any of the avermectins or milbemycins. There are several case reports of the use of ILE to treat overdoses of this class of compounds in companion animals. Criteria for declaring success in these reports usually includes clinical signs resolving quicker than expected, a greater improvement in animals either receiving ILE or a higher dose of ILE than in animals either not receiving ILE or a lower dose of ILE, and a reduction in plasma levels of the toxicant after ILE administration. The latter criterion is especially confusing to the authors. Although it is generally understood that ILE acts through drawing toxicants into the plasma, thus theoretically elevating plasma levels,[81,82] case reports typically report a decrease in toxicant plasma concentrations post-ILE administration. Whether the decreases mean that the theoretic models are incorrect, or there are analytical difficulties in quantifying toxicants sequestered in liposomes, or there is a lack of efficacy in the case reports, is not clear. Not surprisingly, a recent systematic review of human and animal cases and studies characterized the quality of evidence for the efficacy of ILE therapy as "low to very low" for toxicants other than local anesthetics.[83] Both randomized, controlled clinical trials and experimental studies involving set doses of avermectins or milbemycins and ILE, with plasma levels measured at consistent time points, would serve to better define whether ILE therapy is efficacious for treating toxicosis caused by ivermectin and related compounds.

Although uncommon, adverse effects of lipid therapy have been reported in human and animal species in case reports and experimental studies where lipid emulsions were administered on a short-term basis.[82,84,85] Adverse effects include volume overload, fat overload syndrome, anaphylactoid reactions or anaphylaxis, hemolysis, and worsening of respiratory function in patients already experiencing respiratory compromise. Less severe adverse effects include persistent hyperlipemia and reversible corneal lipidosis. The incidence of adverse effects is related to the rate of infusion and the total ILE dose administered.[82]

Rather than discouraging the use of ILE therapy, the previous discussion is intended to encourage the weighing of potential benefits versus the risk of harm caused by ILE therapy, until the point when better evidence regarding efficacy of ILE therapy becomes available. Consider intravenous lipid therapy if pronounced CNS signs, such as severe stupor, coma, or seizures, emerge. Also realize that animals with the *ABCB1-1Δ* or similar gene mutations may not benefit from ILE for the avermectins-milbemycins class of toxicants. The APCC recommends using a 20% lipid solution starting with a 1.5 mL/kg bolus followed by a constant rate infusion of 0.25 mL/kg/min for 30 to 60 minutes, which mirrors the protocol suggested in a recent review of ILE therapy for small animal patients.[84] The initial dose may be repeated every 4 hours as long as serum is not lipemic, but should be discontinued if a positive response is not seen after three treatments.

Physostigmine can cause short-term improvement in patients severely affected by MLs. Administration of physostigmine resulted in 30 to 90 minutes of improvement in moderate to severe CNS depression resulting from ivermectin-sensitive collies being administered 0.2 mg/kg ivermectin.[20] Physostigmine is a cholinergic drug that causes increased amounts of acetylcholine to accumulate at the synapse. Acetylcholine modulates inhibitory GABAergic and excitatory glutamatergic neuronal firing,[86] the net result of which may result in an improvement of clinical signs. Physostigmine is best used either to give an owner visual reassurance that the patient can still recover or to try to arouse a patient enough to encourage it to eat and drink. Frequent administration is not recommended because the effects are temporary and significant cholinergic effects including drooling, urination, and diarrhea, and tremors and seizures, may be seen.[27]

Flumazenil is a $GABA_A$ antagonist that seemed to reverse the effects of ivermectin in an experimental model of drug interactions in rodents.[6,87] However, the use of flumazenil to treat ML toxicosis has not been evaluated clinically. Flumazenil is an antagonist at the benzodiazepine binding site, rather than at the GABA binding site, on $GABA_A$ receptors,[75] so flumazenil prevents benzodiazepines from binding $GABA_A$ receptors rather than directly influencing the effect of GABA. If flumazenil interacts with ML binding sites in an allosteric manner to reduce the effect of ML binding, then flumazenil would be of benefit, but it is unknown if this occurs. If it were beneficial, then it would serve a similar purpose to physostigmine: to improve clinical signs, but only transiently because flumazenil has a short time of effect.[88] Reported dosages for flumazenil in dogs range from 0.04 to 0.25 mg/kg intravenously.[88] Starting at the low end of the dosage range is advised, especially because flumazenil can potentially cause seizures at higher dosages through its effect as a benzodiazepine antagonist.[88]

DIAGNOSTICS

Genotyping in dogs to determine if the *ABCB1-1Δ* gene mutation is present is performed through the Veterinary Clinical Pharmacology Laboratory at Washington State University College of Veterinary Medicine (http://www.vetmed.wsu.edu/depts-VCPL/) using either blood or cells from a cheek swab. Ideally dogs should be tested before using any dose of an ML higher than one for heartworm prevention, especially if the dog is a breed or breed mix of those known to carry the gene defect.

Plasma or stomach contents are submitted to a veterinary diagnostic laboratory to test for levels of MLs to document exposure. Response to physostigmine is also suggestive of ML intoxication if exposure is uncertain.[74] For post-mortem testing, samples to submit include frozen brain, liver, and fat.[74]

OUTCOME

The prognosis is guarded to good depending on the exposure dose and agent involved. Severely affected dogs may require long-term care, which may be a financial burden for some owners. Depending on the dose and half-life of agent involved, recovery can take days to weeks. Reportedly one dog recovered completely after being comatose for 7 weeks.[71] After recovery, long-term sequelae are not expected.[74] Sedation and blindness seem to the longest lasting signs, but even blindness is not expected to be permanent because most dogs seem to recover visual ability (ASPCA APCC, unpublished information, 2011). Two dogs with documented retinal edema did recover well with only residual retinal scarring.[17] Likewise four cats with electroretinogram changes postivermectin exposure were documented to recover by a 1-month recheck.[18]

SUMMARY

Drugs in the avermectin and milbemycin classes have a wide margin of safety between therapeutic and toxic dosages when administered to companion animals at their labeled dosages and dosing frequency. Toxicosis becomes more likely when higher, extralabel dosages are administered to dogs with the *ABCB1-1Δ* gene mutation or when companion animals are inadvertently exposed to, or iatrogenically overdosed with, concentrated ML-containing products intended for large animal use. Drug interactions between MLs and other P-gp substrates, such as spinosad or ketoconazole, might also result in ML toxicosis. Once clinical signs develop, recovery can take days to weeks because of extensive distribution of MLs in the body and their slow elimination. Decontamination measures instituted soon after exposure and good supportive care are the aspects of treatment that are most likely to favorably influence outcome. ILE therapy has been suggested to be a beneficial treatment of ML toxicosis. However, controlled clinical trials are lacking, and questions remain as to whether dogs with defective P-gp is a subpopulation in which lipid therapy is effective.

REFERENCES

1. Vercruysse J, Rew RS, editors. Macrocyclic lactones in antiparasitic therapy. New York: CABI; 2002.
2. Lanusse CE, Lifschitz AL, Imperiale FA. Macrocyclic lactones: endectocide compounds. In: Riviere JE, Papich MG, editors. Veterinary pharmacology and therapeutics. 9th edition. Ames (IA): Wiley-Blackwell; 2009. p. 1119–44.
3. Bloomquist JR. Chloride channels as tools for developing selective insecticides. Arch Insect Biochem Physiol 2003;54:145–56.
4. Sieghart W. Structure, pharmacology, and function of GABAA receptor subtypes. Adv Pharmacol 2006;54:231–63.
5. Sieghart W. Structure and pharmacology of gamma-aminobutyric acid A receptor subtypes. Pharmacol Rev 1995;47:181–234.
6. Trailovic SM, Nedeljkovic JT. Central and peripheral neurotoxic effects of ivermectin in rats. J Vet Med Sci 2011;73:591–9.

7. Mealey KL. Canine ABCB1 and macrocyclic lactones: heartworm prevention and pharmacogenetics. Vet Parasitol 2008;158:215–22.

8. Dean M, Annilo T. Evolution of the ATP-binding cassette (ABC) transporter superfamily in vertebrates. Annu Rev Genomics Hum Genet 2005;6:123–42.

9. Ginn PE. Immunohistochemical detection of P-glycoprotein in formalin-fixed and paraffin-embedded normal and neoplastic canine tissues. Vet Pathol 1996;33: 533–41.

10. Van Der Heyden S, Chiers K, Ducatelle R. Tissue distribution of p-glycoprotein in cats. Anat Histol Embryol 2009;38:455–60.

11. Macdonald N, Gledhill A. Potential impact of ABCB1 (p-glycoprotein) polymorphisms on avermectin toxicity in humans. Arch Toxicol 2007;81:553–63.

12. Mealey KL, Greene S, Bagley R, et al. P-glycoprotein contributes to the blood-brain, but not blood-cerebrospinal fluid, barrier in a spontaneous canine p-glycoprotein knockout model. Drug Metab Dispos 2008;36:1073–9.

13. Bernacki J, Dobrowolska A, Nierwinska K, et al. Physiology and pharmacological role of the blood-brain barrier. Pharmacol Rep 2008;60:600–22.

14. Urquhart BL, Kim RB. Blood-brain barrier transporters and response to CNS-active drugs. Eur J Clin Pharmacol 2009;65:1063–70.

15. Mealey KL, Bentjen SA, Gay JM, et al. Ivermectin sensitivity in collies is associated with a deletion mutation of the mdr1 gene. Pharmacogenetics 2001;11: 727–33.

16. Plumb DC. Plumb's veterinary drug handbook. 5th edition. Stockholm (WI): PharmaVet; 2005.

17. Kenny PJ, Vernau KM, Puschner B, et al. Retinopathy associated with ivermectin toxicosis in two dogs. J Am Vet Med Assoc 2008;233:279–84.

18. Meekins JM, Guess SC, Ranklin AJ. Retinopathy associated with ivermectin toxicosis in five cats. J Am Vet Med Assoc 2015;246:1238–41.

19. Perez R, Cabezas I, Sutra JF, et al. Faecal excretion profile of moxidectin and ivermectin after oral administration in horses. Vet J 2001;161:85–92.

20. Tranquilli WJ, Paul AJ, Seward RL, et al. Response to physostigmine administration in collie dogs exhibiting ivermectin toxicosis. J Vet Pharmacol Ther 1987;10: 96–100.

21. Houston DM, Parent J, Matushek KJ. Ivermectin toxicosis in a dog. J Am Vet Med Assoc 1987;191:78–80.

22. Hadrick MK, Bunch SE, Kornegay JN. Ivermectin toxicosis in two Australian shepherds. J Am Vet Med Assoc 1995;206:1147–50.

23. Merola V, Khan S, Gwaltney-Brant S. Ivermectin toxicosis in dogs: a retrospective study. J Am Anim Hosp Assoc 2009;45:106–11.

24. Hopkins KD, Marcella KL, Strecker AE. Ivermectin toxicosis in a dog. J Am Vet Med Assoc 1990;197:93–4.

25. Mealey KL, Meurs KM. Breed distribution of the ABCB1-1Delta (multidrug sensitivity) polymorphism among dogs undergoing ABCB1 genotyping. J Am Vet Med Assoc 2008;233:921–4.

26. Fassler PE, Tranquilli WJ, Paul AJ, et al. Evaluation of the safety of ivermectin administered in a beef-based formulation to ivermectin-sensitive Collies. J Am Vet Med Assoc 1991;199:457–60.

27. Hopper K, Aldrich J, Haskins SC. Ivermectin toxicity in 17 collies. J Vet Intern Med 2002;16:89–94.

28. Lewis DT, Merchant SR, Neer TM. Ivermectin toxicosis in a kitten. J Am Vet Med Assoc 1994;205:584–6.

29. See AM, McGill SE, Raisis AL, et al. Toxicity in three dogs from accidental oral administration of a topical endectocide containing moxidectin and imidacloprid. Aust Vet J 2009;87:334–7.

30. Crandell DE, Weinberg GL. Moxidectin toxicosis in a puppy successfully treated with intravenous lipids. J Vet Emerg Crit Care (San Antonio) 2009;19:181–6.

31. Snowden NJ, Helyar CV, Platt SR, et al. Clinical presentation and management of moxidectin toxicity in two dogs. J Small Anim Pract 2006;47:620–4.

32. Beal MW, Poppenga RH, Birdsall WJ, et al. Respiratory failure attributable to moxidectin intoxication in a dog. J Am Vet Med Assoc 1999;215:1813–7.

33. Woodward KN. Joint WHO/FAO Expert Committee on Food Additives. 771. Ivermectin (WHO Food Additives Series 31). 1993. Available at: http://www.inchem. org/documents/jecfa/jecmono/v31je03.htm. Accessed June 11, 2018.

34. Tranquilli WJ, Paul AJ, Todd KS. Assessment of toxicosis induced by high-dose administration of milbemycin oxime in collies. Am J Vet Res 1991;52:1170–2.

35. Barbet JL, Snook T, Gay JM, et al. ABCB1-1 Delta (MDR1-1 Delta) genotype is associated with adverse reactions in dogs treated with milbemycin oxime for generalized demodicosis. Vet Dermatol 2009;20:111–4.

36. Kozan E, Sevimli FK, Birdane FM, et al. Efficacy of eprinomectin against *Toxacara canis* in dogs. Parasitol Res 2008;102:397–400.

37. Doscher ME, Wood IB, Pankavich JA, et al. Efficacy of nemadectin, a new broad-spectrum endectocide, against natural infections of canine gastrointestinal helminths. Vet Parasitol 1989;34:255–9.

38. Yas-Natan E, Shamir M, Kleinbart S, et al. Doramectin toxicity in a collie. Vet Rec 2003;153:718–20.

39. Geyer J, Klintzsch S, Meerkamp K, et al. Detection of the nt230(del4) MDR1 mutation in White Swiss Shepherd dogs: case reports of doramectin toxicosis, breed predisposition, and microsatellite analysis. J Vet Pharmacol Ther 2007; 30:482–5.

40. McKellar QA, Benchaoui HA. Avermectins and milbemycins. J Vet Pharmacol Ther 1996;19:331–51.

41. Chittrakarn S, Janchawee B, Ruangrut P, et al. Pharmacokinetics of ivermectin in cats receiving a single subcutaneous dose. Res Vet Sci 2009;86:503–7.

42. Baraka OZ, Mahmoud BM, Marschke CK, et al. Ivermectin distribution in the plasma and tissues of patients infected with Onchocerca volvulus. Eur J Clin Pharmacol 1996;50:407–10.

43. González Canga A, Sahagún Prieto AM, José Diez Liébana M, et al. The pharmacokinetics and metabolism of ivermectin in domestic animal species. Vet J 2009;179:25–37.

44. Gokbulut C, Karademir U, Boyacioglu M, et al. Comparative plasma dispositions of ivermectin and doramectin following subcutaneous and oral administration in dogs. Vet Parasitol 2006;135(3–4):347–54.

45. Al-Azzam SI, Fleckenstein L, Cheng KJ, et al. Comparison of the pharmacokinetics of moxidectin and ivermectin after oral administration to beagle dogs. Biopharm Drug Dispos 2007;28:431–8.

46. Eraslan G, Kanbur M, Liman BC, et al. Comparative pharmacokinetics of some injectable preparations containing ivermectin in dogs. Food Chem Toxicol 2010; 48(8–9):2181–5.

47. Vanapalli SR, Hung YP, Fleckenstein L, et al. Pharmacokinetics and dose proportionality of oral moxidectin in beagle dogs. Biopharm Drug Dispos 2002; 23:263–72.

48. Lallemand E, Lespine A, Alvinerie M, et al. Estimation of absolute oral bioavailability of moxidectin in dogs using a semi-simultaneous method: influence of lipid co-administration. J Vet Pharmacol Ther 2007;30:375–80.

49. Sarasola P, Jernigan AD, Walker DK, et al. Pharmacokinetics of selamectin following intravenous, oral and topical administration in cats and dogs. J Vet Pharmacol Ther 2002;25:265–72.

50. Martinez M, Modric S, Sharkey M, et al. The pharmacogenomics of P-glycoprotein and its role in veterinary medicine. J Vet Pharmacol Ther 2008;31:285–300.

51. Lespine A, Dupuy J, Alvinerie M, et al. Interaction of macrocyclic lactones with the multidrug transporters: the bases of the pharmacokinetics of lipid-like drugs. Curr Drug Metab 2009;10:272–88.

52. Calabrese EJ. P-glycoprotein efflux transporter activity often displays biphasic dose-response relationships. Crit Rev Toxicol 2008;38:473–87.

53. Tranquilli WJ, Paul AJ, Seward RL. Ivermectin plasma concentrations in collies sensitive to ivermectin-induced toxicosis. Am J Vet Res 1989;50:769–70.

54. Coelho JC, Tucker R, Mattoon J, et al. Biliary excretion of technetium-99m-sestamibi in wild-type dogs and in dogs with intrinsic (ABCB1-1Delta mutation) and extrinsic (ketoconazole treated) P-glycoprotein deficiency. J Vet Pharmacol Ther 2009;32:417–21.

55. Mealey KL, Waiting D, Raunig DL, et al. Oral bioavailability of P-glycoprotein substrate drugs do not differ between ABCB1-1Delta and ABCB1 wild type dogs. J Vet Pharmacol Ther 2010;33:453–60.

56. Mealey KL, Munyard KA, Bentjen SA. Frequency of the mutant MDR1 allele associated with multidrug sensitivity in a sample of herding breed dogs living in Australia. Vet Parasitol 2005;131:193–6.

57. Han JI, Son HW, Park SC, et al. Novel insertion mutation of ABCB1 gene in an ivermectin-sensitive Border Collie. J Vet Sci 2010;11:341–4.

58. Bissonnette S, Paradis M, Daneau I, et al. The ABCB1-1Delta mutation is not responsible for subchronic neurotoxicity seen in dogs of non-collie breeds following macrocyclic lactone treatment for generalized demodicosis. Vet Dermatol 2009;20:60–6.

59. Hugnet C, Lespine A, Alvinerie M. Multiple oral dosing of ketoconazole increases dog exposure to ivermectin. J Pharm Pharm Sci 2007;10:311–8.

60. Dunn ST, Hedges L, Sampson KE, et al. Pharmacokinetic interaction of the antiparasitic agents ivermectin and spinosad in dogs. Drug Metab Dispos 2011;39:789–95.

61. Sherman JG, Paul AJ, Firkins LD. Evaluation of the safety of spinosad and milbemycin 5-oxime orally administered to Collies with the MDR1 gene mutation. Am J Vet Res 2010;71:115–9.

62. Saunders NR, Habgood MD, Dziegielewska KM. Barrier mechanisms in the brain, II. Immature brain. Clin Exp Pharmacol Physiol 1999;26:85–91.

63. Leuschen MP, Nelson RM Jr. Telencephalic microvessels of premature beagle pups. Anat Rec 1986;215:59–64.

64. Daood M, Tsai C, Ahdab-Barmada M, et al. ABC transporter (P-gp/ABCB1, MRP1/ABCC1, BCRP/ABCG2) expression in the developing human CNS. Neuropediatrics 2008;39:211–8.

65. Tsai CE, Daood MJ, Lane RH, et al. P-glycoprotein expression in mouse brain increases with maturation. Biol Neonate 2002;81:58–64.

66. Pekcec A, Schneider EL, Baumgartner W, et al. Age-dependent decline of blood-brain barrier P-glycoprotein expression in the canine brain. Neurobiol Aging 2011;32:1477–85.

67. Jourdan G, Boyer G, Raymond-Letron I, et al. Intravenous lipid emulsion therapy in 20 cats accidentally overdosed with ivermectin. J Vet Emerg Crit Care (San Antonio) 2015;25:667–71.

68. Wyse CA, McLellan J, Dickie AM, et al. A review of methods for assessment of the rate of gastric emptying in the dog and cat: 1898-2002. J Vet Intern Med 2003;17:609–21.

69. Cooney DO. Activated charcoal in medical applications. New York: Dekker; 1995. p. 85–8, 310–3, 426–31.

70. Beasley VR, Dorman DC. Management of toxicoses. Vet Clin North Am Small Anim Pract 1990;20:307–37.

71. Lovell RA. Ivermectin and piperazine toxicoses in dogs and cats. Vet Clin North Am Small Anim Pract 1990;20:453–68.

72. Bond GR. The role of activated charcoal and gastric emptying in gastrointestinal decontamination: a state-of-the-art review. Ann Emerg Med 2002;39:273–86.

73. Dorrington CL, Johnson DW, Brant R, et al. The frequency of complications associated with the use of multiple-dose activated charcoal. Ann Emerg Med 2003;41:370–7.

74. Mealey KL. Ivermectin: macrolide antiparasitic agents. In: Peterson ME, Talcott PA, editors. Small animal toxicology. St Louis (MO): Saunders Elsevier; 2006. p. 785–94.

75. D'Hulst C, Atack JR, Kooy RF. The complexity of the GABAA receptor shapes unique pharmacological profiles. Drug Discov Today 2009;14:866–75.

76. Bates N, Chatteron J, Robbins C, et al. Lipid infusion in the management of poisoning: a report of 6 canine cases. Vet Rec 2013;172:339.

77. Clarke DL, Lee JA, Murphy LA, et al. Use of intravenous lipid emulsion to treat ivermectin toxicosis in a Border Collie. J Am Vet Med Assoc 2011;239:1328–33.

78. Wright HM, Chen AV, Talcott PA, et al. Intravenous fat emulsion (IFE) for treatment of ivermectin toxicosis in 3 dogs ACVIM Forum abstract N-1. J Vet Intern Med 2011;25:725.

79. Epstein SE, Hollingsworth SR. Ivermectin-induced blindness treated with intravenous lipid therapy in a dog. J Vet Emerg Crit Care (San Antonio) 2013;23:58–62.

80. Pollio D, Michau TM, Weaver E, et al. Electroretinographic changes after intravenous lipid emulsion therapy in a dog and a foal with ivermectin toxicosis. Vet Ophthalmol 2018;21:82–7.

81. Fernandez AL, Lee JA, Rahilly L, et al. The use of intravenous lipid emulsion as an antidote in veterinary toxicology. J Vet Emerg Crit Care (San Antonio) 2011; 21:309–20.

82. Hayes BD, Gosselin S, Calello DP, et al. Systematic review of clinical adverse events reported after acute intravenous lipid emulsion administration. Clin Toxicol (Phila) 2016;54:365–404.

83. Levine M, Hoffman RS, Lavergne V, et al. Systematic review of the effect of intravenous lipid emulsion therapy for non-local anesthetics toxicity. Clin Toxicol (Phila) 2016;54:194–221.

84. Robben JH, Dijkman MA. Lipid therapy for intoxications. Vet Clin North Am Small Anim Pract 2017;47:435–50.

85. Rothschild L, Bern S, Oswald S, et al. Intravenous lipid emulsion in clinical toxicology. Scand J Trauma Resusc Emerg Med 2010;18:51.

86. Lucas-Meunier E, Fossier P, Baux G, et al. Cholinergic modulation of the cortical neuronal network. Pflugers Arch 2003;446:17–29.

87. Trailovic SM, Varagic VM. The effect of ivermectin on convulsions in rats produced by lidocaine and strychnine. Vet Res Commun 2007;31:863–72.

88. Gwaltney-Brant SM, Rumbeiha WK. Newer antidotal therapies. Vet Clin North Am Small Anim Pract 2002;32:323–39.

89. Mealey KL. Pharmacogenetics. Vet Clin North Am Small Anim Pract 2006;36:961–73.

90. Mealey KL, Northrup NC, Bentjen SA. Increased toxicity of P-glycoprotein-substrate chemotherapeutic agents in a dog with the MDR1 deletion mutation associated with ivermectin sensitivity. J Am Vet Med Assoc 2003;223:1453–5.

91. Balayssac D, Authier N, Cayre A, et al. Does inhibition of P-glycoprotein lead to drug-drug interactions? Toxicol Lett 2005;156:319–29.

92. Joint WHO/FAO Expert Committee on Food Additives. 696. Ivermectin (WHO Food Additives Series 27). 1991. Available at: http://www.inchem.org/documents/jecfa/jecmono/v27je03.htm. Accessed June 11, 2018.

93. Roberts G. Joint WHO/FAO Expert Committee on Food Additives. 854. Doramectin (WHO Food Additives Series 36). 1996. Available at: http://www.inchem.org/documents/jecfa/jecmono/v36je02.htm. Accessed June 11, 2018.

94. Heartgard Plus [package insert]. Duluth, GA: Merial Inc; 2015. Available at: https://heartgard.com/assets/Dog_information.pdf. Accessed June 11, 2018.

95. Novotny MJ, Krautmann MJ, Ehrhart JC, et al. Safety of selamectin in dogs. Vet Parasitol 2000;91:377–91.

96. Paul AJ, Tranquilli WJ, Hutchens DE. Safety of moxidectin in avermectin-sensitive collies. Am J Vet Res 2000;61:482–3.

97. ProHeart 6 [package insert]. Kalamazoo, MI: Zoetis; 2016. Available at: https://www.zoetisus.com/products/dogs/proheart6/img/assets/proheart-6-prescribing-information.pdf. Accessed June 11, 2018.

98. Delucchi L, Castro E. Use of doramectin for treatment of notoedric mange in five cats. J Am Vet Med Assoc 2000;216:215–6.

99. Interceptor plus [package insert]. Greenfield, IN: Elanco US Inc; 2017. Available at: https://assets.ctfassets.net/fistk1blxig0/1tqWcOsDWcCQ08eyACyWeg/70c1a23628bd0503c16ff3df0ecb2a6f/Interceptor_Plus_PA100648X_W1a_CP.pdf. Accessed June 11, 2018.

100. Revolution topical parasiticide for dogs and cats [package insert]. Kalamazoo, MI: Zoetis; 2014. Available at: https://www.zoetisus.com/_locale-assets/mcm-portal-assets/products/pdf/revolution-prescribing-information.pdf. Accessed June 11, 2018.

101. Advantage multi for cats topical solution [package insert]. Shawnee Mission, KS: Bayer HealthCare; 2015. Available at: https://bayer.cvpservice.com/product/view/basic/1040051. Accessed June 11, 2018.

102. Advantage multi for dogs topical solution [package insert]. Shawnee Mission, KS: Bayer HealthCare; 2015. Available at: https://bayer.cvpservice.com/product/view/basic/1040052. Accessed June 11, 2018.

103. Woodward K. Joint WHO/FAO Expert Committee on Food Additives. 855. Moxidectin (WHO Food Additives Series 36). 1996. Available at: http://www.inchem.org/documents/jecfa/jecmono/v36je03.htm. Accessed June 11, 2018.

Toxicology of Newer Insecticides in Small Animals

Tina Wismer, DVM, MS*, Charlotte Means, DVM, MLIS

KEYWORDS

- Insecticides • Toxicity • Insect growth regulators • Spinosads
- Organophosphates/carbamates • Pyrethrins/pyrethroids • Isoxazolines
- Essential oils

KEY POINTS

- Newer insecticides are significantly safer because these insecticides can target physiologic differences between insects and mammals, resulting in greater mammalian safety.
- Emerging therapies, such as intravenous lipid emulsion therapy, offer effective treatment of some older insecticides, such as permethrin.
- Isoxazolines are the newest group of flea and tick preventives and treatments for dogs and cats. Preliminary safety studies indicate a wide margin of safety for this class of insecticides.

In the broadest definition, a pesticide (from fly swatters to chemicals) is a substance used to eliminate a pest. A pest can be insects, mice or other animals, weeds, fungi, or microorganisms such as bacteria and viruses. An ideal pesticide would be specific to, safe, and highly efficacious in eliminating the target pest. Humans, domestic animals, wildlife, and the environment would experience minimal to no impact. This ideal pesticide would have a short half-life and break down into nontoxic components. It would be inexpensive and easy to apply. The ideal pesticide has not yet been discovered.

However, although not perfect, newer insecticides are significantly safer. These insecticides are able to target physiologic differences between insects and mammals, resulting in greater mammalian safety. This article briefly reviews toxicity information of both older insecticides, such as organophosphates (OPs), carbamates, pyrethrins, and pyrethroids, as well as some newer insecticides.

This article originally appeared in *Veterinary Clinics of North America: Small Animal Practice*, Volume 42, Issue 2, March 2012.
The authors have nothing to disclose.
ASPCA Animal Poison Control Center, 1717 South Philo Road, Suite 36, Urbana, IL 61802, USA
* Corresponding author.
E-mail address: tina.wismer@aspca.org

ORGANOPHOSPHATES AND CARBAMATES

OPs and carbamates are used to control insect and nematode infestations. They are available as sprays, pour-ons, oral anthelmintics, baits, collars, dips, dusts, granules, and foggers.[1] OPs and carbamates competitively inhibit acetylcholinesterase (AChE) by binding to its esteric site.[2] With AChE bound, acetylcholine (ACh) accumulates at nerve junctions in muscles, glands, and the central nervous system (CNS). The excessive ACh causes excessive stimulation of smooth muscle and glandular secretions. At skeletal muscle junctions, the excessive ACh is partly stimulatory (fasciculations) and partly inhibitory (muscle weakness).

After binding, the bonds of some compounds strengthen with time, known as aging. This aging renders the enzyme unusable (covalent bonding). Inhibition of AChE by OPs tends to be irreversible, whereas inhibition by carbamates is reversible.[3] Recovery of AChE activity after irreversible binding occurs only through the synthesis of new enzymes.[3]

OPs and carbamates are quickly absorbed after dermal, oral, and inhalation exposures.[1] Clinical signs of toxicosis can occur within minutes to hours of exposure, depending on the dose, route, and toxicity of the compound. OPs and carbamates distribute quickly in the body. Most, with the exception of chlorinated OPs (ie, chlorpyrifos), do not accumulate in fat. OPs and carbamates are hydrolyzed in the body. The toxicity and duration of clinical signs depend on treatment, dose, compound, and species of animal (**Table 1**).[4] Cats are considered more susceptible to AChE inhibitors than are dogs in general.[5] Very young, very old, and debilitated animals are also more susceptible.

OPs and carbamates produce muscarinic, nicotinic, and CNS signs. The muscarinic signs include the SLUDDE (salivation, lacrimation, urination, defecation, dyspnea, emesis) signs as well as miosis and bradycardia. Dyspnea is caused by of increased bronchial secretions. Sympathetic stimulation can override the muscarinic signs and result in mydriasis and tachycardia.[4] The nicotinic effects include muscle tremors, fasciculations, weakness, ataxia, and paresis progressing to paralysis.[6] The CNS signs are characterized by hyperactivity, ataxia, seizures, and coma.[6] CNS signs usually occur with high doses or from the highly toxic compounds. Death is caused by respiratory failure or cardiac arrest.[6]

OP-induced delayed neuropathy in animals is characterized by hind-limb ataxia, hypermetria, and proprioceptive deficits. Clinical signs of delayed neuropathy usually

Table 1 Common acetylcholinesterase inhibitors (organophosphates and carbamates)	
Highly Toxic	
$LD_{50} < 50$ mg/kg	Aldicarb, coumaphos,[a] disulfoton, famphur, methomyl, parathion, phorate, terbufos
Moderately Toxic	
LD_{50} 50–1000 mg/kg	Acephate, carbaryl, chlorpyrifos,[a] diazinon, phosmet, propoxur, trichlorfon[a]
Low Toxicity	
$LD_{50} > 1000$ mg/kg	Dichlorvos,[a] dimethoate, malathion, fenthion,[a] temephos, tetrachlorvinphos

Abbreviation: LD_{50}, dose that is lethal for 50% of a test sample.
[a] Compounds that have caused clinical neuropathy in humans.
Data from Hayes WJ Jr. Pesticides studied in man. Baltimore (MD): Williams & Wilkins; 1982. p. 284–435.

begin 2 to 3 weeks after exposure and are thought to be caused by phosphorylation of neurotoxic esterase (not from inhibition of AChE).[4] Acute pancreatitis (protracted vomiting, diarrhea that can often be hemorrhagic, increased pancreatic enzymes) can follow OP exposure, caused by ACh release from pancreatic nerves and prolonged hyperstimulation of pancreatic acinar cells.[4] The species that are more sensitive to the delayed neurotoxic effects of organophosphorus esters accumulate the esters more rapidly and eliminate them more slowly (chickens>cats>rodents).[7]

If OP/carbamate poisoning is suspected from the clinical signs, a test dose of atropine can be given. Take the baseline heart rate and then administer a preanesthetic dose of atropine sulfate (0.02 mg/kg) intravenously (IV). If the heart rate increases and the pupils dilate, look elsewhere for the cause of the signs because it takes roughly 10 times the preanesthetic dose (0.2 mg/kg) to resolve clinical signs caused by OP/carbamate insecticides.[4]

AChE activity can be measured in serum, plasma, or whole blood. Whole blood is preferred because in most animal species 80% or more of the total blood AChE activity is in the red blood cells. AChE activity varies widely among species of animals, but generally an AChE activity that is less than 50% of normal indicates significant exposure, whereas an AChE activity less than 25% of normal plus the presence of characteristic clinical signs (SLUDDE, nicotinic signs) indicates toxicosis.[4] After death, AChE activity can be checked in the brain or eye (retina). Because AChE activity varies among the regions of the brain, one-half of the brain or whole eye (frozen or chilled) should be submitted for testing.[8] Blood and brain AChE do not always correlate well with the severity of clinical signs.[8] Animals that die rapidly may not have depressed (brain or blood) AChE activity. Carbamates are reversible inhibitors of AChE and the results may be normal even when characteristic clinical signs of toxicosis are present. A definitive diagnosis can be reached by finding an anticholinesterase insecticide in the tissue or body fluids (gastrointestinal [GI] tract, liver, skin, blood, and so forth), presence of clinical signs, and significantly depressed cholinesterase activity (OPs). AChE activity can remain depressed for 6 to 8 weeks with an OP exposure.

If the animal is asymptomatic, decontamination can include emesis (if oral ingestion) and administration of activated charcoal.[4] Because of the quick onset of seizures with the highly toxic AChE inhibitors, do not recommend inducing emesis at home. With dermal exposures to OPs and carbamates, wash the animal with liquid dish detergent and water. Wear gloves and ensure adequate ventilation.

If symptomatic, stabilize the animal and control seizures (diazepam, barbiturates) before proceeding. Oxygen and/or endotracheal intubation may be needed in small animals. A high dose of atropine sulfate (0.2 mg/kg) is given to control the muscarinic signs (SLUDDE). Give one-fourth of the initial dose IV and the rest intramuscularly (IM) or subcutaneously (SQ). Atropine does not reverse nicotinic effects (muscular weakness and so forth) or CNS effects (seizures). Atropine blocks the effects of accumulated ACh at the synapse and should be repeated as needed to control bradycardia and increased bronchial secretions.[4] Glycopyrrolate may also be used to control the muscarinic signs (0.01–0.02 mg/kg IV).

Oximes are used to reverse the neuromuscular blockade and nicotinic signs. Oximes should be given as soon as possible because they cannot reverse binding once aging has occurred. Pralidoxime chloride (2-PAM; Protopam) is the most common oxime used to treat OP toxicosis in the United States (20 mg/kg IM or IV twice a day; continue until nicotinic signs are present; discontinue after 3 or 4 treatments if no response or if aggravation of nicotinic signs is seen). Oximes are not used during carbamate intoxications. Diphenhydramine may also help to combat muscle weakness and tremors, although the usefulness of this treatment has not been established.[5] The prognosis depends on the type of OP/carbamate involved, exposure amount (dose), and treatment measures. Prognosis is considered good unless the animal shows signs of respiratory distress (increased pulmonary secretions, respiratory paralysis) or seizures.

PYRETHRINS/PYRETHROIDS

Pyrethrins are botanic insecticides obtained from *Chrysanthemum cinerariaefolium*. Pyrethrums are plant derived (natural), whereas pyrethroids are synthetic analogues of pyrethrins and have been modified to remain stable in sunlight. Pyrethroids are divided into type I, which do not contain a cyano group, and type II, which contain an alpha cyano group (**Table 2**). Etofenprox is a nonester pyrethroidlike insecticide. Pyrethrins/pyrethroids are often formulated with insect growth regulators (methoprene), synergists, solvents (petroleum distillates, acetone), and other carriers (isopropanol). In some situations, the inert ingredients may cause more adverse effects than the insecticide.[9] Pyrethroids cause a rapid knockdown of insects but, because pyrethroids are rapidly metabolized, some insects may recover. Synergists such as piperonyl butoxide or MGK-264 are frequently added to the products to increase toxicity to insects.[9,10]

Pyrethroids modulate gating kinetics by slowing the closing of sodium gates. Type II pyrethroids cause a longer duration of the sodium current in the axon than type I pyrethroids and pyrethrins. Thus, type 1 pyrethroids tend to cause tremors and seizures. Type II pyrethroids cause depolarizing conduction blocks with weakness and paralysis. Type II pyrethroids are considered more toxic than type I. Paresthesia is thought to result from direct action on sensory nerve endings. Pyrethrins/pyrethroids can be absorbed dermally, orally, and via inhalation. In animals, dermal absorption is limited because of intradermal metabolism. Pyrethrins/pyrethroids are highly lipophilic and distribution to tissues (fat, CNS, peripheral nervous system) is rapid. They are also quickly metabolized and eliminated primarily through the urine. The kinetics vary with the specific agent.[9,11] Pyrethroids are generally considered safe when used per label directions. Oral LD_{50} (the dose that is lethal for 50% of a test sample) varies with specific agents. Cats are especially sensitive to concentrated pyrethrins/pyrethroids available in monthly spot-ons (permethrin, phenothrin, and so forth), although individual sensitivity exists. Some cats are sensitive enough that casual contact with a dog treated with a spot-on containing concentrated permethrin (45%–65% permethrin) can cause clinical signs.

Paresthesia is common in all species of animal following dermal application. Paresthesia includes ear twitching, paw and/or tail flicking, hiding, hyperexcitability, and hyperesthesia. Many topical sprays are formulated with isopropyl alcohol and heavy application can result in clinical signs resembling alcohol toxicity (sedation, lethargy, and ataxia). Presence of alcohol in the formulation also frequently causes a taste reaction (drooling, foaming, excessive licking motions, and vomiting).[9,10]

Table 2 The 2 types of pyrethroids	
Type I	Allethrin, bifenthrin, bioresmethrin, permethrin, phenothrin, resmethrin, sumithrin, tefluthrin, tetramethrin
Type II	Cyfluthrin, cyhalothrin, cypermethrin, cyphenothrin, deltamethrin, fenpropathrin, fenvalerate, flucythrinate, flumethrin, fluvalinate, tralomethrin

Concentrated pyrethroids (monthly spot-ons) are most likely to cause toxicity, especially in cats. Clinical signs of pyrethrin/pyrethroid toxicity in cats include paresthesia, generalized tremors, shaking, ataxia, drooling, seizures, and death. Rarely, myoglobinuria develops (most likely caused by shaking/tremors) resulting in acute renal failure. Dogs typically develop signs of paresthesia (shaking of legs, mild muscle fasciculation, rubbing of application site, agitation, nervousness) after dermal application.[9,12–14] When ingested, granular bifenthrin products designed for lawn use seem to result in vomiting, diarrhea, ataxia, tremors and sometimes seizures in dogs (ASPCA APCC, unpublished data, 2011).

Taste reactions are treated with a taste treat such as milk or tuna. For dermal exposures to spot-ons, bathing multiple times with a liquid dishwashing liquid is important. Paresthesia to spot-ons may be treated by rubbing vitamin E oil on the application area. Corn or olive oil may be used as well. Tremoring or seizing animals should be stabilized before bathing. Methocarbamol (50 mg/kg IV; repeat as needed; maximum dose 330 mg/kg/d) works well for controlling tremors. Diazepam can be tried in mild cases. For severe tremors or seizures, a constant-rate infusion of propofol, barbiturates, or gas anesthesia can also be used. Body temperature should be closely monitored. Many cats present hyperthermic because of muscle activity, but, after bathing and stabilization, the temperature decreases. Intravenous IV fluids are recommended. Intravenous lipid emulsion therapy (see Sharon Gwaltney-Brant and Irina Meadows' article, "Intravenous Lipid Emulsions in Veterinary Clinical Toxicology," in this issue, for dosing instructions) is used for resolving severe tremors and seizures from permethrin toxicosis.

AVERMECTINS

For details, see Valentina M. Merola and Paul A. Eubig's article "Toxicology of Avermectins and Milbemycins (Macrocyclic Lactones) and the Role of P-Glycoprotein in Dogs and Cats," in this issue.

IMIDACLOPRID

Imidacloprid was the first neonicotinoid insecticide registered for use. It is approved as a topical spot-on for dogs and numerous products for agricultural and yard use.[15] Imidacloprid mimics the action of ACh in insects; however, imidacloprid is not degraded by AChE. Imidacloprid binds to the postsynaptic nicotinic ACh receptor. This binding results in persistent activation, preventing impulse transmission and a buildup of ACh and leads to hyperexcitation, convulsions, paralysis, and insect death. The binding affinity of imidacloprid at the nicotinic receptors in mammals is much less compared with the binding affinity in insects. Imidacloprid is most effective against insects with large numbers of nicotinergic ACh receptors. Thus, fleas are susceptible to imidacloprid but ticks are not.[16,17] It has been hypothesized that there are 2 binding sites, based on a rat study, with different affinities for imidacloprid. Based on the study, imidacloprid has both agonistic and antagonistic effects on nicotinic ACh receptor channels.[17]

Imidacloprid is absorbed rapidly and almost completely from the GI tract. It is metabolized in the liver to 6-chloronicotinic acid, an active metabolite. Imidacloprid is widely distributed to tissues but does not accumulate and has poor penetration of the blood-brain barrier, contributing to mammalian safety. Elimination is primarily via urine (70%–80%) and feces (20%–30%). Dermal exposures have practically no systemic absorption. Imidacloprid is spread across the skin via translocation. The product is found in hair follicles and shed with hair and sebum.[15,16]

Dermal hypersensitivity to topical products may occur. Erythema, pruritus, and alopecia may be noted at the application site. Oral ingestions of topical preparations can cause drooling or vomiting. Oral ulcers and gastritis have been seen in cats dosed orally.[16] Large ingestions of agricultural or yard use products, although rare, may result in clinical signs similar to nicotine toxicosis. These signs may include lethargy, drooling, vomiting, diarrhea, ataxia, and muscle weakness.[15]

Imidacloprid has a wide margin of safety. In safety studies, topical applications at 50 mg/kg did not cause adverse effects; the NOEL (no effect level) 1-year feeding study in dogs was 41 mg/kg. Imidacloprid is labeled for use in pregnant animals. Topical products have been labeled for puppies and kittens as young as 7 weeks.[16,18]

Treatment of dermal hypersensitivity includes bathing with a liquid dishwashing detergent or follicle-flushing shampoo. In cases with severe pruritus, antihistamines or corticosteroids may be required. Most oral exposures can be treated by diluting with milk or water. Most cases of vomiting are self-limiting. If massive ingestions occur, treatment of clinical signs is symptomatic and supportive; no specific antidote exists.

NITENPYRAM

Nitenpyram is an insecticide in the neonicotinic class. Nitenpyram is an over-the-counter tablet developed as an oral adult flea insecticide. Nitenpyram is considered safe for pregnant and lactating animals. Nitenpyram works systemically and fleas begin to die within 30 minutes. Off-label use includes treating maggot infestations.[19] The mechanism of action is similar to that of other neonicotinic insecticides (imidacloprid). Neonicotinic insecticides have little to no binding to vertebrate peripheral ACh receptors.[20]

Nitenpyram is rapidly and almost completely absorbed. The peak plasma level is 1.21 hours for dogs and 0.63 hour for cats. The half-life is 2.8 hours in dogs and 7.7 hours in cats. Nitenpyram has almost no tissue accumulation. It is primarily eliminated via the urine unchanged (94%).[21]

Nitenpyram has a wide margin of safety. Adult dogs and cats were dosed up to 10 times a therapeutic dose daily for 1 month without adverse effects.[19] Cats receiving 125 mg/kg (125 times therapeutic dose) did show hypersalivation, lethargy, vomiting, and tachypnea. These clinical signs typically developed within 2 hours of treatment and resolved within 24 hours.[19,21]

Reported clinical signs are generally associated with the flea die-off and are not related to the medication. Reported signs include pruritus, hyperesthesia, hyperactivity, panting, agitation, excessive grooming, trembling, and ataxia. Signs are usually self-limiting and resolve without any treatment.[19]

FIPRONIL

Fipronil is a phenylpyrazole insecticide. Fipronil is approved as a spot-on or spray as well as ant and roach baits and seed and soil treatments.[20] Fipronil binds to gamma-aminobutyric acid (GABA) receptors of insects and blocks chloride passages (GABA antagonist). GABA receptors normally have an inhibitory effect but the net result of fipronil is stimulation of the nervous system and, ultimately, insect death. Fipronil has significantly less binding affinity for mammalian GABA receptors because of differences in receptor configuration.[16,22]

Fipronil does not readily penetrate the skin, although it is lipid soluble. When applied topically, it is found on the hair shaft and in the stratum corneum and epidermis and accumulates in the sebaceous glands.[16] Orally, fipronil is absorbed slowly. It distributes to several tissues, including the GI tract, adrenal glands, and abdominal fat. Fipronil is metabolized by the liver and excreted in the feces and urine.[16]

Fipronil may cause dermal hypersensitivity-type reactions in sensitive animals. Erythema, pruritus, irritation, and alopecia at the application site are the most commonly noted signs from topical exposures. Many of these reactions may be related to the carriers. Typically, dermal hypersensitivity develops within hours to a couple of days of application and lasts 24 to 48 hours. Oral ingestions may cause taste reactions (hypersalivation, foaming, gagging), retching, and vomiting. Gastritis has been reported after ingestion of spot-on products and is most likely related to carriers rather than the fipronil. Rarely, in cases of massive ingestions, ataxia, tremors, and seizures are possible. Extralabel use of fipronil on rabbits is known to cause severe and potentially fatal seizures.[16,23,24]

Fipronil has a wide margin of safety in laboratory animals. There is no reported LD_{50} for dogs and cats. The oral LD_{50} in rats and mice is 97 and 95 mg/kg, respectively. Dogs seem to be more sensitive than cats to fipronil.[23]

Treatment of dermal hypersensitivity includes bathing with a liquid dishwashing detergent by 48 hours after the topical application. Antihistamines and steroids may be used if pruritus is present. After oral exposures, taste reactions are treated by diluting with milk or water. If significant vomiting or gastritis is present, antiemetics and GI protectants may be needed. Fluids and other supportive care should be started, and tremoring or seizing animals should receive methocarbamol, diazepam, or barbiturates as needed.[16]

SPINOSAD

Spinosad is found as granules or sprays for agricultural and lawn use and chewable tablets for dogs to kill fleas.[25] A spot-on containing spinetoram, a related compound, is available for use on cats to kill fleas. Spinosad is a tetracyclic macrolide. It is a combination of spinosyn A and spinosyn D.[25] Spinosyns are produced from the naturally occurring bacterium *Saccharopolyspora spinosa*, an aerobic, nonantibiotic actinomycete. Spinosad activates nicotinic ACh receptors. Treated insects develop involuntary muscle contractions and tremors. Continued hyperexcitation results in prostration, paralysis, and flea death. Spinosad is not known to interact with the binding sites of other nicotinic or GABAergic insecticides (imidacloprid, nitenpyram, fipronil, mibemycin, and so forth). Spinosad is more selective for insect versus vertebrate nicotinic AChRs.[25]

Spinosad is quickly absorbed after oral ingestion and peak blood concentrations occur within 1 to 6 hours depending on the dose.[26] Spinosad is well distributed throughout the body, with the highest concentrations found in fat, liver, kidneys, and lymph nodes.[26] Spinosad is biotransformed with glutathione conjugates and eliminated in the feces (70%–90%) via the bile.[27] Most of the radiolabeled agent is excreted within 24 hours. Elimination from the thyroid is much slower and can result in higher concentrations in the thyroid compared with other tissues. The half-life of spinosad is 25 to 42 hours.[27]

Canine daily doses of 100 mg/kg for 10 consecutive days (16.7 times the maximum recommended monthly dose) caused vomiting and transient mild increases in alanine transaminase level.[25] Phospholipidosis (vacuolation) of the lymphoid tissue was seen in all dogs.[25] Cats dosed at 80 to 120 mg/kg experienced vomiting.[25]

The most common adverse clinical effects seen after ingestion are vomiting and lethargy. These signs usually begin within a few hours of exposure.[25] Ataxia, inactiveness, anorexia, diarrhea, and tremors have also been reported. Concurrent administration of spinosad to animals receiving high doses of ivermectin therapy (eg, demodicosis doses) can result in mild to moderate ivermectin toxicity.[25] It is recommended that dogs receiving extralabel doses of ivermectin not receive concurrent treatment with spinosad.[25] In an overdose situation, induction of emesis and administration of activated charcoal are rarely needed. Most treatment is symptomatic and supportive and includes managing vomiting and diarrhea.

ISOXAZOLINES

Isoxazolines are the newest group of flea and tick preventives and treatments for dogs and cats. Most isoxazolines are given as a chewable tablet and are labeled for dogs only.[28] There is 1 product available as a topical for both dogs and cats.[29] Isoxazolines work by binding the ligand-gated chloride channels (GABA receptor and glutamate-receptor) in insects and acarines. Presynaptic and postsynaptic transfer of chloride ions across the cell membranes results, leading to hyperexcitation and uncontrolled activity of the CNS and, ultimately, the death of the flea or tick. Selective toxicity to insects and acarines is implied by the differential sensitivity of insects' and acarines' GABA receptors versus mammalian GABA receptors.[30,31]

The kinetics (absorption, peak plasma, distribution, and so forth) vary between specific active ingredients. Dosing recommendations, minimum weights and ages, as well as dosing frequencies also vary (**Table 3**).

Elimination is primarily through bile, although afoxolaner does have some urinary excretion as well.[32] Safety studies for all of the isoxazolines indicate a wide margin of safety. Only fluralaner has been studied for safety in breeding, pregnant, and lactating dogs.[33] All of the isoxazolines are effective in controlling fleas and some ticks, and aiding in the control of flea allergy dermatitis in dogs.[34–36]

The most common clinical signs noted are vomiting, diarrhea, lethargy, and anorexia. There are some reports of seizures in dogs and cats. Label inserts generally recommend not using in animals with preexisting seizures or neurologic disease.[28,29] If vomiting occurs within 3 hours of administration of a chewable tablet, the product should be redosed.

Symptomatic animals need symptomatic and supportive care. Confine if ataxic. If an animal is vomiting, an antiemetic such as maropitant (Cerenia), can be dosed at 1 mg/kg SQ. If tremors are present, administer methocarbamol at 50 to 150 mg/kg IV, and titrate up as needed. Most reported seizures are singular, but, if multiple or prolonged, use diazepam (0.5 mg/kg IV) or levetiracetam (60 mg/kg IV). If a topical product was used and the animal is hypersalivating because of taste, give a taste treat (milk, canned food) or rinse mouth. In general, vomiting occurs within minutes to a few hours, and seizures generally occur within an hour to 24 hours later. Signs typically resolve within 24 hours (ASPCA APCC, unpublished data, 2018).

INDOXACARB

Indoxacarb is found in insect baits (ant and roach) for home use and granules and liquids for agricultural use.[37] Recently, a spot-on containing indoxacarb has been introduced for use on dogs and cats. Indoxacarb acts by blocking sodium channels in the nervous system of insects. It is an oxadiazine insecticide, despite its name.[38]

Indoxacarb is metabolized in the liver and excreted in both the feces and urine.[39] Most of the dose was excreted within 96 hours. The oral NOEL in dogs is 40 ppm (1.1 mg/kg/d).[40] The most common clinical signs seen in dogs and cats are vomiting, lethargy, diarrhea, and anorexia[41] There is 1 case of a human developing methemoglobinemia after a massive ingestion of indoxacarb (suicide attempt).[42] Treatment is

Table 3
Isoxazoline insecticides

Active Ingredient	Brand	Species	Minimum Age	Minimum Weight	Dosing Interval	Dosing Comments	Bioavailability (%)	Peak Plasma	T$_{1/2}$
Afoxolaner	Nexgard	Dog	8 wk	>1.8 kg (4 lb)	Monthly, chewable tablet	Can give with or without food	73.9	2–6 h	15.5 ± 7.8 d
Sarolaner	Simparica	Dog	>6 mo	>1.3 kg (2.8 lb)	Monthly, chewable tablet	Can give with or without food	86 starved 107 fed	3 h	10–12 d
Fluralaner	Bravecto	Dog	6 mo	>2.0 kg (4.4 lb)	12 wk Lone Star ticks: 8 wk	Give with food	25	2 h to 3 d	9.3–16.2 d
Fluralaner topical solution	Bravecto	Cat	6 mo	1.2 kg (2.6 lb)	12 wk	—	—	7–21 d	11–13 d
Fluralaner topical solution	Bravecto	Dogs	6 mo	2.0 kg (4.4 lb)	12 wk	—	25	7–42 d	14–29 d

Data from Refs.[28,29,32–35]

symptomatic and supportive. Because of a low concentration of indoxacarb present in most ant and roach baits, ingestion only requires monitoring for signs of stomach upset.

ESSENTIAL OILS

Essential oils are produced by plants. The oils are a mixture of terpenes (complex hydrocarbons) and other chemicals. Essential oils give plants their characteristic odors. They vary widely in toxicity. Although the oils have several uses, some are used as natural flea and tick treatments on pets. **Table 4** lists the common essential oils used for flea treatments.

Essential oils are rapidly absorbed orally and dermally. Oils are typically metabolized in the liver by glucuronide and glycine conjugates. Cytochrome P-450 enzyme systems in the liver can be induced with repeated exposure to some essential oils. Cats seem to be more sensitive to the effects of essential oil than dogs. Essential oils and their metabolites are primarily eliminated in the urine.[43,44]

The most common clinical signs after dermal exposure include ataxia, muscle weakness, and behavioral abnormalities. Oral ingestions can cause vomiting, diarrhea, and CNS depression. Essential oils can cause aspiration pneumonia if inhaled. Mortality has been reported following the use of melaleuca oil in cats (see **Table 4** for clinical signs of specific oils in addition to these common signs).[39,40,45]

All species of animals may be susceptible to essential oils. Animals with preexisting liver disease have an increased risk of toxicosis. The LD_{50} of essential oils varies widely but is typically between 2 and 5 g/kg body weight. Mixing oils with organic solvents such as alcohols or the presence of irritated and reddened skin can potentially increase absorption of essential oils, resulting in toxicity.[46] The specific mechanism of action is not established.

Dermal exposures require bathing with a liquid dishwashing detergent. Emesis, in most cases, is contraindicated because a risk of aspiration pneumonia exists. Activated charcoal can be given if a large ingestion has occurred. Baseline blood work should be obtained because some oils cause hepatic damage and acid-base and electrolyte abnormalities. Body temperature should be monitored and corrected as needed. Intravenous fluids can help maintain pressure and hydration status and also aids in renal elimination. Monitor cardiac and respiratory functions as needed. Seizures and tremors usually respond well to diazepam or methocarbamol. Aspiration

Table 4
Common essential oils used for flea treatments

Common Name and Source of Essential Oil	Specific Clinical Signs
Citrus sp (oranges, limes, grapefruit) D-limonene/linalool	Cats: scrotal dermatitis, profound hypotension (undiluted dips) Rare: immune-mediated dermatopathies (TENS)
Melaleuca alternifolia (tea tree)	Transient hind-limb paresis (spot-on), hepatotoxicity
Mentha pulegium pennyroyal oil, pulegone	Hepatotoxicity
Peppermint, clove, cinnamon, lemongrass, thyme (commercial sprays and spot-ons)	Agitation, tremors, seizures, rarely death

Abbreviation: TENS, toxic epidermal necrolysis syndrome.
Data from Refs.[44,52–55]

pneumonia may require oxygen and broad-spectrum antibiotics. Hepatic damage usually responds to good supportive care. The use of S-adenosyl-L-methionine or milk thistle may be helpful.[40]

LUFENURON

Lufenuron is available as an oral suspension for cats, an injectable for cats, and an oral tablet for dogs. It is approved for use in dogs and cats 6 weeks of age and older for the control of flea populations. It has also been used off label for control of dermatophytosis. Lufenuron, a benzoylphenylurea derivative, is a chitin synthesis inhibitor.[47] By stopping polymerization and deposition of chitin, it prevents the eggs from developing into adults.

Only about 40% of an oral dose of lufenuron is absorbed in the small intestine.[47] Absorption is enhanced if administered with a fatty meal. Lufenuron is stored in fat and is slowly redistributed back into the circulation. Lufenuron is not metabolized but excreted unchanged into the bile and eliminated in the feces.

Dogs dosed at 30 times the therapeutic dose for 10 months did not develop and signs of toxicosis.[47] Cats tolerate oral dosages of up to 17 times the therapeutic dosage with no adverse effects.[47] Cats do require a substantially higher oral dosage per kilogram than do dogs for equivalent efficacy.

Adverse signs seen after ingestion include vomiting, lethargy, and diarrhea. Injection site pain and swelling can occur in cats. Do not give the injectable product to dogs because they will develop a severe local reaction.[47] Most signs are self-limiting, and treatment, if needed, is symptomatic and supportive.

METHOPRENE

Methoprene is available as suspensions, emulsifiable and soluble concentrates, briquettes, sprays, foggers, baits, and spot-ons. Methoprene is labeled for flea control in dogs and cats, aquatic mosquito control, crop pest control, and home pest control.[48] Methoprene is a juvenile hormone analogue. While juvenile hormone concentrations remain high, the insect remains in the same stage and cannot molt.[44] Methoprene is also absorbed by the female flea and affects her ovaries, providing an immediate inhibitory effect.[44]

Methoprene can be absorbed both orally and dermally. It is rapidly excreted, mostly in the urine and feces.[48] Sufficient methoprene is excreted unchanged that the concentration in feces is sufficient to kill some larvae that breed in dung.[48]

Methoprene is considered fairly safe in mammals. The dog oral LD_{50} is greater than 5 g/kg.[48] Younger animals are more susceptible to adverse effects (lethargy, ataxia, rarely tremors) after oral dosing.[43] Oral exposures can cause drooling, vomiting, and lethargy and rarely ataxia or tremors. The ataxia appears within 2 to 8 hours after administration and lasts 6 to 12 hours (ASPCA APCC, unpublished data, 2011). Usually no treatment is necessary if the animal has ingested a small amount. Local dermal hypersensitivity reactions (redness, itching, rubbing) can be seen in some animals. Most of the symptomatic animals recover without treatment. If the animal is ataxic, prevent further stimulation (provide a quiet and dark environment). Methocarbamol may help with muscle tremors.

PYRIPROXYFEN

Pyriproxyfen is used for insect control on pets, in the home, and on agricultural crops. It is available as a spray, fogger, collar, mousse, shampoo, granule, spot-on, powder, and liquid.[49] Pyriproxyfen is a pyridine-based nonneurotoxic carbamate that does not inhibit cholinesterase. It is an insect juvenile hormone analogue. It is both ovicidal and larvicidal.[49]

Pyriproxyfen is quickly absorbed and peak levels are reached in 2 to 8 hours after ingestion.[50] It is metabolized in the liver and excreted mainly in the feces.[49] The oral NOEL in dogs is 100 mg/kg/d for 1 year.[51] Hypersalivation and self-limiting vomiting may be seen with ingestion. Most animals do not need treatment.

SUMMARY

Insecticidal poisoning has become less common in small animal patients because the newer available insecticides are more specific in their mechanisms and target mostly insects, not mammals. This advance has made many of the newer pesticides safer for use on dogs and cats compared with some of the highly toxic OPs and carbamates available earlier. Serious toxicity problems can still occur, especially with inappropriate use of permethrin-containing spot-ons in cats.

REFERENCES

1. Meerdink GL. Anticholinesterase insecticides. In: Plumlee KH, editor. Clinical veterinary toxicology. St Louis (MO): Mosby; 2004. p. 178–80.
2. Hayes WJ Jr, editor. Pesticides studied in man. Baltimore (MD): Williams & Wilkins; 1982. p. 284–435.
3. Osweiler GD. Organophosphorus and carbamate insecticides. In: Toxicology. Philadelphia: Lippincott Williams & Wilkins; 1996. p. 231–6.
4. Fikes JD. Organophosphorus and carbamate insecticides. Vet Clin North Am Small Anim Pract 1990;20:353–67.
5. Nafe LA. Selected neurotoxins. Vet Clin North Am Small Anim Pract 1988;18: 593–604.
6. Humphreys DJ. Veterinary toxicology. 3rd edition. Philadelphia: WB Saunders; 1988.
7. Abou-Donia MB, Graham DG, Ashry MA. Delayed neurotoxicity of leptophos and related compounds: differential effects of subchronic oral administration of pure, technical grade, and degradation products on the hen. Toxicol Appl Pharmacol 1980;53:150–63.
8. Plumlee KH. Total cholinesterase activity in discrete brain regions and retina of normal horses. J Vet Diagn Invest 1997;9:109–10.
9. Volmer PA. Pyrethrins and pyrethroids. In: Plumlee KH, editor. Clinical veterinary toxicology. St Louis (MO): Mosby; 2004. p. 188–90.
10. Proudfoot AT. Poisoning due to pyrethrins. Toxicol Rev 2005;24:107–13.
11. Anadón A, Martínez-Larrañaga MR, Martínez MA. Use and abuse of pyrethrins and synthetic pyrethroids in veterinary medicine. Vet J 2009;182:7–20.
12. Malik R, Ward MP, Seavers A, et al. Permethrin spot-on intoxication of cats: literature review and survey of veterinary practitioners in Australia. J Feline Med Surg 2010;12:5–14.
13. Haworth MD, Smart L. Use of intravenous lipid therapy in three cases of feline permethrin toxicosis. J Vet Emerg Crit Care (San Antonio) 2012;22:697–702.
14. Ceccherini G, Perond F, Lippi I, et al. Intravenous lipid emulsion and dexmedetomidine for treatment of feline permethrin intoxication: a report from 4 cases. Open Vet J 2015;5:113–21.

15. Sheets LP. Imidacloprid: a neonicotinoid insecticide. In: Krieger R, editor. Handbook of pesticide toxicology, volume 2, agents. San Diego (CA): Academic Press; 2001. p. 1123–30.
16. Wismer T. Novel insecticides. In: Plumlee KH, editor. Clinical veterinary toxicology. St Louis (MO): Mosby; 2004. p. 183–6.
17. Nagata K, Song JH, Shono T, et al. Modulation of the neuronal nicotinic acetylcholine receptor channel by the nitromethylene heterocycle imidacloprid. J Pharmacol Exp Ther 1998;285:731–8.
18. Griffin L, Hopkins TJ. Imidacloprid: safety of a new insecticidal compound in dogs and cats. Compend Contin Educ Pract Vet 1997;19:17–20.
19. Hovda LR, Hooser SB. Toxicology of newer pesticides for use in dogs and cats. Vet Clin North Am Small Anim Pract 2002;32:455–67.
20. Vo DT, Hsu WH, Abu-Basha EA, et al. Insect nicotinic acetylcholine receptor agonists as flea adulticides in small animals. J Vet Pharmacol Ther 2010;33:315–22.
21. Witte ST, Luembert LG. Laboratory safety studies of nitenpyram tablets for the rapid removal of fleas on cats and dogs. Compend Contin Educ Pract Vet 2001;23:7–11.
22. Cole LM, Nicholson RA, Casida JE. Action of phenylpyrazole insecticides at the GABA-gated chloride channel. Pestic Biochem Physiol 1993;46:47–54.
23. Gupta RC. Fipronil. In: Gupta RC, editor. Veterinary toxicology basic and clinical principles. New York: Academic Press; 2007. p. 502–4.
24. Stern L. Fipronil toxicosis in rabbits. In: Vet Med. 2015. Available at: http://veterinarymedicine.dvm360.com/fipronil-toxicosis-rabbits. Accessed April 30, 2018.
25. Comfortis™ (Spinosad) chewable tablets prescribing information package insert. Indianapolis (IN): Eli Lilly and Company; 2007.
26. Robertson-Plouch C, Baker KA, Hozak RR, et al. Clinical field study of the safety and efficacy of spinosad chewable tablets for controlling fleas on dogs. Vet Ther 2008;9:26–36.
27. Bartholomaeus A. Toxicological evaluations: Spinosad IPCS INCHEM: pesticide residues in food 2001. Available at: http://www.inchem.org/documents/jmpr/jmpmono/2001pr12.htm. Accessed May 5, 2018.
28. Datz C. Isoxazolines. In: Plumb's therapeutic brief 2018. Available at: https://www.cliniciansbrief.com/article/isoxazolines. Accessed April 30, 2018.
29. Bravecto (fluralaner topical solution) for cats (package insert). Madison (NJ): Merck Animal Health; 2016.
30. Shoop WL, Harline EF, Gould BR, et al. Discovery and mode of action of afoxolaner, a new isoxazoline parasiticide for dogs. Vet Parasitol 2014;201:179–89.
31. Gassel M, Wolf C, Noag S, et al. The novel isoxazoline ectoparasiticide fluralaner, selective inhibition of arthropod γ-aminobutyric acid and L-glutamate-gated chloride channels and insecticidal/acaricidal activity. Insect Biochem Mol Biol 2014; 45:111–24.
32. Letendre L, Huang R, Kvaternick V, et al. The intravenous and oral pharmacokinetics of afoxolaner used as a monthly chewable antiparasitic for dogs. Vet Parasitol 2014;201:190–7.
33. Bravecto [package insert]. Madison (NJ): Merck Animal Health; 2014.
34. Becskei C, De Bock F, Illambas J, et al. Efficacy and safety of a novel oral isoxazoline, sarolaner (Simparica™) in the treatment of naturally occurring flea and tick infestations in dogs presented as veterinary patients in Europe. Vet Parasitol 2016;222:49–55.

35. Cherni JA, Mahabir SP, Six RH. Efficacy and safety of sarolaner (Simparica™) against fleas on dogs presented as veterinary patients in the United States. Vet Parasitol 2016;222:43–8.
36. Walther FM, Roepke AMJ, Nuemberger MC. Safety of fluralaner chewable tablets (Bravecto): a novel systemic antiparasitic drug in dogs after oral administration. Parasit Vectors 2014;7:87.
37. Crop protection handbook. Willoughby (OH): Meister Publishing; 2004. p. C-280.
38. Narahashi T, Zhao X, Ikeda T, et al. Differential actions of insecticides on target sites: basis for selective toxicity. Hum Exp Toxicol 2007;26:361–6.
39. Tomlin CDS, editor. The pesticide manual, a world compendium. Surrey (United Kingdom): British Crop Protection Council; 2009. Indoxacarb (173584-44-6).
40. California Environmental Protection Agency/Department of Pesticide Regulation. Toxicology data review summaries: indoxacarb. Available at: http://www.cdpr.ca. gov/docs/risk/toxsums/pdfs/5331.pdf. Accessed May 4, 2018.
41. Wismer T, Means C. Toxicology of newer insecticides in small animals. Vet Clin North Am Small Anim Pract 2012;42:335–47.
42. Prasanna L, Manimala Rao S, Singh V, et al. Indoxacarb poisoning: an unusual presentation as methemoglobinemia. Indian J Crit Care Med 2008;12:198–200.
43. Means C. Selected herbal hazards. Vet Clin North Am Small Anim Pract 2002;32: 367–82.
44. Means C. Essential oils. In: Plumlee KH, editor. Clinical veterinary toxicology. St Louis (MO): Mosby; 2004. p. 149–50.
45. Khan SA, McLean MK, Slater MR. Concentrated tea tree oil toxicosis in dogs and cats: 443 cases (2002–2012). J Am Vet Med Assoc 2014;244(1):95–9.
46. Wolfe A. Essential oil poisoning. Clin Toxicol 1999;37:721–7.
47. Stansfield DG. A review of safety and efficacy of lufenuron in dogs and cats. Canine Pract 1997;22:34–48.
48. Environmental Protection Agency. R.E.D. facts: methoprene. Washington, DC: Office of Pesticides and Toxic Substances; 1991.
49. Palma KG, Meola SM, Meola RW. Mode of action of pyriproxyfen and methoprene on eggs of Ctenocephalides felis felis (Siphonaptera: Pulicidae). J Med Entomol 1995;30:421–6.
50. Matsunaga H, Yoshino H, Isobe N, et al. Metabolism of pyriproxyfen in rats. 1. Absorption, disposition, excretion, and biotransformation studies with [phenoxy-phenyl-14C]pyriproxyfen. J Agric Food Chem 1995;43:235–40.
51. Gwaltney-Brant S. Atypical topical spot-on products. In: Peterson ME, Talcott PA, editors. Small animal toxicology. 3rd edition. Saint Louis (MO): Elsevier; 2013. p. 751–2.
52. Frank AA, Ross JL, Sawwell BK. Toxic epidermal necrolysis associated with flea dips. Vet Hum Toxicol 1992;34:57–61.
53. Rosenbaum MR, Kerlin RL. Erythema multiforme major and disseminated intravascular coagulation in a dog following application of a d-limonene-based insecticidal dip. J Am Vet Med Assoc 1995;207:1315–9.
54. Lee JA, Budgin JB, Mauldin EA. Acute necrotizing dermatitis and septicemia after application of a d-limonene-based insecticidal shampoo in a cat. J Am Vet Med Assoc 2002;221:258–62.
55. Sudekum M, Poppenga RH, Raju N. Pennyroyal oil toxicosis in a dog. J Am Vet Med Assoc 1992;200:817–8.

Common Rodenticide Toxicoses in Small Animals

Camille DeClementi, VMD[a,b], Brandy R. Sobczak, DVM[b],*

KEYWORDS

- Rodenticide • Anticoagulant • Bromethalin • Cholecalciferol

KEY POINTS

- Understanding the 3 most common types of rodenticides pets may be exposed to, and the importance of confirming the active ingredient.
- Clinical signs that may occur and diagnostic testing, if available.
- Decontamination, treatment, and monitoring parameters for each type of rodenticide.

This article focuses on the 3 most commonly used rodenticide types: anticoagulants, bromethalin, and cholecalciferol. Because there are multiple types of rodenticides available on the market and the color of the bait is not coded to a specific type of rodenticide, it is important to verify the active ingredient in any rodenticide exposure. In addition, many animal owners use the term D-con to refer to any rodenticide regardless of the brand name or type of rodenticide. Rodenticide baits are most typically formulated as bars or blocks. Loose bait such as pellets are no longer produced for consumer sale according to new Environmental Protection Agency (EPA) risk mitigation rules; however, this form (loose bait) may be seen for some time while older products are used up. The EPA released their final ruling on rodenticide risk mitigation measures in 2008 and all the products on the market had to be compliant by June 2011. The purpose of the measures is to reduce exposures to children and nontarget species, including wildlife. After June 2011, consumer products may not contain the second-generation anticoagulants brodifacoum, difethialone, difenacoum, and bromadiolone and instead must contain either first-generation anticoagulants (chlorophacinone, diphacinone) or nonanticoagulants, including bromethalin and cholecalciferol.[1] These regulations are likely to cause an increase in the number of bromethalin and cholecalciferol cases seen in veterinary clinics.

This article originally appeared in *Veterinary Clinics of North America: Small Animal Practice*, Volume 42, Issue 2, March 2012.

The authors have nothing to disclose.

[a] ASPCA Animal Hospital, 424 East 92nd Street, New York, NY 10128, USA; [b] ASPCA Animal Poison Control Center, 1717 South Philo Road, Suite 36, Urbana, IL 61802, USA

* Corresponding author.

E-mail address: brandy.sobczak@aspca.org

ANTICOAGULANT RODENTICIDES

The discovery of the causative agent of sweet-clover poisoning in cattle, dicoumarol, led to the development of the anticoagulant rodenticides. Cattle with this type of poisoning developed internal bleeding; therefore, dicoumarol was tested as a rodenticide. Warfarin, named after the Wisconsin Alumni Research Foundation, was the first compound marketed as an anticoagulant rodenticide. The first-generation anticoagulants were created during the 1940s and 1950s. They required continuous exposure to achieve rodent control. The second-generation anticoagulant rodenticides (SGARs), including brodifacoum, difethialone, difenacoum, and bromadiolone, were developed in the subsequent decades as rodents developed resistance to the first-generation anticoagulants. SGARs were formulated to be more palatable to rodents, more effective, faster, and longer acting.[2] Although chlorophacinone and diphacinone were developed after warfarin like the SGARs listed earlier, they differ structurally and the EPA has not placed the same restrictions on their use.[1,2]

Warfarin and pindone are short-acting anticoagulants with shorter half-lives (<24 hours) compared with the long-acting products whose half-lives are up to 6 days.[3] The long-acting anticoagulants include diphacinone, difethialone, chlorophacinone, brodifacoum, and bromadiolone. Veterinarians are well trained to use their knowledge and judgment to make treatment decisions for their patients according to each unique case. As a general guideline, the American Society for the Prevention of Cruelty to Animals (ASPCA) Animal Poison Control Center (APCC) recommends decontamination if and as needed and monitoring (prothrombin time [PT] or proteins induced by vitamin K deficiency or antagonists [PIVKA]) or treatment with vitamin K_1 (if and as needed) when the ingested dose of warfarin is greater than 0.5 mg/kg and of other anticoagulants is greater than 0.02 mg/kg.

Exposure in domestic pets occurs through ingestion of the product from the bait container or from the environment to which the rodents have carried the bait. Now that the EPA is requiring consumer products be contained in tamper-resistant bait stations and has prohibited the sale of pelleted formulations to consumers, it is hoped that pets will be protected from finding a rodent's hoard of product. For anticoagulants, toxicosis from a pet ingesting rodents poisoned by the bait (also called relay toxicosis) is of limited concern because the amount of rodenticide in the rodent is small. However, if the pet is very small and ingests a large number of the poisoned rodents, relay toxicosis is possible. For example, a barn cat that preys on rodents as its main source of nutrition could become intoxicated if those rodents were poisoned by an anticoagulant rodenticide.[3]

Pathophysiology and Clinical Signs

The anticoagulant rodenticides cause their effects by interfering with the production of the clotting factors II, VII, IX, and X by the liver. In the normal production of these factors, vitamin K_1 is converted to vitamin K_1 epoxide. The enzyme vitamin K_1 epoxide reductase then converts vitamin K_1 epoxide back to the active form of vitamin K_1. This cycle repeats over and over to create active clotting factors. The anticoagulants inhibit vitamin K_1 epoxide reductase, thereby leading to depletion of active vitamin K_1 and the halt of the production of active clotting factors.[3,4]

During the first 36 to 72 hours following ingestion of the anticoagulant, the patient is usually clinically normal as the clotting factors are slowly depleted. Usually within 3 to 5 days, enough clotting factors are depleted for hemorrhage to develop. It is possible in some patients with underlying illnesses (such as preexisting bleeding disorders or hepatic disease) that depletion of coagulation factors may occur sooner, resulting in hemorrhage as early as 24 to 48 hours following exposure.

Many poisoned animals are not presented to a veterinarian until clinical signs develop. It is important to remember that hemorrhage can occur anywhere in the body; however, the most common clinical signs are dyspnea, coughing, lethargy, and hemoptysis.[3] Bleeding into body cavities such as the chest, abdomen, and joints is also common. Many patients present with vague clinical signs of lethargy, weakness, and anemia without any overt external hemorrhage, although some animals present with frank external hemorrhage from surgical or traumatic sites, the gastrointestinal (GI) tract, or orifices. Abdominal distention, exophthalmia, lameness, bruising, hematomas, or muffled heart sounds are also possible. Bleeding into the brain or spinal cord may result in severe central nervous system (CNS) disturbances, seizing, paresis, paralysis, or acute death.[3] Tracheal constriction caused by thymic, peritracheal, or laryngeal bleeding may result in severe dyspnea.[2]

Diagnosis

Because it has the shortest half-life, factor VII is the first to be affected. Depletion of factor VII leads to an increase of the PT. Levels of PIVKA, the collective term for the precursors of the vitamin K–dependent clotting factors, also become increased. The PT may be increased within 36 to 72 hours. Beyond 72 hours, as other factors become depleted, increases in activated partial thromboplastin time and activated clotting time develop. Clinical pathologic abnormalities can include anemia, thrombocytopenia, hypoproteinemia, and decreases in CO_2 and P_{O_2}.[2]

Diagnosis is based on history of exposure, compatible clinical signs, and laboratory results that indicate coagulopathy. Differential diagnoses should include congenital and acquired coagulopathies, and other causes of anemia (eg, trauma). Coagulation panels may aid in the differentiation of anticoagulant rodenticide from other coagulopathies. Serum chemistry profiles to detect hepatic or other systemic disease that might affect blood clotting may be indicated.[4] Anticoagulant toxicosis may be worsened in cases of significant hepatic disease because of impaired ability to synthesize coagulation factors and decreased metabolism of ingested rodenticide.

Treatment

For patients that have recently ingested an anticoagulant rodenticide, decontamination by emesis (with 3% hydrogen peroxide or apomorphine in dogs, dexmedetomidine or xylazine in cats) is indicated as long as the patient does not have any underlying conditions that would make inducing emesis contraindicated (including seizure disorder and significant cardiovascular disease). The bar forms of bait may remain in the stomach for a period of time, allowing for effective emesis as long as 4 to 8 hours after ingestion. If emesis is unsuccessful or contraindicated, the clinician can start on oral vitamin K_1.[3] Activated charcoal is not necessary, because there can be risks for hypernatremia and aspiration. The dosing of oral vitamin K_1 would also need to be delayed at least 4 hours after administering charcoal. Injectable vitamin K_1 is not recommended (discussed later).

In asymptomatic patients, clinicians may choose to either begin prophylactic vitamin K_1 therapy or monitor the PT and only place the patient on vitamin K_1 if the PT becomes increased. If the PT is monitored, a baseline should be run and then repeated at 48 and 72 hours after exposure. The baseline PT is important to determine whether any previous exposures may have occurred of which the owner was not aware. No treatment with vitamin K_1 is necessary if the PT remains normal after 72 hours. However, any increase in the PT warrants full treatment with vitamin K_1.

Clinicians should remember that vitamin K_1 administration could result in falsely normal PT values because new clotting factor synthesis only requires 6 to 12 hours. Therefore, if the PT is being monitored, no vitamin K_1 should be given. The dosage of vitamin K_1 is 3 to 5 mg/kg divided twice a day and given orally with a fatty meal to enhance absorption. For the short-acting anticoagulant rodenticides (warfarin and pindone), the duration of treatment with vitamin K_1 is 14 days; for bromadiolone, 21 days; and for the other SGARs, 4 weeks.[2] Sometimes, if the ingested dose of anticoagulant is very high, more than 4 weeks of treatment with vitamin K_1 may be necessary (discussed later).

For symptomatic patients, stabilization is critically important. Oxygen may be needed for dyspnea. Transfusions with whole blood or fresh or fresh frozen plasma may be necessary to replace blood and clotting factors. Once the patient is bleeding, decontamination is not indicated because the exposure would have occurred multiple days prior. Once stabilized, the patient should be started on oral vitamin K_1. Vitamin K_1 should not be given by injection because of the risk of hematoma formation or risk of bleeding at the venipuncture and possible risk of anaphylactic reaction. Oral administration is ideal, because vitamin K_1 will be delivered directly to the liver, where the clotting factors are activated through the portal circulation. The patient should be hospitalized until the PT is normal, and the patient can then be sent home to continue oral vitamin K_1 therapy for the durations recommended earlier. If the active ingredient of the anticoagulant product is unknown, continue vitamin K_1 therapy for at least 4 weeks.

For all patients, it is advisable to check PT at 48 to 72 hours following the last dose of vitamin K_1. Vitamin K_1 should be continued for 1 additional week or longer if the PT is still increased, which may happen when the pet ingests large amounts of bait. If possible, avoid the use of other highly protein-bound drugs (corticosteroids, nonsteroidal antiinflammatory drugs, and so forth) during the treatment, and instruct the owner to restrict exercise during this time. The prognosis is excellent in patients treated before clinical signs develop. If the patient presents after bleeding has started, the prognosis depends on the severity and the location of the bleeding. For example, a patient that bled into the brain and presented seizing has a much more guarded prognosis than a patient that bled into a joint and presented with lameness.[3]

BROMETHALIN

Bromethalin is a neurotoxin that inhibits mitochondrial energy (ATP) production within the brain.[5] It is available in pelleted forms such as place packs, blocks or bars of bait, and baited worms. The pellets and bait bars/blocks are 0.01% bromethalin. Usually the place packs are 0.75 oz (21.2 g) of pelleted bait, and the bars/blocks are 0.5 oz (15 g) and 1 oz (30 g), which is equivalent to 2.13 mg/pack and 1.42 or 2.84 mg/bar of bromethalin, respectively. The baited worms are 0.025% bromethalin and weigh 5 g, which is 1.25 mg of bromethalin per worm.

Pathophysiology and Clinical Signs

Bromethalin is readily absorbed from the GI tract and can peak in the plasma within several hours after ingestion (4 hours within the rat). It is metabolized in the liver via mixed-function oxygenases. The N-demethylated metabolite desmethyl bromethalin is much more toxic than the parent compound. Both bromethalin and desmethyl bromethalin have a wide distribution within the body. The highest levels are found within the fat and brain because of the highly lipophilic nature of bromethalin. Excretion is very slow and occurs through the bile, with evidence of some enterohepatic recirculation. The plasma half-life in rats is approximately 5 to 6 days.[5,6]

Bromethalin and desmethyl bromethalin uncouple oxidative phosphorylation, which is critical for brain and cellular function. As a result, cellular and tissue ATP are decreased and sodium-potassium ion channel pumps are affected. This process leads to electrolyte imbalances and a fluid shift into myelinated areas of the brain and spinal cord.[6] Cerebral lipid peroxidation may also occur, which then damages organelles and cellular membranes. A chain reaction of progressive and irreversible cellular damage and necrosis can then develop.[7]

Clinical signs of bromethalin toxicosis are often dose dependent and can manifest as 2 different syndromes. High doses of bromethalin can cause a convulsant syndrome, which usually is seen at doses greater than or equal to the LD_{50} for a species. In both dogs and cats, clinical signs may include hyperesthesia, hyperexcitability, tremors, seizures, vocalization, moderate to severe CNS depression, hypothermia, and death. Signs may occur within 4 to 18 hours of ingestion.

Lower doses of bromethalin (less than the LD_{50}) lead to a paralytic syndrome. With these exposures, the onset of clinical signs is slower and sometimes delayed. Signs may take 1 to 7 days to develop, initially manifesting as ataxia, CNS depression, paresis of the hind limbs, then progressing to recumbency.[5,8] Additional findings may include upper motor neuron signs: proprioceptive deficits, loss of deep pain, and exaggerated pelvic limb reflexes. Animals with a dull mentation may progress to a comatose or semicomatose state.[6] Cats occasionally exhibit abdominal distention and ileus. Ileus has also been seen in dogs, especially after large ingestions of bait (ASPCA APCC Database, unpublished data, 2002–2018). Other clinical signs in dogs and cats may include vomiting, diarrhea (often with bait), tremors, weakness, hyperesthesia, hypersalivation, vocalization, hypothermia, extensor rigidity, nystagmus, anisocoria, tachypnea, absent menace response, abnormal papillary light reflex, and opisthotonus. A decerebrate posture and seizures may occur in the terminal stages, and death may be from respiratory depression.[5,8,9]

Cats are much more sensitive to bromethalin, and the guinea pig is the most resistant, because this species has much lower N-demethylase activity. The LD_{50} in guinea pigs is greater than 1000 mg/kg orally, and 13 mg/kg in rabbits. For dogs, the oral LD_{50} is 3.65 mg/kg, with a minimum lethal dose (MLD) of 2.5 mg/kg. The LD_{50} in cats is much lower: 0.54 mg/kg, with an MLD of 0.45 mg/kg.[6]

Animals have developed clinical signs of toxicosis at even lower doses, because some individuals may be more sensitive than others.[5] Juveniles seem to be more sensitive than adults. Based on clinical cases reported to the ASPCA APCC, clinical signs and death have been reported in dogs exposed to bromethalin at doses as low as 0.36 mg/kg (ASPCA APCC Database, unpublished data, 2001–2018). Cats have developed clinical signs after doses as low as 0.24 mg/kg (ASPCA APCC Database, unpublished data, 1998–2018).[10] The risk for relay toxicosis after ingesting an animal that died of bromethalin is low. However, it is theoretically possible in cats that feed mainly on rodents that have died of bromethalin poisoning, because cats are much more sensitive than other species.

Diagnosis

An antemortem diagnosis is most often made based on the history of bait ingestion and the development of clinical signs. Frequently, owners do not know the bait was consumed until they notice that the stool is discolored (often green). Performing a rectal examination may aid in determining how recent the ingestion was or whether there are multiple animals involved. Clinical laboratory tests are often unremarkable and nondiagnostic. An increase in cerebrospinal fluid (CSF) pressure may or may not be present in symptomatic animals. If it is increased, it is usually not as high as that in animals with head trauma. The reason for this may be that the edema is confined within the myelin sheaths. Analysis of the CSF is often normal, without any evidence of inflammation.[5]

Postmortem diagnosis is often based on histologic changes in the CNS and possible detection of residues. Grossly in dogs, cerebral edema is usually mild. In fatal ingestions, histologic lesions include spongy degeneration of the white matter in the optic nerve, cerebrum, cerebellum, brain stem, and spinal cord. Myelin and cellular edema and vacuolization are also seen.[5,8] Although the white matter is primarily affected, vacuolization can occasionally be seen in the cerebral cortical gray matter. No peripheral nerve lesions occur.[9] Detection of bromethalin in the stomach contents, ascites, fat, liver, kidney, and brain may also be performed at select veterinary laboratories.[6,8]

Treatment

In asymptomatic animals, decontaminate by inducing emesis if the exposure was within the past 4 hours. If the ingestion was more than 4 hours earlier, single or repeated doses of activated charcoal may be indicated, depending on the amount consumed (**Table 1**). Cats may need longer treatment and multiple charcoal doses because of their greater sensitivity to bromethalin.[5]

For animals that are given activated charcoal, especially those given repeated doses, obtaining baseline serum sodium levels is recommended before administration because of the potential for development of hypernatremia. Intravenous fluid administration and monitoring in the clinic for 4 hours may also be warranted with

Table 1
The American Society for the Prevention of Cruelty to Animals Animal Poison Control Center's decontamination recommendations for bromethalin ingestion

Time Since Exposure (h)	Dose Ingested (mg/kg)[a]	Action
Dogs		
<4	0.1–0.49	Emesis or 1 dose of activated charcoal
>4	0.1–0.49	One dose of activated charcoal
<4	0.5–0.75	Emesis and 3 doses of activated charcoal over 24 h
>4	0.5–0.75	Three doses of activated charcoal over 24 h
<4	>0.75	Emesis and 3 doses of activated charcoal a day for 48 h
>4	>0.75	Three doses of activated charcoal a day for 48 h
Cats		
<4	0.05–0.1	Emesis[b] or 1 dose of activated charcoal
>4	0.05–0.1	One dose of activated charcoal
<4	0.1–0.3	Emesis and 3 doses of activated charcoal over 24 h
>4	0.1–0.3	Three doses of activated charcoal over 24 h
<4	>0.3	Emesis and 3 doses of activated charcoal a day for 48 h
>4	>0.3	Three doses of activated charcoal a day for 48 h

[a] 1 oz of 0.01% bromethalin bait contains 2.84 mg of bromethalin.
[b] Emesis in cats can be induced with xylazine 0.4 to 0.5 mg/kg intramuscular (IM) or intravenous (IV), or dexmedetomidine 7 μg/kg IM, and reversed with yohimbine (0.1 mg/kg IV); emesis success with xylazine in cats is approximately 43% (ASPCA APCC, unpublished data, 2009).

administration of a single dose of charcoal. Serum sodium should be closely monitored for patients receiving repeated charcoal doses. Some animals can have an osmotic fluid shift after charcoal administration (with or without sorbitol), and the risk of hypernatremia may increase after multiple doses. Development of hypernatremia can cause CNS signs within the first 4 to 6 hours of dosing activated charcoal (ataxia, tremors, depression, seizures), which could be mistaken for bromethalin toxicosis. If these signs develop, repeat a serum sodium level and compare it with the baseline. If repeated charcoal is needed, it is recommended to reduce the subsequent doses by half after giving the initial dose (eg, if a 4.5-kg [10-lb] dog is given 30 mL of activated charcoal, the rest of the doses should be decreased to 15 mL). The first dose can be given with a cathartic such as sorbitol, and the subsequent doses without a cathartic, to reduce the risk of electrolyte derangements. The charcoal can be repeated at 8-hour intervals. If it is not being passed in the stools before the next dose, give the animal a warm-water enema to move the charcoal out of the GI tract. This enema can also provide electrolyte-free water to the body, if the sodium level is starting to become increased.

Symptomatic bromethalin patients are difficult to treat successfully, especially if the patient is showing serious CNS effects. If signs are less severe, such as ataxia or depression, some animals may recover with supportive care over a period of 1 to 4 weeks. However, some animals may have permanent neurologic dysfunction. In patients with tremors, seizures, coma, or paralysis, the prognosis is poor to grave.

Cerebral edema can be treated with mannitol and corticosteroids, but often signs return once therapy is discontinued. Side effects of mannitol are dehydration, hypernatremia, hyperkalemia, hypotension, pulmonary edema, and renal failure. Rehydrating these animals may worsen the CNS signs. Furosemide may be an alternative to mannitol to reduce these risks and may be combined with dexamethasone. Tremors and seizures can be treated with methocarbamol, benzodiazepines, barbiturates, propofol, or levetiracetam. Recumbent animals may need nutritional support and good nursing care to prevent decubital ulcers and pneumonia.[5,6] Although bromethalin is lipophilic, intralipid emulsion (ILE) therapy is not considered a standard of care, because there are no studies to prove it is effective with symptomatic bromethalin patients. Once there is damage to the neurons, ILE is not expected to reverse these changes. There is also the risk of pulling more bromethalin into systemic circulation with ILE, especially if there is still bait in the GI tract. A prokinetic agent, such as metoclopramide, may also help to move any bait out of the GI tract and decrease ileus. It may also move the charcoal out of the GI tract, reducing the risk of hypernatremia.

CHOLECALCIFEROL

The chemical name of vitamin D_3 is cholecalciferol. Vitamin D_3 is required by the body and is acquired in mammals as part of the diet or by dermal exposure to ultraviolet light.[11,12] An understanding of the metabolic pathway of cholecalciferol is important to a discussion of intoxication by cholecalciferol rodenticides. In the liver, cholecalciferol is metabolized to calcifediol (25-hydroxycholecalciferol). This conversion has limited negative feedback; therefore, a large ingestion of cholecalciferol leads to a significant increase in calcifediol level.[13] Calcifediol is then metabolized by the kidney to calcitriol (1,25-dihydroxycholecalciferol), which is the most active metabolite. As calcitriol concentrations increase, a negative feedback mechanism halts the production of calcitriol; however, calcifediol continues to be produced in high enough amounts to lead to clinical effects.[13] Because calcifediol has a very long half-life,[12] poisoned patients may require treatment for an extended period of time.

Pathophysiology and Clinical Signs

The metabolites of cholecalciferol cause their effects by increasing serum calcium and phosphorus levels.[13] They act to increase intestinal absorption of calcium, stimulate calcium and phosphorus transfer from bones into the plasma, and enhance renal tubular reabsorption of calcium. Within 48 hours of exposure, patients may develop vomiting, lethargy, and muscle weakness as a result of the increased plasma concentration on the cells in the body.[13] Prolonged increases of serum calcium and phosphorus levels can lead to tissue mineralization. Tissue mineralization in the kidneys can lead to acute renal failure. Decreased functioning of the GI tract, skeletal and cardiac muscles, blood vessels, and ligaments can result from mineralization in these areas.[13]

The literature suggests that clinical signs can be seen at cholecalciferol doses of 0.5 mg/kg.[11] This dose corresponds with a 23-kg (50-lb) dog ingesting only 14.2 g (0.5 oz) of a typical 0.075% cholecalciferol bait; therefore, even small ingestions may warrant treatment. The ASPCA APCC recommends decontamination when the ingested dose is greater than 0.1 mg/kg.

Clinical signs typically occur within 12 to 36 hours of ingestion of the rodenticide. The common clinical signs seen with cholecalciferol toxicosis include vomiting, anorexia, depression, polyuria, and polydipsia. Acute renal failure can develop within 24 to 72 hours. If the patient survives the initial clinical signs, they may have long-term effects relating to mineralization of their tissues and organs.[13]

Diagnosis

Often the diagnosis is made based on the history of ingestion and the development of clinical signs. Some owners also notice bait in the stool. A rectal examination may help confirm ingestion and rule in or rule out other pets in the household that may also have been exposed. Clinical laboratory tests to perform include serum phosphorus, calcium (total and ionized), blood urea nitrogen (BUN), and serum creatinine levels. A urinalysis may show isosthenuria.[12] Be certain that the blood sample is not hemolyzed or lipemic, because this can lead to a falsely increased total calcium level. Young animals also have increased calcium levels from normal bone growth. Ionized calcium (iCa) is affected by the pH of blood or serum. An acidic pH dissociates calcium from protein and increases iCa. An alkaline pH occurs when samples are exposed to air. With loss of carbon dioxide, calcium binds to protein and decreases iCa, so samples should be collected and handled anaerobically.[14] A reference laboratory is ideal for testing iCa, because some in-house analyzers are not accurate.[15]

After acute exposures, the serum phosphorus level is often the first laboratory increase that is seen (>7–8 mg/dL). This increase is then followed by an increase in serum calcium level (13–20 mg/dL), and these changes can occur within 24 to 72 hours after ingestion. Radiography or ultrasonography occasionally help in diagnosing soft tissue mineralization in symptomatic animals.[11,14]

Specific antemortem testing includes serum levels of 25-hydroxycholecalciferol (also called calcifediol), which is the primary circulating metabolite of cholecalciferol. Ionized calcium and serum intact parathyroid hormone (PTH) levels may also be of value. In animals that have ingested cholecalciferol, the 25-hydroxycholecalciferol levels are increased at least 15 times more than normal. In some patients, levels remain increased for weeks to months. The iCa is also increased, and the PTH level is low.[12,14] Testing for 1,25-dihydroxycholecalciferol (calcitriol) and other vitamin D_3 analogues such as calcipotriene is not readily available.[11] Calcitriol has a short half-life and often peaks within the serum on the fourth day after ingestion, then rapidly declines. The homeostatic negative control mechanism for calcium is not triggered until 4 days after exposure.[16]

Postmortem diagnosis is more difficult. The kidney is the best organ to use for detecting 25-hydroxycholecalciferol levels. Plasma and serum samples can be used as well. On gross necropsy, the stomach may be empty from vomiting and anorexia, and animals are often dehydrated. Gastric ulceration with hemorrhage may also be present, and the gastric mucosa may be hyperemic and swollen. The kidneys may be normal in appearance or look mottled. The lungs may look hemorrhagic, edematous, or normal.[12] In addition, there is soft tissue mineralization within the heart, kidneys, GI tract, skeletal muscles, ligaments, and tendons. Azotemic ulcers may be evident in the oral cavity.[11] Histopathologic findings may include soft tissue mineralization of the great vessels, stomach, kidneys, and lungs but these are not pathognomonic. Within the heart and arteries, the atria and aorta have the most evidence of mineralization. Within the vessels, it is often within the smooth muscles. Myocardial degeneration may be present within the heart, including mineralized and necrotic myocytes. The stomach may have mineralization within the smooth muscles and the lamina propria. The stomach wall is often congested, with the mucosal epithelium showing erosion, necrosis, sloughing, and hemorrhage. These lesions are often located near bands of mineralization. The kidneys often have evidence of mineralization within the glomerulus, convoluted tubules, and the blood vessels, resulting in epithelial cell necrosis and cellular debris. Protein cast formation may also be observed. Within the lungs, the alveolar septae are often thickened, with hemorrhage and mineralization.[11,12]

Treatment

In asymptomatic animals, decontaminate by inducing emesis if the exposure was within the past 4 hours. If the ingestion was more than 4 hours earlier, administer activated charcoal if the animal has not been vomiting before presentation. There is evidence of enterohepatic recirculation of cholecalciferol, so repeated doses of activated charcoal may be needed[11] (see treatment recommendations for bromethalin for charcoal administration suggestions). The use of cholestyramine resin has shown some benefit in reducing vitamin D_3 levels in humans. Cholestyramine can be given as an adjunct treatment in dogs at 0.3 to 0.5 g/kg by mouth 3 times a day for 4 days. If activated charcoal is given as a single dose, then start the cholestyramine 8 hours later. Baseline serum chemistries of total calcium, ionized calcium, phosphorus, BUN, and creatinine should be obtained and monitored every 24 hours for 4 days. If these remain normal, no additional treatment is needed.

In symptomatic animals, treatment is designed to correct the hypercalcemia. Often animals have been vomiting and are anorexic; therefore, rehydration and diuresis should be instituted first with 0.9% sodium chloride (NaCl) at 2 to 3 times maintenance fluid rate. After the animal is rehydrated, loop diuretics and glucocorticoids can be instituted.[14,17,18] Sodium ions enhance calcium excretion by reducing tubular calcium reabsorption and enhancing calciuresis. Furosemide enhances calcium renal excretion by decreasing sodium and chloride reabsorption across the loop of Henle, which diminishes the positive potential across the tubule. Thiazide diuretics should be avoided, because these can decrease calciuresis. Monitoring hydration status is critical with diuretic use. Prednisone aids in suppression of bone resorption. It also reduces the absorption of calcium by the intestines and increases the urinary excretion of calcium by reducing absorption by the distal tubules. If the patient is acidotic, sodium bicarbonate may decrease iCa as calcium ions bind to plasma proteins and bicarbonate. The dose is 1 to 4 mEq/kg slowly intravenously, and effects may last up to 3 hours. If the serum phosphorus is increased, phosphate binders such as aluminum hydroxide given orally are beneficial. A diet low in phosphorus and calcium should be fed for at least 4 weeks[11,12,14] (**Box 1** shows medication doses).

Box 1

American Society for the Prevention of Cruelty to Animals Animal Poison Control Center recommended management of hypercalcemia associated with cholecalciferol and vitamin D analogues (revised November 2017)

Stabilize animal as needed (fluids, antiemetics, antiseizure medications, and so forth)
Decontamination

- Less than 4 hours after ingestion: emesis. Dogs: 3% hydrogen peroxide, 2.2 mL/kg by mouth, maximum 3 tablespoons (may repeat once); or use apomorphine 0.03 mg/kg IV. Cats: xylazine 0.4–0.5 mg/kg intramuscular (IM) or intravenous (IV), or dexmedetomidine 7 μg/kg IM. Activated charcoal (6–12 mL/kg by mouth, repeat half of the initial dose every 8–12 hours for 2–3 doses). Monitor for hypernatremia in patients receiving activated charcoal.
- Greater than 4 hours after ingestion: activated charcoal. Use caution to avoid aspiration; contraindicated in vomiting animals; monitor serum calcium and phosphorous levels for 4 days (discussed later).
- Cholestyramine has been shown to be effective in laboratory animals and humans to enhance excretion of vitamin D by binding to bile acids. Dose: 0.3 to 1 g/kg by mouth 3 times a day for 4 days.

Laboratory monitoring

- Baseline calcium, phosphorus, BUN, creatinine; complete serum biochemistry is recommended, especially in older animals or animals with previously existing health problems.
- If Ca, P, BUN, Cr are normal on presentation, monitor Ca, P, BUN, Cr every 12 to 24 hours for at least 4 days. Phosphorus level tends to increase before calcium. Treatment may be discontinued if 96-hour values are normal.
- If Ca, P, BUN, and/or Cr are abnormal on presentation, go to the hypercalcemia management protocol (below).
- Monitor Ca × P product; if greater than 60 in adult animals, then chances of soft tissue mineralization increase. To compute, take Ca level (in mg/dL) and multiply by P level (in mg/dL); for example, if Ca = 14 and P = 5, then Ca × P = 70 and there is risk of soft tissue mineralization; some laboratories report values in units other than mg/dL so be sure to convert to mg/dL before calculating the product. Young dogs may have higher baseline serum calcium and phosphorous levels. In these dogs, Ca × P product between 60 and 95 may be normal. Do not just look at this value only; other trends (increase in serum calcium and phosphorous levels and comparison with baseline values) should also be considered when interpreting the results. Most dogs with persistent significant hypercalcemia show signs of anorexia, lethargy, and some GI signs. Some increase in Ca × P product in the absence of clinical signs or other electrolyte changes may not be significant.

Hypercalcemia management protocol I (preferred): pamidronate is a bisphosphonate used in humans to treat hypercalcemia of malignancy.

- IV normal saline (0.9% NaCl); twice maintenance; forced diuresis; maintain diuresis until calcium levels have decreased.
- Furosemide: 2.5 to 4.5 mg/kg by mouth 3 to 4 times a day or 0.5 mg/kg/h via continuous intravenous (IV) infusion; avoid thiazide diuretics because they reduce renal excretion of calcium.
- Prednisone: 1 to 3 mg/kg by mouth divided twice a day.
- Pamidronate (Aredia): 1.3 to 2 mg/kg; dilute in normal saline and administer intravenously over a 2-hour period.

Hypercalcemia management protocol II: the authors think that this protocol is less desirable, because calcitonin is not consistent in its ability to decrease serum calcium, and some dogs become refractory to calcitonin. In addition, in experimental dogs, concurrent use of pamidronate and calcitonin resulted in greater soft tissue mineralization than when either drug was used alone.

- IV normal saline; twice maintenance; forced diuresis; maintain diuresis until calcium levels have decreased.
- Furosemide: 2.5 to 4.5 mg/kg by mouth 3 to 4 times a day or 0.5 mg/kg/h via continuous IV infusion; avoid thiazide diuretics because they reduce renal excretion of calcium.
- Prednisone: 1 to 3 mg/kg by mouth divided twice a day.
- Salmon calcitonin (Calcimar): 4 to 6 U/kg subcutaneously 2 to 3 times a day.

Once Ca levels have stabilized:
- Wean off fluids and monitor Ca, P, BUN, and Cr at least every 24 hours. If BUN and Cr levels are increased, treat for acute renal failure (ie, maintain fluid diuresis). If calcium level starts to increase, reinstitute fluid therapy and consider another dose of pamidronate (generally expect this to occur within 5–7 days after first dose). In our experience, most dogs given pamidronate have required only 1 dose, although some have needed repeated doses.
- Switch to an oral corticosteroid and furosemide; if laboratory values remain normal 5 to 7 days after discontinuing IV fluids, gradually wean off of these medications over 1 to 2 weeks.
- Aluminum hydroxide: 30 to 90 mg/kg/d by mouth in divided doses as needed if phosphorus level remains increased.
- Closely monitor appetite, and for GI signs: development of anorexia or vomiting may be an indication that the calcium level has increased. Monitor Ca and P for a minimum of 5 to 7 days after those values have returned to normal, then 2 to 3 times a week for 2 weeks, and then weekly for 2 weeks. Feed a low-Ca diet during this time period.
- Monitor for hypocalcemia.

Patients that are severely affected or whose calcium levels continue to increase despite therapy need more aggressive treatment. The preferred drug to use is pamidronate disodium, which is a bisphosphonate that inhibits bone resorption. It is administered slowly intravenously in 0.9% NaCl. The drug can inhibit bone resorption for a long duration, but some animals do need a second infusion. Increases in BUN and creatinine levels can occur after administration, so animals should be maintained on intravenous fluids during this time and until calcium levels normalize. The pamidronate treatment may need to be repeated in 5 to 7 days after the initial dose. The cost of pamidronate may be high, but it often reduces the calcium level within 24 to 48 hours after dosing. Monitoring renal values is important when using this drug, and caution should be used in animals with azotemia.[11,12,19] In humans, side effects of pamidronate include hypocalcemia, hypophosphatemia, hypokalemia, and hypomagnesemia.[17] Monitoring these parameters in veterinary patients is recommended.

If pamidronate is unavailable, another option is calcitonin salmon but it is less effective. It also has a very short half-life (2–4 hours) and must be given intramuscularly multiple times a day for several weeks. It works by reducing the activity and formation of osteoclasts, and the decrease in calcium level is rapid. Vomiting and anorexia are often side effects, and animals often become refractory to treatment within a few days. Combining pamidronate and calcitonin is used in human medicine but is not recommended in veterinary patients because studies do not show any benefit when used together in dogs, and it potentially worsens the outcome.[14,20]

Saline diuresis should be continued until the serum calcium levels return to normal. Fluid therapy in symptomatic patients may be needed for 1 week or longer because the half-life of cholecalciferol is very long (29 days). Furosemide and prednisone may need to be continued for 1 to 2 weeks after the animal is off fluids and then gradually tapered. After fluid therapy has stopped, the calcium levels should be monitored every 24 hours for 96 hours, then twice a week for 2 weeks, then once a week for 2 weeks, to make sure there is not a relapse.[11,14,20]

SUMMARY

This article covers the pathophysiology, clinical signs, diagnosis, and treatment of the 3 most commonly encountered rodenticides: anticoagulants, bromethalin, and cholecalciferol. Anticoagulants cause coagulation abnormalities and bleeding, bromethalin is a neurotoxin, and cholecalciferol leads to increased serum calcium and phosphorus levels, which result in tissue mineralization and possibly renal failure. Risk mitigation policies implemented by the EPA beginning in June 2011 are likely to cause an increase in the number of bromethalin and cholecalciferol cases seen in veterinary clinics.

REFERENCES

1. US Environmental Protection Agency. Final risk mitigation decision for ten rodenticides. Available at: http://www.epa.gov/opp00001/reregistration/rodenticides/finalriskdecision.htm. Accessed May 11, 2011.
2. Murphy MJ. Anticoagulant rodenticides. In: Gupta RC, editor. Veterinary toxicology basic and clinical principles. New York: Elsevier; 2007. p. 525–47.
3. Merola V. Anticoagulant rodenticides: deadly for pests, dangerous for pets. Vet Med 2002;97:716–22.
4. Sheafor SE, Couto CG. Clinical approach to a dog with anticoagulant rodenticide poisoning. Vet Med 1994;94:466–71.
5. Dorman DC. Bromethalin. In: Peterson ME, Talcott PA, editors. Small animal toxicology. 2nd edition. St Louis (MO): Elsevier Saunders; 2006. p. 609–18.
6. Dorman D. Bromethalin. In: Plumlee KH, editor. Clinical veterinary toxicology. St Louis (MO): Mosby; 2004. p. 446–8.
7. Osweiler GD. The action of poisons. In: Osweiler GD, Nieginski EA, Cann M, et al, editors. Toxicology. Baltimore (MD): Williams and Wilkins; 1996. p. 17–22.
8. Dorman DC, Simon J, Harlin KA, et al. Diagnosis of bromethalin toxicosis in the dog. J Vet Diagn Invest 1990;2:123–8.
9. Dorman DC, Zachary JF, Buck WB. Neuropathologic findings of bromethalin toxicosis in the cat. Vet Pathol 1992;29:139–44.
10. Dunayer E. Bromethalin: the other rodenticide. Vet Med 2003;98:732–6.
11. Morrow CK, Volmer PA. Cholecalciferol. In: Plumlee KH, editor. Clinical veterinary toxicology. St Louis (MO): Mosby; 2004. p. 448–51.
12. Rumbeiha WK. Cholecalciferol. In: Peterson ME, Talcott PA, editors. Small animal toxicology. 2nd edition. St Louis (MO): Elsevier Saunders; 2006. p. 629–42.
13. Morrow C. Cholecalciferol poisoning. Vet Med 2001;96:905–11.
14. Rosol TJ, Chew DJ, Nagode LA, et al. Disorders of calcium: hypercalcemia and hypocalcemia. In: DiBartola SP, editor. Fluid therapy in small animal practice. 2nd edition. Philadelphia: WB Saunders; 2000. p. 108–62.
15. Tappin S, Rizzo F, Dodkin S, et al. Measurement of ionized calcium in canine blood samples collected in prefilled and self-filled heparinized syringes using the i-STAT point-of-care analyzer. Vet Clin Pathol 2008;37(1):66–72.
16. Rumbeiha WK, Braselton WE, Nachreiner RF, et al. The postmortem diagnosis of cholecalciferol toxicosis: a novel approach and differentiation from ethylene glycol toxicosis. J Vet Diagn Invest 2000;12:426–32.
17. Kadar E, Rush JE, Wetmore L, et al. Electrolyte disturbances and cardiac arrhythmias in a dog following pamidronate, calcitonin, and furosemide administration for hypercalcemia of malignancy. J Am Anim Hosp Assoc 2004;40:75–81.
18. Jensterle M, Pfeifer M, Sever M, et al. Dihydrotachysterol intoxication treated with pamidronate: a case report. Cases J 2010;3:78–93.
19. Gwaltney-Brant SM, Rumbeiha WK. Newer antidotal therapies. Vet Clin Small Anim 2002;32:323–39.
20. Rumbeiha WK, Kruger JM, Fitzgerald SF, et al. Use of pamidronate to reverse vitamin D_3-induced toxicosis in dogs. Am J Vet Res 1999;60:1092–7.

Toxicology of Explosives and Fireworks in Small Animals

Patti Gahagan, DVM[a], Tina Wismer, DVM, MS[b],*

KEYWORDS

- Explosives • Nitrates • Explosive detection dogs/working dogs • Fireworks
- Barium • Chlorates

KEY POINTS

- Exposure to explosives and fireworks in dogs can result in variable severity of clinical signs depending on the presence of different chemicals and the amount.
- The risk can be lessened by proper education of dog handlers and owners about the seriousness of the intoxications.
- Most animals will recover within 24 to 72 hours with supportive care.

EXPLOSIVES

An explosive is any material that can undergo rapid and self-propagating decomposition, resulting in the liberation of heat and the production of energy, most commonly through the expansion of gases. The released energy has several potential uses. These uses include commercial applications, such as blasting in mines and quarries, demolition in the construction industry, military applications, and firearms applications.

There are more than 300 materials classified by the Bureau of Alcohol, Tobacco, Firearms, and Explosives (ATF) as explosive materials.[1] It is beyond the scope of this article to deal with each of these materials from a toxicity standpoint. However, explosive materials can be grouped according to similarity of chemical structure, which makes evaluation of the toxicity potential much easier to understand.

Explosives are classified based on the rapidity of the decomposition and resultant energy wave as either low-order explosives or high explosives. Examples of low-order explosives include pipe bombs, gunpowder, and petroleum-based bombs.

This article originally appeared in *Veterinary Clinics of North America: Small Animal Practice*, Volume 42, Issue 2, March 2012.

The authors have nothing to disclose.

[a] Novartis Animal Health US, Inc, 3200 Northline Avenue, Suite 300, Greensboro, NC 27408, USA; [b] ASPCA Animal Poison Control Center, 1717 South Philo Road, Suite 36, Urbana, IL 61802, USA

* Corresponding author.

E-mail address: tina.wismer@aspca.org

High explosives propagate a supersonic shockwave when the explosive material decomposes into hot, rapidly expanding gases. Examples of high explosives include trinitrotoluene (TNT), cyclonite (RDX), and pentaerythritol tetranitrate (PETN). (**Table 1** provides a glossary of abbreviations.)

Explosives can also be classified as primary, secondary, or tertiary based on how easily the decomposition process can be initiated. Primary explosives are used to ignite secondary explosives. Examples of primary explosives include lead azide (LA), lead styphnate (LS), and nitroglycerin (NG). Blasting caps contain primary explosives and are used to ignite secondary explosives to initiate the decomposition process. Secondary explosives are much more stable than primary explosives and detonate only under specific circumstances. Examples of secondary explosives include TNT and RDX. Tertiary explosives are quite insensitive to shock and cannot be reliably detonated by primary explosives. Typically, a small amount of a secondary explosive (ignited by a small amount of a primary explosive) is used to detonate tertiary explosives. Ammonium nitrate and fuel oil (ANFO) is an example of a tertiary explosive.[1]

Most explosives are tightly regulated, with access limited by various agencies, most notably the ATF. Exposure of small animals to explosive materials is limited primarily to dogs and will most commonly result from improper or negligent storage of materials, stolen materials no longer being handled appropriately, and training aids used to train explosives detection dogs.

Explosives detection dogs working in actual field conditions (not in training scenarios) are unlikely to suffer from toxic ingestions, as they are trained extensively not to touch or otherwise interfere with explosives. A working dog that violates this training in actual field conditions is more likely to be seriously injured or killed by an explosion than to suffer any toxicosis. Therefore, dogs in training are most likely to consume explosive agents. Careful training techniques that limit the novice dog's ability to come in contact with and consume training aids make oral exposures uncommon.

Although the specific odors that explosives detection dogs are trained to detect may vary based on specific needs, these dogs are commonly trained to alert on 6 specific odors: black powder or smokeless powder; commercial dynamite containing ethylene glycol dinitrate (EGDN) or NG; RDX; PETN; TNT (military dynamite); and

Table 1	
Glossary of explosives	
Abbreviation	**Definition**
ANFO	Ammonium nitrate/fuel oil
Black powder	Potassium nitrate + carbon + sulfur
C4	RDX + plasticizer
EGDN	Ethylene glycol dinitrate
NC	Nitrocellulose
NG	Nitroglycerine
PETN	Pentaerythritol tetranitrate
RDX	Research Department Explosive; cyclotrimethylenetrinitramine, also known as cyclonite, hexogen, and T-4
Semtex	RDX + PETN
Smokeless powder	Nitrocellulose-based propellant (gunpowder)
TNT	Trinitrotoluene

slurries/water gel explosives.[2] Therefore, these are the explosives most likely to be encountered by a training dog in a clinical setting.

Many low explosives are also tightly regulated and not likely to be ingested by dogs. However, some agents used in explosives are readily available without restriction and pose toxic concerns to companion animals. These agents include the petroleum distillates and nitrates, including fertilizers. Although most commonly thought of in its use as an explosive, NG is also available as a medicine (vasodilator) and could potentially be ingested in households as well.

Nitroaromatics

TNT is a nitroaromatic compound most commonly used by the military as a booster for other high explosives. It is also used in commercial mining operations. TNT and other nitroaromatic compounds easily penetrate the skin. Dermal exposure can cause methemoglobinemia, anemia, local dermal irritation, and hepatic injury. Urinary bladder tumors have been associated with chronic dermal TNT exposure in humans.[3] Dermal exposures are rare in dogs. If dermal exposure does occur, decontamination by bathing with a liquid dishwashing detergent should be instituted. Gloves should be worn to protect the bather. Any dermal lesions should be treated symptomatically and supportively.

An acute inhalation exposure in dogs can cause mild and transient respiratory irritation. Removal to fresh air is usually the only treatment needed. If significant respiratory signs do occur, institute symptomatic and supportive care.

Dogs are more likely to be exposed via ingestion of negligently handled or stored materials. Acute oral single-dose median lethal dose (LD_{50}) values have not been established for TNT in dogs; but short-term (90 days) oral LD_{50} values were 1320 and 794 mg/kg in male and female rats, respectively, and 660 mg/kg in male and female mice. The animals developed tremors followed by mild seizures 1 to 2 hours after dosing. Dosages of 20 mg/kg/d for 13 weeks caused anemia with reduced erythrocytes, hemoglobin, and hematocrit in dogs. Other effects included splenomegaly with hemosiderosis, hepatomegaly, elevated serum cholesterol levels, and depressed serum glutamic pyruvic transaminase (alanine aminotransferase) activity in dogs. The no-observable-effect level for dogs was 0.2 mg/kg/d.[4] A 6-month oral toxicity study of TNT in dogs demonstrated the major toxic effects to be hemolytic anemia, methemoglobinemia, hepatic injury, splenomegaly, and death at doses ranging from 0.5 to 32.0 mg/kg/d. Because all doses caused effects, a no-observable-effect level was not established, although only the highest dose (32 mg/kg) was lethal.[5]

Dogs known to have ingested TNT that present to a clinic should undergo decontamination because the amounts needed to cause significant signs in an acute oral exposure are not known. If the ingestion is within 4 hours of exposure and the dog is asymptomatic, emesis induction with apomorphine is a reasonable option. Depending on the amount recovered, N-acetylcysteine (140 mg/kg by mouth or intravenously [IV] then 70 mg/kg by mouth every 8 hours for 5–7 treatments), which helps maintain or restore glutathione levels, may be prudent to help prevent/treat methemoglobinemia. It has been shown to reduce chemically induced methemoglobinemia in vitro.[6] However, there is some question as to whether it will be effective in treating methemoglobinemia formation resulting from nitrite toxicosis.[7] In human medicine, methylene blue is the preferred agent for treating methemoglobinemia secondary to nitrate toxicosis.[8] In dogs, methylene blue is not commonly used because it is not readily available to veterinarians. It can be administered IV as a 1% solution at 1.5 mg/kg. Repeat in 30 minutes once if needed. Monitoring liver values for animals showing significant clinical signs is also recommended.

Nitramines

The most prominent nitramine explosive in use today is cyclonite, also known as RDX or hexhydro-1,3,5-trinitro-1,3,5-triazine. It exhibits a high degree of stability, so it poses little risk for spontaneous detonation. It is commonly combined with plasticizers to make C-4. It is also commonly combined with PETN to form Semtex. PETN is a nitrate ester (discussed in the next section).

Although inhalation of cyclonite can cause numerous signs, including seizures, this is not likely clinically relevant in dogs, as they are more commonly exposed to the plasticized form rather than the crystalline form found in manufacturing plants.[9] Similarly, there is little concern for significant dermal absorption in dogs exposed to the plasticized form.[10]

Following ingestion of cyclonite, absorption is slow.[11] The peak plasma level in humans is 24 hours.[12] In rats, a plateau was reached within several hours but remained stable for 24 hours.[13] The elimination half-life in humans is 15 hours.

There is conflicting information regarding the LD_{50} of cyclonite, probably because of the wide variability of granulation. The LD_{50} of coarse granular cyclonite is 3 times higher than that of fine powder.[14] One study lists the LD_{50} for dogs as 6 mg/kg, whereas another lists the no-observable-effect level at 10 mg/kg/d for 3 months.[15] In a study of 7 female dogs fed a diet of cyclonite at 50 mg/kg/d for 6 days per week for 6 weeks, one dog died at the end of the fifth week of excessive congestion of the walls of the small intestines.[14]

Despite being an organic nitrate–based explosive, cyclonite does not seem to cause nitratelike toxicosis. It is a corrosive irritant of the eyes, skin, mucous membranes, and respiratory tract but mainly acts as a neurotoxicant. There is some evidence that limbic structures in the central nervous system (CNS) may be involved in cyclonite-induced seizure susceptibility.[16] In dogs ingesting cyclonite, seizures are the most common clinical sign and may occur minutes to hours after ingestion. In published case reports, 100% of exposed dogs outside of a research setting experienced seizures. In the American Society for the Prevention of Cruelty to Animals Animal Poison Control Center's database, 11 of 13 symptomatic dogs experienced seizures. Metabolic acidosis is a possible sequelae. Vomiting is also a commonly reported clinical sign in dogs. Development of minor methemoglobinemia in humans has been suggested, but this has not been reported in dogs ingesting cyclonite. There has been one documented case of elevated hepatic enzymes in dogs and one reported case of elevated renal values.[12]

Decontamination via emesis (with apomorphine or 3% hydrogen peroxide) induction is reasonable in asymptomatic dogs ingesting cyclonite. Some explosives detection dog handlers are taught to immediately induce vomiting in the field with any ingestion that occurs during training scenarios (P. Gahagan, personal communication, 2009). Although there may be some concern for inducing vomiting with an agent known to possess some corrosive potential, the corrosive potential of cyclonite is relatively mild compared with the risk of seizure activity. If cyclonite is mixed with more corrosive materials, the risk of significant corrosive injury should be considered in determining whether to induce vomiting. Activated charcoal may be helpful in reducing absorption. Because of slow and delayed absorption of cyclonite, activated charcoal may be beneficial when there is a delay between ingestion and seeking medical assistance. The addition of a cathartic, such as sorbitol or magnesium sulfate, to activated charcoal may decrease the gastrointestinal (GI) transit time and lessen the absorption of cyclonite.

Clinically affected dogs should be treated supportively. Seizures are typically well controlled with diazepam (0.5–2.0 mg/kg IV).[11] Other antiseizure medication, such as levetiracetam, phenobarbital, or propofol, can also be tried. IV fluids for general support are indicated for seizing dogs. Cessation of seizures generally corrects resultant metabolic acidosis, but acid-base status should also be monitored. GI protectants, such as omeprazole or famotidine along with sucralfate, should be given to protect the GI mucosa. Antiemetics, such as maropitant or metoclopramide, can be used to control vomiting.

Most dogs recover with good supportive care. Depending on the dose, the duration of signs can range between 24 and 72 hours. Outside of a research setting, there are no reported deaths from ingestion of cyclonite.

Nitrate Esters

There are 4 nitrate esters commonly used in explosives applications: nitrocellulose (NC), NG, PETN, and EGDN. Both NG and PETN are also used pharmacologically as potent vasodilators.

NC is a highly flammable compound used as a propellant or low-order explosive. By itself it is considered nontoxic. The toxic concern when NC is ingested is more related to compounds with which it may be combined rather than the NC itself. If ingested as a sole agent, the only expected signs would be mild, self-limiting GI upset secondary to dietary indiscretion.

NG is used in the manufacture of dynamite, gunpowder, and rocket propellants. In addition to its uses in the fields of weapons and explosives, it is also used in human medicine to alleviate the pain associated with angina pectoris and in veterinary medicine as a vasodilator.

With ingestion of NG, the most common sign is hypotension. As with most agents with toxic potential, the dose determines the severity of hypotension. When considering NG as an explosive agent, it would be rare for a dog to ingest just NG. It would be much more common for there to be a coingestion of other agents. The other agent would likely be responsible for the main clinical signs, but with NG as a component, blood pressure monitoring would be important. For most symptomatic dogs that have ingested explosive materials containing NG, the use of IV fluids may be adequate to treat the risk for hypotension in such ingestions.

Because of its nitrate contents, NG has the potential for causing methemoglobinemia. However, this rarely occurs in dogs, as monogastrics compared with ruminants are less likely to convert nitrate to nitrite, which is responsible for oxidizing hemoglobin to methemoglobin. There are some human case reports involving methemoglobinemia, but these involved chronic use of NG and often resulted only in clinically insignificant methemoglobinemia. In dogs, mild methemoglobinemia was induced with a daily dose of 25 mg/kg for 12 months.[17] Significant methemoglobinemia is not expected with acute ingestions of NG in dogs. Dogs ingesting explosive materials containing NG should be treated symptomatically. Most signs in affected dogs will likely be from the non-NG components of the material ingested.

PETN is another nitrate ester commonly used in explosives applications. It is a major component of the detonating cord and is also used in blasting caps and other types of detonators. It is also mixed with cyclonite to form the explosive Semtex. Structurally, PETN resembles NG. Therefore, it also has pharmacologic uses for the treatment of angina pectoris and for its vasodilatory effects in humans. The pharmacologic formulation includes a lactose stabilizer. Removing this stabilizer creates its explosive potential.

In one study, dogs were given 5 mg/kg of PETN via an orogastric tube. A gradual decrease in blood pressure occurred, but it spontaneously resolved.[18] PETN is also absorbed via the respiratory tract in dogs with similar changes in blood pressure.[18]

These studies were conducted with pharmacologic preparations of PETN. Ingestion and inhalation of the less stable explosive formulations may yield different results. As with NG, there is a potential for hypotension following ingestion of PETN containing explosive materials; but the bulk of the clinical signs will likely be more related to the other components. For example, ingestion of Semtex will primarily cause signs related to the cyclonite component, although monitoring of blood pressure as part of the treatment is prudent.

EGDN is the fourth nitrate ester used in explosives applications. The only commercial use is in the production of dynamite, most commonly as an EGDN/NG mixture. Ingestion of dynamite will most likely cause GI upset. With sufficient ingestions, there may be a potential for hypotension, depression, bradycardia, and respiratory depression due to the combined effects of EGDN and NG.

Dogs ingesting dynamite may spontaneously decontaminate themselves by vomiting. For those who do not vomit spontaneously, induction of emesis is prudent. With larger ingestions, activated charcoal following emesis induction is reasonable, followed by monitoring of heart rate and blood pressure. Fluids will help support the blood pressure, lessening the risk for hypotension.

Ammonium Nitrate and Fuel Oil

ANFO has largely replaced dynamite in many commercial mining operations. It also has many military applications. Many explosive slurries and gels are ANFO based. Technically, ANFO is a blasting agent, a combination of an inorganic nitrate and a carbonaceous fuel. Adding an explosive ingredient, such as TNT, changes the classification to an explosive.

Ammonium nitrate when ingested will primarily cause GI signs. Vomiting and diarrhea are both common. Even with large ingestions, GI signs tend to predominate. Methemoglobinemia is rare with nitrate ingestion in dogs compared with the more sensitive ruminants.

Fuel oils used in ANFO are hydrocarbon-based petroleum distillates. Ingestion of petroleum distillates most commonly causes GI signs. When vomiting occurs, there is also the risk of aspiration. The risk for aspiration is related to the volatility of the particular petroleum distillate. The upright stance of humans puts them at higher risk for aspiration following ingestion of petroleum distillates compared with quadrupeds like dogs. Although possible, ingestion of less volatile petroleum distillates by dogs does not commonly cause aspiration. Ingestion of petroleum distillates may also cause CNS signs, including depression, ataxia, seizure, or coma. The mechanisms involved are not fully understood, but theories include hydrocarbons having direct CNS toxic effects.

Because of the explosive potential for ANFO, the individual components are not stored together. Therefore, dogs are more likely to ingest the individual components than ingesting the mixed ANFO products. Ingesting a mixture rather than single petroleum distillate will lower the risk for aspiration, as solids are less likely to be aspirated than volatile liquids. Treatment is symptomatic and supportive. In most cases it is best to avoid inducing vomiting. However, if other, more toxic substances were ingested concurrently with ANFO, inducing vomiting should be considered.

Lead-Based Explosives

The lead-based explosives include LA and LS. Neither of these is currently produced in the United States because of toxic and environmental concerns. There are, however, still stockpiles of LA and LS left over from the Vietnam era and used by the military to make primers.[19] Although highly toxic because of their lead content, because LA and LS are both primary explosives, an animal attempting to ingest them is more likely to suffer extensive trauma from detonation than to safely ingest enough to cause lead toxicosis.

The toxic potential of lead is well known in small animal medicine. When ingested, lead affects the CNS and stability of the red blood cell membrane and causes neuronal damage, cerebral edema, demyelination, and decreased nerve conduction. Several veterinary toxicology books have excellent discussions on lead poisoning and its treatment. The readers are encouraged to seek advice from these articles if they suspect lead poisoning from ingestion of lead-based explosive.

FIREWORKS

Fireworks are low-explosive pyrotechnic devices.[20] Fireworks are divided into 2 main classes: consumer and professional. Consumer fireworks can be purchased by the general public and include firecrackers, rockets, and smoke bombs. Professional (display) fireworks are restricted use and are paper or pasteboard tubing filled with combustible materials.[20] Fireworks contain multiple ingredients that produce noise, light, smoke, or floating materials. These ingredients include fuel (usually black powder), oxidizers (nitrates, chlorates, or perchlorates), color-producing compounds, binders, and reducing agents (sulfur, charcoal).[20] Colors in fireworks are produced by a combination of different metals. The toxicity will vary depending on the compounds contained in the firework. Spent (used) fireworks can have a different composition from unused, and the kinetics and toxicity can vary (increased or decreased).[21]

Laboratory testing is available for most components of fireworks. However, because of the time needed to get results, most laboratory tests are not clinically useful. Emesis may be induced if the animal is asymptomatic and only if noncorrosive agents were ingested. Milk or water can be used to dilute corrosive agents. A gastric lavage can be performed if many noncorrosive agents were ingested. If corrosive compounds have been ingested, gastroprotectants should be started. The animal may need an esophagostomy or gastrostomy tube if severe oral or esophageal burns are evident. Silver sulfadiazine can be used topically for dermal burns. Activated charcoal does not bind to chlorates or heavy metals and should also not be used if corrosive agents were ingested.

The exact composition of the firework is often unknown, so treatment is tailored toward supportive care. Monitoring of renal and liver values may be needed in affected animals for up to 72 hours after ingestion. Oxygen should be administered if the animal appears cyanotic. IV fluids should be used to maintain normal blood pressure and urine production. Ingestion of wood, plastic, metal, or paper components can lead to foreign body obstruction or perforation of the digestive tract.

Aluminum

Aluminum salts are commonly used in sparklers because they produce silver and white flames and sparks.[20] Aluminum is poorly absorbed from the GI tract. Acute aluminum toxicity is unlikely in healthy patients.[22]

Antimony

Antimony (antimony sulfide) is used to produce glitter effects. Antimony compounds are poorly absorbed from the GI tract, but they are locally corrosive.[23] Antimony toxicosis is very rare. Ingestion can cause oral ulcers, vomiting, and bloody diarrhea. GI protectants may help reduce GI irritation.

Barium

Barium salts (barium chloride, barium nitrate) are added to fireworks to produce green colors and to help stabilize other volatile elements.[20] Oral absorption of barium depends on the solubility of the particular barium salt but is generally rapid. Barium can cause severe hypokalemia by blocking the exit of potassium from skeletal muscle.[24] Barium stimulates skeletal, smooth, and cardiac muscle, causing vomiting, diarrhea, salivation, hypertension, and arrhythmias within hours after exposure.[24] Peak serum concentrations are reached usually within 2 hours.[25] Signs can progress to tremors, seizures, paralysis, mydriasis, tachypnea, respiratory failure, and cardiac shock.[24] If no signs develop within 6 to 8 hours of exposure, none are expected. Barium is radiopaque, and magnesium sulfate can be used to precipitate barium in the GI tract and prevent further absorption.[24] Potassium chloride can be used to correct hypokalemia and related cardiac arrhythmias.[24] Antiemetics, fluids, and vasodilators may all be needed for symptomatic and supportive care.

Beryllium

Beryllium produces white sparks when used in fireworks. It is very poorly absorbed from the GI tract, but inhalation can be problematic.[26] Inhaled beryllium is cytotoxic to alveolar macrophages, causing cell death and interstitial fibrosis.[23] Pneumonitis, dyspnea, and pulmonary edema can develop; but exposure to beryllium through inhalation in dogs is very unlikely. Beryllium is also known to be carcinogenic. Oral exposure in dogs may result in self-limiting vomiting.

Calcium

The addition of calcium to fireworks can produce orange colors or can be added to deepen other colors.[20] Calcium salts are poorly absorbed from the GI tract. Most acute oral ingestions of calcium salts produce mild vomiting and diarrhea. Calcium chloride is corrosive and can cause GI hemorrhage. Hypercalcemia is not likely. Sodium chloride diuresis along with furosemide can be used to enhance calcium excretion.[27]

Cesium

Cesium (cesium nitrate) produces indigo colors in fireworks. The toxicity of cesium salts is rarely of importance.[28] The metal can cause dermal burns due to its reactivity with water and oxygen.

Chlorates

Chlorates are found in fireworks as a component of many oxidizers and are used to strengthen the color of the flame. Chlorates are locally irritating and can cause vomiting and diarrhea.[29,30] Orally, chlorates are well absorbed with slow excretion through the kidney (unchanged). Chlorates cause direct damage to the proximal renal tubular cells and severe renal vasoconstriction.[30] Chlorates are also potent oxidizing agents. The oxidation of red blood cells causes hemolysis and methemoglobinemia. Development of methemoglobinemia can be delayed for 1 to 10 hours after exposure. The oral LD_{50} in dogs is 1 g/kg.[29] Elevations in renal values and hyperkalemia can be seen.[21]

Gastric lavage with mineral oil has been suggested to prevent absorption of chlorates.[29] The mineral oil can be mixed with 1% sodium thiosulfate for increased efficacy. Methylene blue (1% injectable solution at 1.0–1.5 mg/kg IV, repeat once in 30 minutes if needed) can be used to convert chlorate-induced methemoglobin back to hemoglobin, although methylene blue is not readily available in most veterinary clinics.[29] If no methylene blue is available, *N*-acetylcysteine (140 mg/kg IV or by mouth then 70 mg/kg by mouth every 8 hours for 5–7 treatments) and ascorbic acid can be tried (20–30 mg/kg intramuscularly every 8 hours) to reverse methemoglobinemia. Do not use ascorbic acid if aluminum has been ingested, as it can enhance aluminum absorption and brain aluminum accumulation. Sodium thiosulfate can also be used to inactivate chlorate ions. On necropsy, chocolate-colored blood and tissues (methemoglobinemia), dark kidneys, and renal tubular necrosis indicate chlorate intoxication.[29]

Copper

Copper salts (copper chloride, copper halides) are used to produce blue colors in fireworks.[31] Copper salts are locally corrosive but have minimal absorption.[31] Gastric protectants should be started. Absorbed copper can cause hemolysis. Metallic copper has little to no toxicity.

Iron

Iron provides gold sparks in fireworks.[20] Iron absorption is a regulated process and excess iron has a corrosive effect on the GI tract.[32] Vomiting, diarrhea, and severe GI irritation/ulcers can result. Excess absorbed iron causes free radical formation and lipid peroxidation. The liver is the most affected organ. Peak serum iron concentrations occur in 2 to 6 hours after ingestion. Large iron ingestions can cause CNS depression, acidosis, liver failure, and shock before death. Magnesium hydroxide will combine with iron to form FeOH, which is poorly absorbed. GI protectants should be started. Deferoxamine is an iron chelator (ascorbic acid increases effectiveness), but it can potentially cause blindness and ototoxicity.[33] Care should be taken if giving deferoxamine to working or service dogs.

Lithium

Lithium carbonate can be used to add red coloration to the fireworks.[20] Soluble lithium salts are quickly absorbed from the GI tract. Lithium affects neuronal metabolism in the CNS, nerve excitation, and synaptic transmission.[34] Peak plasma levels are reached within 2 to 5 hours. Vomiting is common; higher doses can cause tremors, ataxia, and seizures. Diuresis with 0.9% sodium chloride will increase excretion of lithium.

Magnesium

Adding magnesium to fireworks gives white sparks and improved brilliance. Magnesium absorption occurs in the small intestine. Magnesium salts stimulate GI motility and fluid secretions, leading to diarrhea. Large amounts of absorbed magnesium can cause neuromuscular blockade by inhibiting the release of acetylcholine, resulting in flaccid paralysis, hypotension, respiratory depression, and electrocardiographic changes (bradycardia, prolonged PR and QRS interval).[35] Elevations in renal values can also be seen (rare). IV calcium gluconate can reverse respiratory depression induced by hypermagnesemia.[36] Animals with ileus are more at risk for developing magnesium toxicosis.

Nitrates

Nitrates are oxidizing compounds found in fireworks.[20] Sodium nitrate can be added to make gold or yellow colors. Nitrates are converted in vivo to nitrites. Nitrites cause methemoglobinemia. Monogastric animals have a limited ability to perform this action, so they usually do not develop methemoglobinemia with acute ingestions.[37]

Phosphorus

Phosphorus can be found in the fuel part of the firework or can be added for glow-in-the-dark effects. Phosphorus can be absorbed orally, dermally, or by inhalation. The white phosphorus found in fireworks can cause severe hemorrhagic gastroenteritis, abdominal pain, muscular weakness, and possible cardiovascular collapse.[38] When serum phosphorus levels increase, it binds with calcium (calcium phosphate), leading to hypocalcemia, which can be treated with IV calcium gluconate. Hepatic and renal injury can also be seen. N-acetylcysteine can be used to protect against phosphorus-induced liver injury.[39] Phosphorus can also cause electrocardiographic changes (QRS or QT interval changes, ventricular arrhythmias). Decontamination with a copper sulfate (20–100 mL of 0.2% to 0.4% copper sulfate) or potassium permanganate (2–4 mL/kg, 1:10,000 solution) gastric lavage has been suggested to decrease absorption of phosphorus. Phosphorus absorption is enhanced when given with alcohols or fats, so do not dilute with milk. Treatment may include the use of GI protectants, IV fluids, and monitoring of hepatic and renal functions.

Potassium

Potassium (potassium nitrate, potassium perchlorate) plays many roles in fireworks. It provides a violet color and is part of the black powder explosive and oxidative mixture. Potassium is quickly absorbed from the proximal GI tract. Excess potassium causes depolarization of cardiac muscle and increases cardiac muscle excitability, leading to hypotension or hypertension, cardiac dysrhythmias (peaked T waves, small P waves, QRS widening becoming progressively prolonged), heart block, and cardiac arrest.[40] However, animals with normal renal function usually have minimal toxicosis consisting of GI signs only. If animals become symptomatic and show evidence of hyperkalemia, the use of IV sodium bicarbonate will help patients' hyperkalemia by shifting potassium intracellularly. Other measures to treat hyperkalemia can be used as needed (0.9% saline, 5% dextrose, insulin-dextrose combination, and so forth).

Rubidium

Rubidium (rubidium nitrate) is used in fireworks for its violet color and as an oxidizer.[41] Rubidium is considered to be of low toxicity.

Strontium

Strontium (strontium carbonate) is added to fireworks for its brilliant red color and ability to stabilize firework mixtures.[42] It is commonly used because it is inexpensive. Acute ingestions are not expected to cause serious health problems. Signs of mild stomach upset can be seen in dogs.

Sulfur

Sulfur (sulfur dioxide) is found in black powder and reducing agents.[20] Vomiting and diarrhea are common following ingestion.[43] Sulfur can be converted to hydrogen sulfide in the colon by bacteria. Hydrogen sulfide can cause ataxia, arrhythmias, collapse, unconsciousness, pulmonary edema, and death; but these signs from sulfur ingestion are not expected.

Titanium

Titanium is added to fireworks to produce silver sparks. Titanium is biologically inert and practically nontoxic.[44] There is poor GI absorption, and the unchanged metal is excreted in the feces.

Zinc

Zinc produces smoke effects in fireworks. Zinc salts are corrosive and produce vomiting, diarrhea, and GI ulcers.[45] Absorption of soluble zinc salts is highly variable. Zinc metal can be ionized in the stomach and absorbed. Once absorbed, zinc causes hemolytic anemia and secondary renal failure. Zinc may be chelated with calcium disodium EDTA, British Anti-Lewisite (BAL), or D-penicillamine once it is no longer in the GI tract.[45] Most cases of zinc toxicosis do not require treatment with a chelating agent. Zinc toxicosis in dogs usually requires administration of IV fluids and monitoring for hemoglobinuria and renal functions.

SUMMARY

Exposure to explosives and fireworks in dogs can result in variable severity of clinical signs depending on the presence of different chemicals and the amount. The risk can be lessened by proper education of dog handlers and owners about the seriousness of the intoxications. Most animals will recover within 24 to 72 hours with supportive care. Cyclonite, barium, and chlorate ingestion carries a risk of more severe clinical signs.

REFERENCES

1. Commerce in explosives; list of explosive materials. US Federal Register 2010;75: 70291–3.
2. Police K-9 Certification Standards of the National Tactical Police Dog Association, Inc. (NTPDA) for Tracking/Trailing, Patrol, Narcotics Detection, Explosive Detection, Article Search. Certification Standards. Available at: www.tacticalcanine. com/certification-standards/. Accessed May 8, 2018.
3. Explosives: Nitroaromatics. Available at: GlobalSecurity.org Web site; www. globalsecurity.org/military/systems/munitions/explosives-nitroaromatics.htm Accessed May 8, 2018.
4. Dilley JV, Tyson CA, Spanggord RJ, et al. Short-term oral toxicity of 2,4,6-trinitrotoluene in mice, rats, and dogs. J Toxicol Environ Health 1982;9:565–85.
5. Levine BS, Rust JH. Six month oral toxicity study of trinitrotoluene in beagle dogs. Toxicology 1990;63:233–44.
6. Wright RO, Magnani B, Shannon MW, et al. N-Acetylcysteine reduces methemoglobin in vitro. Ann Emerg Med 1996;28:499–503.
7. Tanen DA, LoVecchio F, Curry SC. Failure of intravenous N-acetylcysteine to reduce methemoglobin produced by sodium nitrite in human volunteers: a randomized controlled trial. Ann Emerg Med 2000;35:369–73.
8. Herman MI, Chyka PA, Butlse AY. Methylene blue by intraosseous infusion for methemoglobinemia. Ann Emerg Med 1999;33:111–3.
9. Explosives: Nitramines. Available at: GlobalSecurity.org Web site; www. globalsecurity.org/military/systems/munitions/explosives-nitramines.htm. Accessed May 8, 2018.
10. US Dept of Health and Human Services. Occupational Safety and Health Guideline for Cyclonite. 1995. Available at: www.cdc.gov/niosh/docs/81-123/pdfs/0169. pdf. Accessed May 8, 2018.
11. Bruchim Y, Saragusty J, Weisman A, et al. Cyclonite (RDX) intoxication in a police working dog. Vet Rec 2005;157:354–6.
12. Fishkin RA, Stanley SW, Langston CE. Toxic effects of cyclonite (C-4) plastic explosive ingestion in a dog. J Vet Emerg Crit Care (San Antonio) 2008;18: 537–40.

13. Faust RA. Toxicity summary for hexahydro-1,3,5-trinitro-1,3,5-triazine (RDX). Oak Ridge (TN): Oak Ridge National Laboratory; 1994.
14. Bingham E, Cohrssen B, Powell CH. 5th edition. Patty's toxicology, vols. 1–9. New York: John Wiley & Sons; 2001. p. 616.
15. De Cramer KG, Short RP. Plastic explosive poisoning in dogs. J S Afr Vet Assoc 1992;63:30–1.
16. Burdette LJ, Cook LL, Dyer RS. Convulsant properties of cyclotrimethylenetrinitramine (RDX): spontaneous audiogenic and amygdaloid kindled seizure activity. Toxicol Appl Pharmacol 1988;93:436–44.
17. Ellis HV 3rd, Hong CB, Lee CC, et al. Subacute and chronic toxicity studies of trinitroglycerin in dogs, rats, and mice. Fundam Appl Toxicol 1984;4(Pt 1):248–60.
18. von Oettingen WF, Donahue DD. Acute toxic manifestations of PETN. US Public Health Bull 1944;282:23–30.
19. Oyler KD, Cheng G, Mehta N, et al. Green explosives: potential replacements for lead azide and other toxic detonator and primer constituents. Available at: www.researchgate.net/publication/265224862_GREEN_EXPLOSIVES_POTENTIAL_REPLACEMENTS_FOR_LEAD_AZIDE_AND_OTHER_TOXIC_DETONATOR_AND_PRIMER_CONSTITUENTS. Accessed May 8, 2018.
20. Gondhia R. The chemistry of fireworks. Available at: www.ch.ic.ac.uk/local/projects/gondhia/composition.html. Accessed May 8, 2018.
21. Wismer TA. Matches and fireworks. In: Osweiler GD, Hovda LR, Brutlag AG, editors. Blackwell's Five-minute veterinary consult clinical companion small animal toxicology. Ames (IA): Wiley-Blackwell; 2011. p. 568–73.
22. Henry DA, Goodman WG, Nudelman RK. Parenteral aluminum administration in the dog: IPlasma kinetics, tissue levels, calcium metabolism, and parathyroid hormone. Kidney Int 1984;25:362–9.
23. Gwaltney-Brant SM. Heavy metals. In: Haschek WM, Rousseaux CG, Wallig MA, editors. Handbook of toxicologic pathology. 2nd edition. San Diego (CA): Academic Press; 2002. p. 701–33.
24. Roza O, Berman LB. The pathophysiology of barium: hypokalemic and cardiovascular effects. J Pharmacol Exp Ther 1971;177:433–9.
25. Johnson CH, VanTassell VJ. Acute barium poisoning with respiratory failure and rhabdomyolysis. Ann Emerg Med 1991;20:1138–42.
26. Hathaway GJ, Proctor NH, Hughes JP, editors. Proctor and Hughes' chemical hazards of the workplace. 4th edition. New York: Van Nostrand Reinhold Company; 1996. p. 77–8.
27. Suki WN, Yium JJ, Von Minden M. Acute treatment of hypercalcemia with furosemide. N Engl J Med 1970;283:836–40.
28. ATSDR (Agency for Toxic Substances & Disease Registry). Cesium. Available at: www.atsdr.cdc.gov/ToxProfiles/TP.asp?id=578&tid=107. Accessed May 8, 2018.
29. Sheahan BJ, Pugh DM, Winstanley EW. Experimental sodium chlorate poisoning in dogs. Res Vet Sci 1971;12:387–9.
30. Lee DBN, Brown DL, Baker LRI. Haematological complications of chlorate poisoning. Br Med J 1970;2:31–2.
31. Thompson LJ. Copper. In: Gupta RC, editor. Veterinary toxicology. New York: Elsevier; 2007. p. 427–9.
32. Hooser SB. Iron. In: Gupta RC, editor. Veterinary toxicology. New York: Elsevier; 2007. p. 433–7.
33. Chen SH, Liang DC, Lin HC, et al. Auditory and visual toxicity during deferoxamine therapy in transfusion-dependent patients. J Pediatr Hematol Oncol 2005;27:651–3.

34. Brent J, Klein LJ. Lithium. In: Brent J, Wallace KL, Burkhart KK, editors. Critical care toxicology: diagnosis and management of the critically poisoned patient. Philadelphia: Elsevier Mosby; 2005. p. 523–32.

35. Cumpston KL, Erickson TB, Leikin JB. Poisoning in pregnancy. In: Brent J, Wallace KL, Burkhart KK, editors. Critical care toxicology: diagnosis and management of the critically poisoned patient. Philadelphia: Elsevier Mosby; 2005. p. 134.

36. Brühwiler H, Häfliger M, Lüscher KP. Severe accidental magnesium poisoning in a twins pregnancy in the 32nd week of pregnancy. Geburtshilfe Frauenheilkd 1994;54:184–6.

37. Casteel SW, Evans TJ. Nitrate. In: Plumlee KH, editor. Clinical veterinary toxicology. St Louis (MO): Mosby; 2004. p. 127–30.

38. Thompson LJ. Phosphorus. In: Gupta RC, editor. Veterinary toxicology. New York: Elsevier; 2007. p. 473–4.

39. Panganiban LR. Value of N-acetylcysteine in the management of "Watusi"-induced hepatotoxicity. Vet Hum Toxicol 1993;35:348 [abstract: 127].

40. Mattu A, Brady WJ, Robinson DA. Electrocardiographic manifestations of hyperkalemia. Am J Emerg Med 2000;18:721–9.

41. Lenk W, Prinz H, Steinmetz A. Rubidium and rubidium compounds. Ullmann's Encyclopedia of industrial chemistry. Weinheim (Germany): Wiley-VCH Verlag GmbH & Co; 2010. Available at: http://onlinelibrary.wiley.com/doi/10.1002/14356007.a23_473.pub2/full. Accessed May 8, 2018.

42. Patnaik P. Handbook of inorganic chemicals. New York: McGraw-Hill; 2002. p. 884.

43. Hall JO. Sulfur. In: Gupta RC, editor. Veterinary toxicology. New York: Elsevier; 2007. p. 465–9.

44. Goyer RA, Clarkson TW. Toxic effects of metals. In: Klaassen CD, editor. Casarett & Doull's toxicology: the basic science of poisons. 6th edition. New York: McGraw-Hill; 2001. p. 857.

45. Garland T. Zinc. In: Gupta RC, editor. Veterinary toxicology. New York: Elsevier; 2007. p. 470–2.

Mushroom Poisoning Cases in Dogs and Cats
Diagnosis and Treatment of Hepatotoxic, Neurotoxic, Gastroenterotoxic, Nephrotoxic, and Muscarinic Mushrooms

Birgit Puschner, DVM, PhD[a],*, Colette Wegenast, DVM[b]

KEYWORDS

- Amanita • Amanitins • Hepatotoxic mushrooms • Gastrointestinal irritation
- Liver failure • Neurotoxicosis • Psilocin • Toxicosis

KEY POINTS

- Mushrooms of the genus *Amanita* sp are responsible for most deaths in dogs from mushroom poisoning.
- The toxic compounds in mushrooms can affect the gastrointestinal tract, nervous system (muscarinic, hallucinogenic, excitation), kidneys, and liver.
- Early diagnosis and identification of the mushrooms are important for optimal therapeutic intervention.
- Management is primarily supportive, aimed at decontaminating patients and addressing the clinical problems.

There is no simple test that distinguishes poisonous from nonpoisonous mushrooms, and accurate mushroom identification will require consultation with an experienced mycologist. Although it is estimated that only a few species are lethal, it is not clear how many of the mushrooms worldwide contain potentially toxic compounds. New species are being discovered continuously; for many species, toxicity data are unavailable. In the United States, mushroom poisonings of humans and animals continue to

This article originally appeared in *Veterinary Clinics of North America: Small Animal Practice*, Volume 42, Issue 2, March 2012.
The authors have nothing to disclose.
[a] Department of Molecular Biosciences, School of Veterinary Medicine, University of California, 1120 Haring Hall, Davis, CA 95616, USA; [b] Animal Poison Control Center, American Society for the Prevention of Cruelty to Animals (ASPCA), ASPCA Midwest Office, 1717 South Philo Road, Suite 36, Urbana, IL 61802, USA
* Corresponding author.
E-mail address: bpuschner@ucdavis.edu

be a medical emergency and demand extensive efforts from clinicians and toxicologists. It is challenging to establish a confirmed diagnosis of mushroom poisoning in animals because of limited diagnostic assays for toxin detection. Currently, only the detection of amanitins, psilocin, and psilocybin is available at select veterinary toxicology laboratories. Thus, only limited data on confirmed mushroom poisonings in animals exist. Because the risk of animals ingesting toxic mushrooms, particularly in dogs because of their indiscriminate eating habits, is much greater than the risk for humans, mushroom poisoning in animals is likely underreported.

Human and animal mushroom poisoning cases can be reported to the North American Mycological Association's Mushroom Poisoning Case Registry. Reports may be submitted online at https://www.namyco.org/poisonings.php. In addition, the Web site provides a list of volunteers (http://www.namyco.org/mushroom_poisoning_identifiers.php) willing to assist in the identification of mushrooms. The volunteers are listed by region. Alternatively, many universities have lists of mycologists available for assistance.

INCIDENCES

The American Society for the Prevention of Cruelty to Animals (ASPCA) Animal Poison Control Center (APCC) received 2980 incident reports of potential mushroom exposures in animals between January 1, 2013, and December 31, 2017. Those incidents involved 3085 canine, 49 feline, 3 porcine, and 1 avian single agent mushroom exposure (some incidents involved multiple animals). The months of September and October had the highest number of cases reported to the APCC (**Fig. 1**). Regionally, in the continental United States (**Fig. 2**), 40% of incidents were reported from the Northeast region, followed by the West (23%) with California accounting for most cases (n = 427), Southeast (17%), Midwest (13%), and Southwest (7%). In most (97%) of the reported exposures, the type of mushroom ingested was unknown at the time of the original call to the APCC; thus, the agent was classified as an unknown mushroom. In those cases whereby a specific mushroom was identified, *Psilocybe* spp attributed 69%. These data reflect overall trends; but because of reporting and

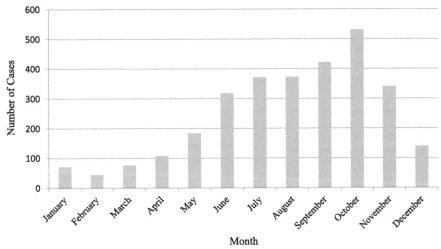

Fig. 1. ASPCA APCC average number of reported mushroom exposure cases by month (January 1, 2013–January 1, 2018).

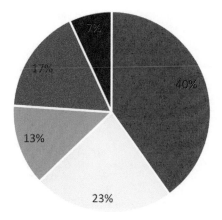

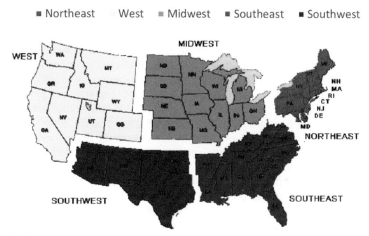

Fig. 2. ASPCA APCC average annual number of reported mushroom exposures by region (January 1, 2013–January 1, 2018).

identification constraints, they are not representative of confirmed exposures/diagnoses of mushroom poisonings. Improved identifications and reporting in small animals may increase the accuracy of incidence data in the future.

HEPATOTOXIC MUSHROOMS

Most confirmed mushroom poisoning cases in animals are caused by hepatotoxic mushrooms that contain cyclopeptides. Although several mushroom genera (*Amanita, Galerina, Lepiota, Cortinarius, Conocybe* spp) contain the hepatotoxic cyclopeptides,[1] *Amanita phalloides* is considered the most toxic worldwide.[2] *A phalloides*, also known as death cap (**Fig. 3**), is found throughout North America with 2 distinct ranges: one on the West Coast from California to British Columbia and one on the East Coast from Maryland to Maine.[3] The mushroom grows commonly in association with oaks, birch, and pine and is the species most frequently resulting in fatalities in humans[4] and probably also in dogs. *A phalloides* is particularly common in the San Francisco Bay area and is most abundant in warm, wet years. The large fruiting bodies appear in the late

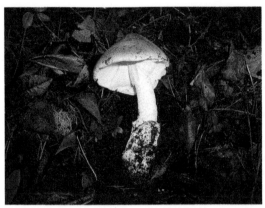

Fig. 3. *Amanita phalloides.* (*Courtesy of* Dr R. Michael Davis, Plant Pathology, University of California, Davis.)

summer and fall and have a smooth, yellowish-green to yellowish-brown cap, white gills, a white ring around the upper part of the stem (veil), and a white cuplike structure around the base of the stem (volva). *A ocreata,* also referred to as the Western North American destroying angel (**Fig. 4**), grows exclusively along the Pacific Coast from Baja California to Washington and is found in sandy soils under oak or pine. *A ocreata* is common in California. The fruiting bodies are found in later winter and spring and have a white or cream-colored cap; white, short gills; a white stem with a white, thin, broken, partial veil; and a white, thin volva. *Amanita bisporigera* is native to Eastern and Midwestern North America and, although genetically very diverse, should be considered highly toxic.[2]

These toxic species contain several different toxins, most notably the amatoxins, which include the hepatotoxic amanitins responsible for most poisonings and fatalities. In humans, the estimated oral median lethal dose (LD_{50}) of α-amanitin is 0.1 mg per kilogram of body weight, which is similar to an oral LD_{50} for methyl-γ-amanitin in dogs of 0.5 mg per kilogram of body weight.[5] On average, species of *A phalloides* and *A ocreata* contain 1.5 to 2.3 mg amanitins per gram of mushroom

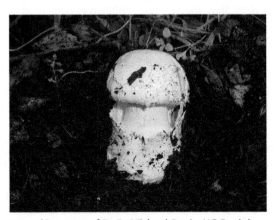

Fig. 4. *Amanita ocreata.* (*Courtesy of* Dr R. Michael Davis, UC Davis.)

dry weight.[6] Therefore, one mushroom cap can contain a lethal dose for an animal or a human.

Amanitins inhibit RNA polymerase II, which shuts down transcription and leads to decreased protein synthesis.[7] Cells with a high metabolic rate, including hepatocytes, crypt cells, and proximal convoluted tubules of the kidneys, are most prone to the toxic effects. Apoptosis of hepatocytes[8,9] and amanitin-induced insulin release[10] are additional effects that contribute to the pathogenesis.

Differences in bioavailability account for differences in species sensitivities. The rate of gastrointestinal (GI) absorption of amanitins is estimated to be much greater in dogs than in mice and rabbits; rats seem relatively resistant to the toxic effects of amanitins. Absorption into the systemic circulation is rapid after which amanitins are distributed to the extravascular space.[11] In the liver, α-amanitin is taken up by hepatocytes via OATP1B3, an organic anion-transporting polypeptide.[12] Amanitins do not undergo metabolism and are primarily excreted unchanged in urine with a small amount (up to 7%) eliminated in bile. In dogs, urinary amanitin concentrations are highest on day 1 but can be detected up to 4 days after exposure.[11] Amanitins are detectable in serum and urine well before any clinical sign of poisoning, whereas routine laboratory tests, such as complete blood count and serum chemistry profiles, are unremarkable until liver or kidney damage has occurred. In humans with *A phalloides* exposure, α- and β-amanitins are present in plasma for up to 36 hours and in urine for up to 72 hours after exposure.[13] In dogs, α- and β-amanitins are detected in plasma within 1 hour of exposure with a plasma half-life ranging from 25 to 50 minutes.[11] Plasma and urine amanitin concentrations do not seem to correlate with the clinical severity or outcome.

Amanitin poisoning is clinically divided into 4 phases, although not all cases present with those 4 consecutive stages.[14] The initial phase is a latency period of approximately 6 to 12 hours, during which no clinical signs of illness occur after the ingestion.[11] During the second phase, poisoned animals develop GI signs (vomiting, diarrhea, evidence of abdominal pain, lethargy, anorexia) between 6 and 24 hours after ingestion. After a period of false recovery of 12 to 24 hours, which signifies the third phase of poisoning, fulminant liver failure develops. During this third phase, close monitoring of liver and kidney function is essential to prevent misdiagnosis. After the GI phase, severe hypoglycemia as a result of the breakdown of liver glycogen can occur.[15] Fifty percent of dogs given lethal doses of amanitins or pieces of *A phalloides* died of hypoglycemia 1 to 2 days after exposure.[5] The fourth and final phase begins 36 to 48 hours after exposure and is characterized by fulminant hepatic failure with subsequent coagulation disorders, encephalopathy, and renal failure. Significant elevations in serum of aspartate aminotransferase, alanine aminotransferase, alkaline phosphatase, and bilirubin are commonly observed.[16] Puppies, or dogs that ingest large amounts of amanitins, can die of amanitin poisoning rapidly, within 24 hours.[17] In a porcine model, decreased albumin and total plasma protein concentrations in the early intoxication phase indicated a lethal outcome.[18]

A tentative diagnosis of hepatotoxic mushroom toxicity can be made based on a history of exposure (witness or suspected exposure), a latency period of 6 to 12 hours before clinical signs are seen, and the types of clinical signs present. Confirmatory diagnosis is made by detection of α-amanitin in serum, urine, gastric contents, suspect mushroom, liver, or kidneys.[19] This testing is provided by select veterinary toxicology laboratories. The well-known Meixner test (also known as the newspaper test of Wieland) should not be relied on alone for amanitin identification.[20] Rapid confirmation of amanitins in suspected exposures assists in the early recognition of exposure and timely therapeutic intervention, whereas a negative result can prevent unnecessary hospitalization. Serum and urine samples should be collected and frozen at various time points beginning as early after exposure as possible. Amanitin has been detected in livers and kidneys of dogs dying of amanitin poisoning. In humans, amanitin concentrations have been detected in livers and kidneys up to 22 days after ingestion and at later time points. Kidneys seem to contain higher concentrations than livers. At necropsy, the liver is often swollen, without any other significant gross abnormalities. Histologically, the liver shows massive hepatocellular necrosis with collapse of hepatic cords[15] and acute tubular necrosis in dogs with renal failure.

There is no specific antidote to treat amanitin intoxication. Despite the evaluation of numerous treatment options, no specific therapy has proved to be effective and the mortality rate in dogs is high. The key elements of treatment are close monitoring, fluid replacement, and supportive care. Activated charcoal at 1 to 2 g/kg by mouth with or without a cathartic like sorbitol (do not use a cathartic if diarrhea is present) followed by 2 or 3 half doses within 24 hours of exposure is recommended. In the past, multidose activated charcoal was recommended. However, recent data indicate that interruption of the enterohepatic circulation of amanitin is unlikely to be effective after 24 hours.[21] Dextrose, vitamin K_1, blood products, and intravenous (IV) fluids must be considered as beneficial therapeutic agents for case management. In Europe, a silibinin-containing product (Legalon-Sil) is a well-established and approved treatment of amanitin poisonings in humans.[22] Silibinin, or silybin, the main component of silymarin, which is extracted from the common milk thistle, *Silybum marianum*, reduces the uptake of amanitins into hepatocytes.[23] In dogs, 50 mg/kg of silibinin IV given at 5 and 24 hours after exposure to *A phalloides* was shown to be effective.[24] Resveratrol (30 mg/kg) given intraperitoneal at 12 and 24 hours after a lethal amanitin exposure to mice prevented and healed hepatotoxicity[25] showing promise as a new treatment approach. Other options include the use of nonspecific hepatoprotective agents like *N*-acetylcysteine (Mucomyst) or *S*-adenosylmethionine (SAMe), although their efficacy remains undetermined. Penicillin G at 1000 mg/kg IV given at 5 hours after dogs were exposed to *A phalloides* was also effective in reducing amanitin uptake into the hepatocytes. However, the efficacy of penicillin G in humans with amanitin poisoning is questionable. Manage vomiting as needed with metoclopramide (0.2–0.4 mg/kg subcutaneously or intramuscularly (IM) every 6 hours or maropitant 1 mg/kg subcutaneously once a day). Extracorporeal decontamination has been used in humans[26]; but efficacy data vary, and no data exist in the veterinary literature. Biliary drainage has been proposed, but therapeutic efficacy must be evaluated.

Hydrazines

Hydrazines are toxins in false morels, *Gyromitra* spp, which are found throughout North America, especially under conifers and aspens. Gyromitrin, the toxin, is estimated at 0.12% to 0.16% in fresh *Gyromitra esculenta*. Although the estimated lethal dose of gyromitrin in humans is 20 to 50 mg/kg for adults and 10 to 30 mg/kg for children,[27] such data are unavailable for dogs or cats. But gyromitrin poisoning is rarely reported in veterinary medicine; only one case report, in a 10-week-old dog, exists.[28] The dog vomited 2 to 3 hours after chewing on a mushroom later identified as *G esculenta*, became lethargic and comatose 6 hours after ingestion, and died 30 minutes later. Gyromitrin is a direct irritant resulting in vomiting and diarrhea within 6 to 12 hours of exposure. The toxin is hydrolyzed in the stomach to monomethylhydrazine, which depletes pyridoxal 5-phosphate resulting in decreased γ-aminobutyric acid (GABA) concentrations and increased glutamic acid concentrations.[29] Clinically, seizures can develop. Additional metabolites of gyromitrin can also result in hemolysis and liver and kidney failure. Diagnosis of gyromitrin poisoning is based on the identification of the mushroom, as detection of gyromitrin is not routinely available. Treatment of gyromitrin poisoning is supportive, including correction of fluid and electrolyte imbalances. Pyridoxine can be given via IV to dogs at 75 to 150 mg per kilogram of body weight during acute phases of seizure activity.[30] Diazepam can also be considered for seizure control at 0.5 to 1.0 mg/kg IV to effect.

Isoxazoles

Ibotenic acid and muscimol are chemically classified as isoxazoles, which are most commonly associated with exposures to *Amanita pantherina* (panther cap, panther agaric) and *Amanita muscaria* (fly agaric). These mushrooms are found throughout the United States but are most abundant in the Pacific Northwest in the summer and fall, where they are often found in coniferous and deciduous forests. Clinical signs of poisoning in humans occur with exposures greater than 6 mg of muscimol or 30 to 60 mg of ibotenic acid.[31] The concentration of ibotenic acid in *A muscaria* is estimated to be at 100 mg/kg fresh, whereas the concentration of muscimol is less than 3 mg per kilogram of fresh weight. Therefore, an average-size, 60- to 70-g fruiting body of *A muscaria* can contain a toxic concentration of isoxazoles. Although the toxicity of isoxazoles is not well documented in dogs, postmortem examination of puppies indicated that ingestion of a single *A pantherina* can be lethal.[32] Although both muscimol and ibotenic acid are present in the mushrooms, muscimol is further derived from ibotenic acid by spontaneous decarboxylation, which can occur during drying of the mushroom, during digestion in the stomach, or after absorption in a variety of tissues. Therefore, muscimol is considered the major toxin responsible for causing clinical signs of toxicosis. Muscimol increases the membrane permeability for anions resulting in a slight, short-lasting hyperpolarization and associated decreased excitability of the receptive neuron. Muscimol also acts on $GABA_A$ receptors and has a depressant action.[33] Neurologic signs in animals include disorientation, opisthotonus, paresis, seizures, paddling, chewing movements, miosis, vestibular signs (ataxia, head tilt, nystagmus, circling, and so forth), respiratory depression, and, in severe cases, coma. In humans, muscimol intoxication is referred to as the pantherine-muscaria syndrome, which is characterized by mydriasis, dryness of the mouth, ataxia, confusion, euphoria, dizziness, and tiredness within 0.5 to 2.0 hours of ingestion, followed by full recovery within 1 to 2 days. Similar clinical signs have been described in cats,[34] while favorable[35] and lethal outcomes have been described in dogs with isoxazole exposure.[32,36] Diagnosis of isoxazole poisoning is based on the history of exposure to a mushroom, quick onset of clinical signs (within hours of exposure), the type of clinical signs (hallucinations and other central nervous system [CNS] effects), and identification of the mushroom. Although muscimol and ibotenic acid are excreted in urine shortly after exposure, routine diagnostic tests are not available. Treatment of isoxazole poisoning is supportive, with focus on seizure control. Early decontamination (induction of emesis and administration of activated charcoal) can be tried in asymptomatic animals. Because of the GABAergic effects of muscimol and ibotenic acid, medications with GABA agonist effects, such as diazepam or phenobarbital, should be used with caution. The use of these medications in a poisoned animal to control seizures may further aggravate CNS and respiratory depression. Thus, if such drugs are used, the animal's respiration should be carefully monitored for need of mechanical ventilation.

Psilocin and Psilocybin

Mushrooms in the genera *Psilocybe*, *Panaeolus*, *Conocybe*, and *Gymnopilus* contain primarily psilocybin, with some also containing psilocin. These mushrooms grow predominantly in fields and animal pastures in the Northwestern and Southeastern United States. The toxin concentrations depend on location, growing conditions, storage conditions, and species. Species common to the Pacific Northwest contain between 1.2 and 16.8 mg/kg psilocybin on a dry weight basis.[37] Oral doses of 10 to 20 mg of psilocybin result in hallucinations in people. Toxicity data for domestic animals do not exist. Psilocin is pharmacologically the most active metabolite of psilocybin after dephosphorylation in plasma, livers, and kidneys.[38] Psilocin is structurally similar to serotonin and activates some serotonin receptors in the CNS,[39] leading to lysergic acid diethylamine–like clinical effects. In the United States, United Kingdom, and Germany, psilocybin and psilocin are classified as controlled substances; mushrooms containing those substances are called magic or hallucinogenic mushrooms. People consuming those mushrooms generally have hallucinations for approximately 1 hour and have full recovery within 12 hours. In dogs, exposure to psilocybin-containing mushrooms can result in aggression, ataxia, vocalization, nystagmus, seizures, and increased body temperature.[40] Exposure can be confirmed by detection of psilocin and psilocybin in urine by select veterinary diagnostic laboratories. Because of the short-lasting effects, mild cases may resolve themselves without treatment. Symptomatic and supportive treatment may be necessary when severe clinical signs are present. Seizures can be controlled with diazepam or phenobarbital.

MUSCARINE-CONTAINING MUSHROOMS

The most common muscarine-containing mushrooms include *Inocybe* spp and *Clitocybe* spp. The largest numbers of mushroom species that contain significant amounts of muscarine belong in these 2 genera.[41] These mushrooms are nondescript little brown mushrooms, although some may be other colors such as white or cream.[34] They can be found in forests, lawns, and parks and fruit in summer and fall, although some fruit year round.[42] Several other genera, such as *Mycena*, *Boletus*, *Entoloma*, and *Omphalotus*, are suspected to contain significant muscarine levels.[41,42] Muscarine is also present in low concentrations in other mushrooms, such as *Amanita muscaria*.[41]

Muscarine is a thermostable muscarinic receptor agonist that binds to acetylcholine receptors in the peripheral nervous system.[41] Stimulation of postganglionic neurons results in parasympathomimetic effects. Unlike acetylcholine, it is not degraded by acetylcholinesterase; toxicity results from unregulated stimulation at the receptors.[41,43] Organophosphates and carbamates can produce similar muscarinic signs; however, they act by inhibition of acetylcholinesterase, which increases the amount of acetylcholine at the receptors. There may also be muscarinic compounds that produce a histaminic effect resulting in flushing, hypotension, and wheezing.

Clinical signs can occur rapidly (often within 5–30 minutes) and mostly within 2 hours of ingestion.[41,43,44] Signs include salivation, lacrimation, urination, diarrhea, dyspnea, and emesis (often described by the acronym SLUDDE). Dyspnea develops in response to increased bronchial secretions and bronchoconstriction. Bradycardia, miosis, hypotension, and abdominal pain are also possible. In the authors' experience, dogs suspected of ingesting muscarinic mushrooms often present with a history of acute onset of vomiting, severe diarrhea, and ptyalism. The saliva may be described as thick and ropey. Differential diagnoses include exposure to pesticides, such as organophosphates, and carbamates and mycotoxins like slaframine. Exposure to cholinesterase-inhibiting pesticides, such as organophosphates and carbamates, may also result in nicotinic signs, such as tremors, muscle weakness, and seizures. Unlike these pesticides, muscarine does not stimulate nicotinic receptors or cross the blood-brain barrier.[41,43] Consequently, nicotinic and direct CNS effects are not expected. Depression may develop as a result of hypotension or hypoxia.[41]

Diagnosis is based on the rapid onset of clinical signs, the type of clinical signs (SLUDDE), and response to treatment. Muscarine has been detected in urine, and analysis could be considered for confirmation of exposure. Identification of the mushrooms from the environment and/or vomitus may also be used to support the diagnosis.

Decontamination includes induction of emesis and administration of activated charcoal in asymptomatic animals following ingestion of mushrooms. The rapid onset of signs (which may include vomiting) following muscarinic mushroom ingestion often makes decontamination unfeasible. Atropine competes with muscarine at the receptors and is the recommended treatment. In dogs and cats, the beginning dosage is 0.04 mg/kg with one-fourth of the dose given via IV and the remainder given subcutaneously or IM.[45] The dosage can be titrated up and repeated if needed to control severe signs. Overatropinization should be avoided and can result in anticholinergic signs, including tachycardia, hyperthermia, behavior changes, and GI stasis. Signs typically respond well to atropine and resolve within 30 minutes of administration. Without treatment, signs may persist for several hours. Supportive care (IV fluids) should be provided as needed. Patients can be provided oral electrolyte supplement and oral probiotics for up to 3 days after discharge.[44] The prognosis, in most cases, is good and long-term effects are not expected.

MUSHROOMS RESULTING IN GASTROINTESTINAL IRRITATION

Mushrooms that result in primarily GI signs are grouped under this category. Specific genera include *Agaricus, Boletus, Chlorophyllum, Entoloma, Gomphus, Hebeloma, Lactarius, Naematoloma, Omphalotus, Ramaria, Rhodophyllus, Russula, Scleroderma, Tricholoma*, and others. These mushrooms have a wide distribution and variation in appearance and substrate.

The toxins in most species have not been identified. Illudin S is thought to be a toxic component in some *Omphalotus* and *Lampteromyces* species.[46] Illudins are cytotoxic and produced hemorrhagic lesions in animal studies.[46] *Omphalotus illudens* also produces a muscarinelike effect, although muscarine has not been isolated.[47] Suspected toxins in other species include monoterpenes, norcaperatic acid, hebelomic acid A, cucurbitane-type triterpene glycosides, lectins, marasmane/lactarane sesquiterpenes, and phenethylamines. Proposed mechanisms include hypersensitivity, idiosyncratic reactions, some enzyme deficiencies, and local GI irritation.[47] Some of the mushrooms in this category are edible, although even the edible species can result in GI signs in sensitive individuals. Some of the toxins are inactivated by cooking.

The onset of clinical signs is fairly fast, and signs are expected within 15 minutes to several hours after ingestion.[48] Vomiting, diarrhea, and abdominal discomfort are common signs. Other signs may include lethargy, hypersalivation, hematemesis, and hematochezia. Secondary electrolyte abnormalities and hypovolemia may develop. A 1-year-old cat ingested one-half of an *Agaricus* spp cap and developed foaming, vomiting, diarrhea, and disorientation. Hematemesis developed in another cat that ingested an unknown species of *Russula*. The mushroom was described as having a shellfish odor, which may have attracted the cat.[49] There is also a report of a 7-month-old potbellied pig that developed vomiting, weakness, hypothermia, abdominal pain, tachycardia, and tachypnea within 1 hour of ingestion of *Scleroderma citrinum*. The pig died within 5 hours despite treatment with fluids and dexamethasone.[50] Differential diagnoses for GI irritant mushrooms include many other causes of acute gastroenteritis, such as dietary indiscretion, garbage poisoning, foreign body ingestion, pancreatitis, bacterial or viral gastroenteritis, ingestion of corrosive or irritating agents, and ingestion of GI irritant plants.

Diagnosis is supported by the history, clinical signs, and evidence of mushrooms in the vomitus. The mushrooms should be saved for identification. It is important to note that GI upset is also an initial sign following ingestion of more dangerous hepatotoxic and nephrotoxic mushrooms, although the onset is typically more delayed. A complete blood count, chemistry panel, and radiographs may be performed to assess the clinical picture and help rule out other causes for the signs. In severe cases, electrolyte and acid-base status should be monitored and corrected as needed.

Decontamination includes emesis and activated charcoal in asymptomatic animals following ingestion of mushrooms. The potential rapid onset of vomiting may make decontamination following ingestion of GI irritant mushrooms less feasible. Treatment is symptomatic and supportive and depends on the extent of signs. IV fluids are recommended to maintain hydration. Sucralfate, H2 blockers (famotidine), and/or proton pump inhibitors (omeprazole) may be used to reduce mucosal irritation. Vomiting should be controlled with antiemetics, such as maropitant and metoclopramide. Many cases are self-limiting and resolve without treatment. The severity of signs depends on the type of mushroom, amount ingested, and individual sensitivity. In most cases, the prognosis is good and full recovery is expected within a few hours to days.

NEPHROTOXIC MUSHROOMS

Some species of mushrooms in the genus *Cortinarius* are nephrotoxic. These mushrooms were first noted to be toxic in Poland in the 1950s.[41,51] Although they are found throughout Europe and North America, reports of toxicity have been rare in North America. There is a report of a woman who developed renal failure after ingesting *Cortinarius orellanosus* mushrooms from under an oak tree in Michigan.[52] *Cortinarius armillatus* is found in the Northeastern United States.[53] To the authors' knowledge, there have been no confirmed cases of accidental animal poisoning resulting from nephrotoxic mushrooms in North America.

The mushrooms are often a rusty or reddish brown color. Webcap is a common name used because of the presence of a cortina or spiderweb-like veil that connects the edge of the cap to the stem in the immature stages. The cortina is not recognizable in adult mushrooms.[42] *Cortinarius* sp grows in forests and mountains and is rare in urban areas.[41] These mushrooms most commonly fruit between August and October.[54]

The bipyridyl toxin orellanine is thought to be the main toxin in *Cortinarius* sp mushrooms. Orelline and orellinine are 2 thermal and photodegradation products that have been identified. These toxins are thought to inhibit protein synthesis in renal tubular epithelium. Another theory is that the toxins reduce cellular NADPH, which results in free radical damage, lipid peroxidation, and membrane destruction.[41] There is a lag time between ingestion and development of signs, which suggests metabolism to an active form of the toxin. Another toxin, a cyclopeptide named cortinarin, has been isolated from some species. Cortinarins A, B, and C have been described. In the liver, cortinarin A is thought to be metabolized to cortinarin B, which is then converted to its sulfoxide form via cytochrome P450 enzymes. Cortinarins A and B sulfoxide are nephrotoxic. Females seem to be more resistant to the toxin than males. This difference may be due to differing binding capacities in the cytochrome P450 system.[41] There is still some controversy over the toxins present in *Cortinarius* sp and their relationship to each other and the nephrotoxicity associated with these mushrooms. Toxicity is not affected by cooking, canning, or drying of the mushrooms.

Interestingly, experimentation in rats has shown significant individual variation in susceptibility. In one study, 20% to 30% of rats were resistant to toxicity even at high dosages.[55]

There is a latent phase between ingestion and the onset of signs. GI signs may occur within 72 hours. Within 3 to 20 days, signs of renal failure may develop. In humans, increased thirst, flank pain, chills, and night sweats have been described. Oliguria followed by diuresis and recovery or chronic renal failure may occur. *Cortinarius orellanus* resulted in signs similar to those noted in humans when given orally to the cat, guinea pig, and mouse experimentally. The main damage was to the renal tubular epithelium.[51,56] In animals, vomiting, diarrhea, polyuria, polydipsia, abdominal pain, and depression may be noted. Differential diagnoses include other causes for GI upset and acute renal failure, such as grape or raisin ingestion, nonsteroidal antiinflammatory drugs, ethylene glycol, lily ingestion (cats), and leptospirosis.

Diagnostic tests to monitor renal values and a complete clinical assessment include a complete blood count and serum chemistry. In addition, urinalysis may reveal isosthenuria, glucosuria, pyuria, proteinuria, cylindruria, and hematuria. Acid-base status and electrolytes should also be monitored. Liver enzymes are expected to remain normal. Orellanine can be detected in mushrooms,[53] stomach contents, and urine within 24 hours of the exposure. Unfortunately, because of the lag time between ingestion and onset of signs, this may not be clinically useful.[41] The clinical signs and laboratory findings are not specific for *Cortinarius* sp ingestion. Because of the rarity of animal poisoning in North America, diagnosis should be made based on the history, mushroom identification if possible, and ruling out more likely causes of renal failure/damage. Renal biopsy may also be useful. In humans, renal biopsies have revealed interstitial edema, interstitial nephritis, and acute tubular necrosis.[52] Thin-layer chromatography has detected orellanine in renal biopsy samples up to 6 months after ingestion. Orellanine has also been measured in human plasma.

Decontamination includes emesis and activated charcoal in asymptomatic animals following ingestion of mushrooms. However, because of the long latent period, patients may not be presented until days after the exposure and the opportunity for decontamination is missed. Treatment consists of supportive care for renal failure and GI signs. IV fluids, GI protectants (sucralfate, famotidine, ranitidine, or omeprazole), and antiemetics (maropitant, metoclopramide) may be used. In humans, chronic hemodialysis is often necessary; in some cases, renal transplant is performed. In humans, forced diuresis is not recommended because of increased renal damage.[57] Furosemide increased toxicity in rats when injected before *Cortinarius orellanoides* ingestion.[55] In animals, peritoneal or hemodialysis could be considered. Experimental treatments, in humans, include use of corticosteroids, *N*-acetylcysteine, and selenium. The results have not been conclusive.[36]

The prognosis following ingestion of nephrotoxic *Cortinarius* sp varies. There seems to be a dosage-dependent aspect as well as individual variation. In humans, renal failure has been reported to occur in 30% to 40% of cases. This effect may be followed by a slow return to normal function or development into chronic renal failure, which requires hemodialysis and/or transplantation. A shorter latent period usually indicates a worse prognosis.[36]

SUMMARY

There are numerous types of mushrooms that are ingested by small animals, mostly dogs. Although many are not toxic, some mushrooms can result in hepatotoxic, neurologic, cardiovascular, hemolytic, muscarinic, GI, and/or nephrotoxic effects. Gross identification by nonmycologists is often not effective, so it is safest to assume that any mushroom ingested may potentially be toxic until or unless identification is accomplished. It should also be assumed that more than one kind of mushroom could be ingested in a single exposure.

Following ingestion of an unknown mushroom in small animals, decontamination should consist of induction of emesis in dogs with 3% hydrogen peroxide (2.2 mL/kg by mouth) or apomorphine (0.03 mg/kg IV, or a crushed tablet dissolved in saline solution, instilled in the conjunctival sac) and in cats with dexmedetomidine (7.0 μg of dexmedetomidine per kilogram IM or 3.5 μg of dexmedetomidine per kilogram IV or xylazine [0.44 mg/kg IM] followed by administration of activated charcoal [1–2 g/kg]) orally in asymptomatic animals. The vomitus should be examined for the presence of mushrooms. Mushroom specimens from the vomitus and/or other similar mushrooms from the animal's environment should be saved for identification. Do not save mushrooms in plastic bags. Instead, place them in a paper bag, towel, or a newspaper. Refrigerate the specimen until shipped out for identification. Specimens should be labeled and dated properly. Information regarding a brief history of exposure, chronology of onset time and types of clinical signs, blood and chemistry changes, treatment used, and response to treatment should be sent to the veterinary diagnostic laboratory when needed.

Baseline complete blood count and chemistry panels should be obtained and repeated as needed. The animal should be monitored at the clinic for several hours for the onset of CNS, cardiovascular, muscarinic, and GI signs. Also, during this time, the animal can be monitored for hypernatremia that may occur following administration of activated charcoal. If signs develop, or are present at the time of presentation, the animal should be treated accordingly. If no signs develop, the animal can be monitored on an outpatient basis for the development of delayed (often beyond 6–8 hours) GI signs that often precede more severe effects associated with the hepatotoxic, hemolytic, and nephrotoxic mushrooms. Typically signs are expected within 4 hours following ingestion of isoxazoles, GI irritants, muscarine, and psilocybins. If the onset of vomiting, diarrhea, and abdominal pain are delayed beyond 6 to 8 hours, it increases the suspicion that the more serious amatoxin, gyromitrin, or orellanine (rare) toxins have been ingested. In asymptomatic animals, serum chemistries could be monitored daily for up to 4 days after ingestion. SAMe could be initiated as a potential liver protectant in case amatoxin was ingested.

REFERENCES

1. Lincoff G, Mitchel D. Cyclopeptide poisoning. Toxic and hallucinogenic mushroom poisoning. A handbook for physicians and mushroom hunters. London: Van Nostrand Reinhold Company; 1977. p. 25–48.
2. Walton J. Distribution and taxonomic variation in the amanita cyclic peptide toxins. the cyclic peptide toxins of amanita and other poisonous mushrooms. Cham (Switzerland): Springer International Publishing; 2018. p. 59–91.
3. Wolfe BE, Richard F, Cross HB, et al. Distribution and abundance of the introduced ectomycorrhizal fungus Amanita phalloides in North America. New Phytol 2010;185(3):803–16.
4. Mitchel DH. Amanita mushroom poisoning. Annu Rev Med 1980;31(1):51–7.
5. Faulstich H, Fauser U. The course of Amanita intoxication in beagle dogs. In: Faulstich H, Kommerell B, Wieland T, editors. Amanita toxins and poisoning. Baden-Baden (Germany): Verlag Gerhard Witzstrock; 1980. p. 115–23.

6. Duffy TJ. Toxic fungi of Western North America. Secondary Toxic fungi of Western North America 2008. Available at: http://www.mykoweb.com. Accessed May 16, 2018.

7. Lindell TJ, Weinberg F, Morris PW, et al. Specific inhibition of nuclear RNA polymerase II by alpha-amanitin. Science 1970;170(3956):447–9.

8. Magdalan J, Ostrowska A, Piotrowska A, et al. alpha-Amanitin induced apoptosis in primary cultured dog hepatocytes. Folia Histochem Cytobiol 2010;48(1):58–62.

9. Garcia J, Costa VM, Carvalho A, et al. Amanita phalloides poisoning: mechanisms of toxicity and treatment. Food Chem Toxicol 2015;86:41–55.

10. De Carlo E, Milanesi A, Martini C, et al. Effects of Amanita phalloides toxins on insulin release: in vivo and in vitro studies. Arch Toxicol 2003;77(8):441–5.

11. Sun J, Niu Y-M, Zhang Y-T, et al. Toxicity and toxicokinetics of Amanita exitialis in beagle dogs. Toxicon 2018;143:59–67.

12. Letschert K, Faulstich H, Keller D, et al. Molecular characterization and inhibition of amanitin uptake into human hepatocytes. Toxicol Sci 2006;91(1):140–9.

13. Jaeger A, Jehl F, Flesch F, et al. Kinetics of amatoxins in human poisoning: therapeutic implications. J Toxicol Clin Toxicol 1993;31(1):63–80.

14. Stein CM, Wu PE, Scott JA, et al. Fulminant hepatic failure following ingestion of wild mushrooms. Can Med Assoc J 2015;187(11):822–4.

15. Puschner B, Rose HH, Filigenzi MS. Diagnosis of Amanita toxicosis in a dog with acute hepatic necrosis. J Vet Diagn Invest 2007;19(3):312–7.

16. Kallet A, Sousa C, Spangler W. Mushroom (Amanita phalloides) toxicity in dogs. Calif Vet 1988;42(1):9–11, 22, 47.

17. Cole FM. A puppy death and amanita-phalloides. Aust Vet J 1993;70(7):271–2.

18. Thiel K, Schenk M, Sipos B, et al. Acute liver failure after amanitin poisoning: a porcine model to detect prognostic markers for liver regeneration. Hepatol Int 2014;8(1):128–36.

19. Filigenzi MS, Poppenga RH, Tiwary AK, et al. Determination of alpha-amanitin in serum and liver by multistage linear ion trap mass spectrometry. J Agric Food Chem 2007;55(8):2784–90.

20. Beuhler M, Lee DC, Gerkin R. The Meixner test in the detection of alpha-amanitin and false-positive reactions caused by psilocin and 5-substituted tryptamines. Ann Emerg Med 2004;44(2):114–20.

21. Thiel C, Thiel K, Klingert W, et al. The enterohepatic circulation of amanitin: kinetics and therapeutical implications. Toxicol Lett 2011;203(2):142–6.

22. Karlson-Stiber C, Persson H. Cytotoxic fungi–an overview. Toxicon 2003;42(4):339–49.

23. Abenavoli L, Capasso R, Milic N, et al. Milk thistle in liver diseases: past, present, future. Phytother Res 2010;24(10):1423–32.

24. Vogel G, Tuchweber B, Trost W, et al. Protection by silibinin against Amanita phalloides intoxication in beagles. Toxicol Appl Pharmacol 1984;73(3):355–62.

25. Sahin A, Arici MA, Yilmaz Y, et al. A comparison of the effectiveness of silibinin and resveratrol in preventing alpha-amanitin-induced hepatotoxicity. Basic Clin Pharmacol Toxicol 2018;122(6):633–42.

26. Mullins ME, Horowitz BZ. The futility of hemoperfusion and hemodialysis in Amanita phalloides poisoning. Vet Hum Toxicol 2000;42(2):90–1.

27. Schmidlin-Mészáros J. Gyromitrin in Trockenlorcheln (Gyromitra esculenta sicc.). Mitt Geb Lebensmittelunters Hyg 1974;65(4):453–65.

28. Bernard MA. Mushroom poisoning in a dog. Can Vet J 1979;20(3):82–3.

29. Lheureux P, Penaloza A, Gris M. Pyridoxine in clinical toxicology: a review. Eur J Emerg Med 2005;12(2):78–85.

30. Villar D, Knight MK, Holding J, et al. Treatment of acute isoniazid overdose in dogs. Vet Hum Toxicol 1995;37(5):473–7.

31. Halpern JH. Hallucinogens and dissociative agents naturally growing in the United States. Pharmacol Ther 2004;102(2):131–8.

32. Hunt RS, Funk A. Mushrooms fatal to dogs. Mycologia 1977;69(2):432–3.

33. Chebib M, Johnston GA. The 'ABC' of GABA receptors: a brief review. Clin Exp Pharmacol Physiol 1999;26(11):937–40.

34. Ridgway RL. Mushroom (Amanita pantherina) poisoning. J Am Vet Med Assoc 1978;172(6):681–2.

35. Martin JG. Mycetism (mushroom poisoning) in a dog. Vet Med 1956;51:227–8.

36. Naude TW, Berry WL. Suspected poisoning of puppies by the mushroom Amanita pantherina. J S Afr Vet Assoc 1997;68(4):154–8.

37. Smolinske SC. Psilocybin-containing mushrooms. In: Spoerke DG, Rumack BH, editors. Handbook of mushroom poisoning. diagnosis and treatment. Boca Raton (FL): CRC Press; 1994. p. 309–24.

38. Grieshaber AF, Moore KA, Levine B. The detection of psilocin in human urine. J Forensic Sci 2001;46(3):627–30.

39. Halberstadt AL, Koedood L, Powell SB, et al. Differential contributions of serotonin receptors to the behavioral effects of indoleamine hallucinogens in mice. J Psychopharmacol 2011;25(11):1548–61.

40. Kirwan AP. 'Magic mushroom' poisoning in a dog. Vet Rec 1990;126(6):149.

41. Benjamin DR. Mushrooms: poisons and panaceas. New York: WH Freeman and Co; 1995.

42. Turner NJ, Szczawinski AF. Common poisonous plants and mushrooms of North America. Timber Press Inc; 1991.

43. Goldfrank L. Mushrooms. In: Nelson SL, Lewin AN, Howland MA, editors. Goldfrank's toxicologic emergencies. 9th edition. New York: McGraw-Hill; 2011. p. 1522–34.

44. Seljetun KO, Krogh A. Acute Inocybe mushroom toxicosis in dogs: 5 cases (2010–2014). J Vet Emerg Crit Care (San Antonio) 2017;27(2):212–7.

45. Papich MG. Saunders handbook of veterinary drugs-e-book: small and large animal. Elsevier Health Sciences; 2015.

46. Bresinsky A, Besl H. A colour atlas of poisonous fungi. A handbook for pharmacists, doctors, and biologists. London: Wolfe Publishing Co; 1990.

47. Rumack BH, Spoerke DG. Handbook of mushroom poisoning: diagnosis and treatment. Boca Raton (FL): CRC press; 1994.

48. Puschner B. Chapter 62-Mushrooms A2-Peterson, Michael E. In: Talcott PA, editor. Small animal toxicology. 3rd edition. St Louis (MO): W.B. Saunders; 2013. p. 659–76.

49. Shaw M. Reported case of Russula ingestion in a cat. In: Cochran KW, editor. North American mycological association report. 1986–87 annual progress report. Grand Rapids (MI): Grand Rapids Poison Center; 1986.

50. Galey FD, Rutherford JJ, Wells K. A Case of Scleroderma-Citrinum Poisoning in a Miniature Chinese Potbellied Pig. Vet Hum Toxicol 1990;32(4):329–30.

51. Michelot D, Tebbett I. Poisoning by Members of the Genus Cortinarius - a review. Mycol Res 1990;94:289–98.

52. Judge BS, Ammirati JF, Lincoff GH, et al. Ingestion of a newly described North American mushroom species from Michigan resulting in chronic renal failure: cortinarius orellanosus. Clin Toxicol 2010;48(6):545–9.

53. Shao D, Tang S, Healy RA, et al. A novel orellanine containing mushroom Cortinarius armillatus. Toxicon 2016;114:65–74.

54. Berger KJ, Guss DA. Mycotoxins revisited: part II. J Emerg Med 2005;28(2): 175–83.
55. Nieminen L, Pyy K. Individual variation in mushroom poisoning induced in the male rate by Cortinarius speciosissimus. Med Biol 1976;54(2):156–8.
56. Gerault A. Intoxication collective de type orellanien provoquée par Cortinarius splendens R Hy. Bull Trimest Soc Mycol Fr 1981;97:67–72.
57. Michelot D, Toth B. Poisoning by Gyromitra esculenta–a review. J Appl Toxicol 1991;11(4):235–43.

Differential Diagnosis of Common Acute Toxicologic Versus Nontoxicologic Illness

Safdar A. Khan, DVM, MS, PhD[a,b,]*

KEYWORDS

- Differential diagnosis • Small animal poisoning • Toxicologic illness
- Nontoxicologic illness

CASE HISTORY

Upon presentation of an acutely ill animal, a veterinary professional must consider poisoning as a potential cause among the differentials. A complete and thorough case history in this regard is essential for differentiating a poisoning situation from a naturally occurring disease. Obtaining a clear recent history may sometimes be quite challenging, especially in situations where the pet was unsupervised before the initiation of clinical signs. History questions must include animal signalment (breed, sex, and age) and weight, previous medical history, vaccination history, type of feed used (brand; home-made or commercial) and any medications the pet is taking. Initial information about any other animals present in the household, timeline of clinical signs, types of clinical signs reported by the owner, number of affected animals, pet's environment (indoor vs. outdoor; fenced or free roaming), location (urban vs. rural), time of the year (summer vs. winter), recent renovations/updates (construction material; lead in older farms/houses), recent visitors, availability of human medications in the pet's environment (antidepressants, pain killers, stimulants, nutritional supplements), presence or recent use of chemicals (insecticides, herbicides, rodenticides) in the house/yard, information about neighboring animals (outbreaks; illnesses; death) and information about indoor/outdoor plants may help provide clues to the clinician to narrow down the search for a possible

This article was adapted and modified with permission from Khan SA. Intoxication versus Acute, Nontoxicologic Illness: Differentiating the Two. In: Ettinger SJ, Feldman EC, Côté E, editors. Textbook of Veterinary Internal Medicine. 8th Edition. St. Louis (MO): Saunder Elsevier; 2017. Chapter 13, p. 63–68.

The author has nothing to disclose. The views and opinions expressed in this article are those of author and do not necessarily reflect policy or position of the editors or their employer or the publisher.

[a] ASPCA Animal Poison Control Center, 1717 South Philo Road, Suite 36, Urbana, IL 61802, USA;
[b] Global Pharmacovigilance, Zoetis, 333 Portage Street, Kalamazoo, MI 49007-9970, USA
* Corresponding author. Global Pharmacovigilance, Zoetis, 333 Portage Street, Kalamazoo, MI 49007-9970.
E-mail address: Safdar.Khan@zoetis.com

cause for the pet's illness. A good case history can help speed up the process of narrowing down a potential cause; eliminate several unnecessary steps, save time, and money.

STABILIZING THE PATIENT

Before obtaining a complete case history, the first goal should be to stabilize the patient and preserve life of the acutely ill animal irrespective of the cause. Relying too much on specific antidotal treatment may be dangerous. A majority of clinical cases on presentation are treated supportively as only a very few specific antidotes are available or needed for treating specific poisonings. Therefore, on presentation, make sure the animal has a patent airway and adequate ventilation. Support and maintain cardiac functions. Monitor heart rate, rhythm, and blood pressure, and treat cardiac arrhythmias and blood pressure changes as needed. Hydration status, fluids, electrolytes, and acid-base balance should be checked and corrected accordingly. Treat central nervous system abnormalities (excitation, depression, seizures) as required, and maintain body temperature within the normal range (treat hypothermia or hyperthermia). After stabilizing the vital functions, obtain a history; then, provide other necessary treatment such as decontamination (administration of activated charcoal, gastric lavage, bathing, dilution), supportive care, and carrying out other diagnostics (complete blood count, chemistries, urinalysis, radiographs, ultrasound) as needed. Collect samples for toxicologic analyses if required. Toxicology testing performed in a diagnostic laboratory can be expensive and time consuming and mostly, results are not available immediately. Therefore, to rule in or out a suspected cause, first perform commonly used in-house diagnostics before ordering toxicology analysis. For example, monitoring prothrombin time or clotting times can be useful in anticoagulant poisoning cases. Other samples for toxicology testing in a diagnostic laboratory include whole blood for heavy metal analysis (lead), blood cholinesterases (organophosphate poisoning), and presence of pesticides (anticoagulant rodenticides). Similarly serum/plasma can be used for some metal analysis (zinc), drugs, alkaloids, and electrolytes (useful in sodium chloride poisoning or water intoxication). Stomach contents (vomitus; freeze upon collection) can be used for detecting pesticides, metals, baits, alkaloids, and drugs. Urine (chilled or frozen) can be used for some metal analysis, drugs and their metabolites, and alkaloids (strychnine).

TOXICOLOGIC VERSUS NONTOXICOLOGIC

Table 1 outlines some important toxicologic versus nontoxicologic rule-outs based on clinical abnormalities one must consider in an acutely ill animal. Where necessary, with each rule-out, along with major clinical abnormality, a brief description of other clinical signs is also provided. An acutely ill animal with sudden onset of clinical effects may often have multiple major clinical signs/abnormalities present. The purpose here is to provide an initial guideline for considering toxicologic versus nontoxicologic rule-out. Once a reasonable etiology has been narrowed down or established, the reader is encouraged to review a more detailed discussion on management of the particular poisoning or disease listed in this reference (see **Table 1**).

Table 1
Toxicologic versus Nontoxicologic Rule-Outs

Major Clinical Abnormality	Common Toxicologic Rule Outs	Nontoxicologic Rule Outs
CNS abnormalities (excitation and seizures)	*Strychnine* (rapid onset, rigidity, hyperesthesia, wooden horse–like stance)	*Trauma/head trauma* (outdoor animal, external or internal wounds/injuries)
	Metaldehyde (hyperthermia, tremors)	*Meningitis* (fever, hyperesthesia, neck stiffness and pain; fundic lesions possible if optic nerve affected)
	Amphetamines or cocaine (ingestion in dogs: sympathomimetic effects and hyperthermia)	
	Tremorgenic mycotoxins (Penitrem A, roquefortine) from eating moldy foods (GI signs, hyperthermia, and tremors)	*Hydrocephalus* (large, rounded head; divergent strabismus; seizures; brain ultrasound exam possible if open fontanelle)
	Cold medications: pseudoephedrine, ephedrine, some antihistamines (sympathomimetic effects, hyperthermia)	*Intracranial neoplasia* (primary or secondary brain tumor; typically older animals; neurologic deficits almost always asymmetrical)
	Organophosphate or carbamate pesticides (cholinergic crisis; SLUD signs)	
	Pyrethrin/pyrethroid-type pesticides (especially permethrin in cats: tremors, shaking, ataxia, seizures, GI signs)	
	Organochlorine pesticides (tremors, shaking, ataxia, seizures)	*Congenital portosystemic shunts* (more common in certain breeds, <6 mo of age, small liver)
	Chocolate: caffeine, theobromine, methylxanthines (polydipsia, polyuria, GI and CV effects)	*Rabies* (acute behavior changes, excitation, paralysis, endemic region)
	Zinc phosphide: mole or gopher baits (GI signs, shaking, dyspnea due to pulmonary edema)	*Canine distemper* (young dogs: history of fever, respiratory, and/or GI signs usually precede CNS signs)
	Bromethalin toxicosis: rat or mouse bait (paresis, weakness, ataxia, tremor)	*Hypocalcemia or hypercalcemia* (hypocalcemic tremor/ tetany; hypercalcemia-induced kidney injury can cause uremic signs)
	Lead (GI signs, hematologic abnormalities [nucleated RBCs, basophilic stippling, anemia])	*Hypoglycemia* (disorientation, ataxia, seizures, serum glucose <60 mg/dL)
	Metronidazole toxicosis (in dogs with repeated use and/ or high dosage: nystagmus, ataxia, weakness, paresis, seizures)	*Idiopathic epilepsy* (dogs 1– 5 years of age: diagnosis of exclusion)

(continued on next page)

	Table 1 (continued)	
Major Clinical Abnormality	**Common Toxicologic Rule Outs**	**Nontoxicologic Rule Outs**
	Nicotine: tobacco or cigarettes (ingestion in dogs: spontaneous vomiting, tremors, CV effects) *Tricyclic antidepressant toxicosis:* amitriptyline, clomipramine, imipramine, nortriptyline (agitation, nervousness, ataxia, CV effects)	*Primary or secondary erythrocytosis* (causing hyperviscosity), PCV 65% to >80%, brick red mucous membranes *Uremia* (secondary to AKI or CKD) *Endotoxemia/septic shock* (hemorrhagic GI signs, progressive weakness, abdominal pain)
CNS abnormalities (eg, CNS depression and/or seizures)	*Ivermectin, moxidectin, and other avermectin* toxicosis (ataxia, weakness, depression, tremors, seizures, blindness) *Marijuana ingestion* (ataxia, hypothermia, urinary incontinence) *Benzodiazepines ingestion:* alprazolam, clonazepam, diazepam, lorazepam (hyporeflexia, ataxia, CNS excitation: paradoxical reaction) *Barbiturate overdose:* short acting or long acting (coma, hypothermia, weakness, ataxia) *Ethylene glycol* (ataxia, disorientation, GI signs) *Methanol or ethanol ingestion* (GI signs, ataxia, weakness, depression) *Propylene glycol:* antifreeze (depression, ataxia, GI signs) *Baclofen* or other centrally acting muscle relaxant ingestion in dogs (vocalization, ataxia, disorientation, coma, hypothermia) *Amitraz insecticide* exposure (depression, ataxia, CV effects, paralytic ileus)	*Thiamine deficiency in cats* (cats fed mainly raw fish diet) *Polyradiculoneuritis/ Coonhound paralysis* (ascending flaccid paralysis; often, evidence of muscle pain; occasionally, raccoon exposure within preceding 2 weeks) *Feline infectious peritonitis:* (blepharospasm due to iritis, fever, weight loss, ataxia, seizures) *Feline leukemia* (lymphadenopathy, nonregenerative anemia) *Feline panleukopenia* (fever, GI signs, ataxia, neutropenia)
Muscle weakness, paresis, paralysis	*Black widow spider bite* (cats: swelling, pain) *2,4-D and other phenoxy herbicides* (dogs: ataxia, weakness, GI signs) *Metronidazole* (see Seizures, above)	*Polyradiculoneuritis/ Coonhound paralysis* (see above) *Botulism* (ascending paresis and paralysis; muscles of pharynx can be affected) *Tick paralysis* (flaccid

(continued on next page)

Table 1
(continued)

Major Clinical Abnormality	Common Toxicologic Rule Outs	Nontoxicologic Rule Outs
	Bromethalin rodenticide (see Seizures, above) *Coral snake* envenomation (cats: local swelling, pain, puncture wound) *Macadamia nuts* ingestion in dogs (weakness, ataxia) *Concentrated tea tree oil* exposure: Melaleuca oil (cats and dogs: weakness, ataxia, CNS depression)	ascending paralysis; rapid improvement of signs [<24 hours] after tick removal if North American [*dermacentor* spp.], longer if Australian [*Ixodes* spp.]) *Aortic thromboembolism* (cold extremities, weakness, firm and painful gastrocnemius muscles [cats]) *Profound anemia* (measure PCV) *Severe hypokalemia, hyponatremia, hypovolemia, hypo- or hyperthermia* (measure parameter) *Degenerative spinal cord diseases* (mentation, cranial nerve function intact)
Acute blindness	*Lead* (see Seizures, above) *Ivermectin, moxidectin,* and other avermectin toxicosis; see Seizures, above *Salt poisoning* (in dogs: polydipsia, GI signs, tremors, ataxia, seizures, serum sodium >160 mEq/L is strongly supportive)	*Retinal detachment or hemorrhage* (fundic exam; ocular ultrasound) *Glaucoma* (measure intraocular pressure) *Trauma* (penetrating injury of head, face) *Acute cataract* (ophthalmic exam) *Optic neuritis* (fundic exam) *Other visual pathway disorders (optic chiasm, optic radiation, occipital cortex)* *Sudden acquired retinal degeneration* (hyperadrenocorticism-like signs; electroretinogram to confirm)
ARF	*Ethylene glycol toxicosis* (ataxia, altered mentation/ depression, GI signs, urine may fluoresce with Wood's lamp; azotemia, calcium oxalate monohydrate crystalluria appear after kidney injury has occurred) *Easter lily (Lilium longiflorum), Tiger lilies (Lilium tigrinum, Lilium lancifolium), Rubrum or*	*Renal infiltration* (lymphoma; usually symmetrical nephromegaly; CNS signs common due to brain metastases) *Renal thromboembolism (evidence of peripheral thromboembolism common) Infectious* (pyelonephritis, leptospirosis, Rocky Mountain spotted fever,

(continued on next page)

Table 1 (continued)		
Major Clinical Abnormality	**Common Toxicologic Rule Outs**	**Nontoxicologic Rule Outs**
	Japanese show lilies (Lilium speciosum), Day lilies (Hemerocallis sp) (ingestion in cats: initially GI signs, azotemia in generally 24–72 h after ingestion)	borreliosis, feline infectious peritonitis: cats) *Urinary tract obstruction* (bladder palpation; abdominal ultrasound to evaluate kidneys, ureters)
	Cholecalciferol rodenticide and other vitamin D₃ analogs: calcipotriene, calcitriol (initial GI signs, then CV, CNS signs; azotemia; hypercalcemia with hyperphosphatemia differentiates from hypercalcemia of malignancy or hyperparathyroidism)	*Chronic kidney disease* (end stage)
	Grapes and raisins ingestion in dogs (initial GI signs, then azotemia in >24 h, possible pancreatitis) *NSAIDs: ibuprofen, naproxen, nabumetone, piroxicam, carprofen, diclofenac, ketoprofen, indomethacin, ketorolac, oxaprozin, etodolac, flurbiprofen, sulindac* (initially GI signs, azotemia in 24–74 h after acute ingestions) *Zinc toxicosis* (see Acute Hemoglobinemia, below) *Melamine and cyanuric acid contamination* (outbreak in the United States in 2007 from contaminated dog and cat food: crystaluria, azotemia, GI signs)	*Ischemic kidney injury and uremia* (hypotension, trauma, shock, anaphylaxis, myoglobinuria; uyrinalysis for renal casts, discoloration) *Amyloidosis* (notably Shar-Pei dogs, Abyssinian cats) *Hypercalcemia* (lymphadenopathy, hepatosplenomegaly possible with lymphoma, rectal palpation for anal sac mass with anal sac adenocarcinoma; malignancy a nd primary hyperparathyroidism typically cause concurrent hypophosphatemia) *Transfusion reactions* (history)
Acute hepatic damage	*Mushrooms:* amanita type (delayed onset GI signs [12 hours after ingestion], acute liver injury in 1–3 days) *Blue-green algae: Microcystis sp* (exposure to stagnant body of water; acute onset GI signs, hypovolemic shock, acute liver injury in 1–2 days) *Iron:* multivitamin ingestion (GI signs, hypovolemic shock, acute liver injury in 1–2 days)	*Hepatic lipidosis* (cats: period of stress, anorexia, obesity) *Hepatic neoplasia* (primary or metastatic, acute or gradual; abdominal ultrasound and biopsy to confirm) *Infectious hepatitis* (leptospirosis, infectious canine hepatitis, canine herpes virus, feline cholangiohepatitis, liver abscess, histoplasmosis, coccidiomycosis, babesiosis, toxoplasmosis, some

(continued on next page)

Table 1 (continued)		
Major Clinical Abnormality	**Common Toxicologic Rule Outs**	**Nontoxicologic Rule Outs**
	Sago palm or cycad palm: *Cycas* sp (ingestion: GI signs, liver injury in 1–3 d, seizures) *Acetaminophen toxicosis* (methemoglobinemia within a few hours, GI signs, increased liver enzymes in 1–3 d) *Aflatoxicosis* (dogs: mostly from contaminated dog food, several outbreaks reported in the United States) *Copper storage* (breed: bedlington Terrier, others) *Xylitol* (see Hypoglycemia) *Other drugs* (carprofen: GI signs, increased ALT days after starting treatment; cortidosteroids: steroid hepatopathy after weeks/ months of use; phenobarbital: chronic hepatopathy after months of use)	rickettsial diseases, feline infectious peritonitis; identify other characteristic features of individual diseases) *Septicemia/endotoxemia* (vomiting, diarrhea, hypothermia, collapse) *Heat stroke* (high body temperature) *Shock* (weak pulse, poor capillary refill time, progressive weakness)
Presence of acute oral lesions/ ulcers	*Acid ingestion* (corrosive lesions on lips, gums, tongue, salivation, vomiting, fever) *Alkali ingestion* (same as with acid, esophageal perforation more likely) *Cationic detergents*: present in several disinfectants (oral burns, salivation, vomiting, fever) *Alkaline battery chewing/ ingestion* (oral burns, salivation, vomiting) *Potpourri ingestion* (cats > dogs: oral burns, salivation, vomiting, tongue protrusion, fever) *Bleaches*: sodium or calcium hypochlorite (bleach-like smell, salivation, vomiting, wheezing, gagging) *Ingestion of phenolic compounds* (especially in cats: oral ulcers/lesion may be present; Heinz body anemia and hemolysis may be seen)	*Uremic stomatitis* (uremic halitosis, azotemia, GI signs) *Periodontal disease* (associated with dental calculus; gingival lesions) *Trauma* (presence of foreign body, recent tooth fracture) *Electrical cord chewing* (sharply demarcated ulcers, dyspnea due to noncardiogenic pulmonary edema) *Systemic lupus erythematosus* and other autoimmune diseases (lesions are characteristically at the mucocutaneous junction; joint pain, other systemic signs can be present) *Infectious* (feline calicivirus infection, FeLV, FIV, nocardiasis, ulcerative necrotizing stomatitis, *Fusobacterium* spp. infection; identify other characteristic features of individual diseases)

(continued on next page)

Table 1
(continued)

Major Clinical Abnormality	Common Toxicologic Rule Outs	Nontoxicologic Rule Outs
Acute methemoglobinemia, Heinz body anemia, hemolysis, or blood loss (anemia)	*Acetaminophen* (chocolate-brown colored mucous membrane within hours, dyspnea) *Naphthalene mothball* ingestion (moth ball-like odor in the breath, hemolysis) *Onions and garlic* toxicosis (hemolysis in 2–3 d, anemia, coffee-color urine) *Zinc toxicosis* (metallic object in the GI tract, gastritis, pancreatitis, hemolysis, hemoglobinuria) *Iron* (see Acute Hepatic Injury) *Anticoagulant rodenticides*: brodifacoum, bromadiolone, chlorophacinone, difethialone, diphacinone, pindone, warfarin (lethargy, dyspnea due to pulmoney hemorrhage, persistent bleeding at venipuncture site; increased PT +/− aPTT) *Rattlesnake* envenomation (swelling, pain, +/− fang puncture marks in skin; endemic region) *Other Drugs* (local anesthetic toxicosis [lidocaine, benzocaine, tetracaine, dibucaine]: methemoglobinemia, CV and CNS effects; phenazopyridine and other azo dyes toxicosis [methemoglobinemia, hemoglobinuria])	*Trauma* (overt blood loss) *Immune-mediated hemolytic anemia* (spherocytosis +/− autoagglutination on blood smear) *Thrombocytopenia* (immune-mediated or infectious, uncommonly drug-induced; platelet count) *Chronic Kidney Disease* (smaller kidneys, azotemia, uremic halitosis, oral ulcers) *Infectious* (ehrlichiosis, FeLV hookworms, *Mycoplasma hemofelis*, babesiosis; serologic testing, fecal flotation, blood smear) *Disseminated intravascular coagulation* (secondary to shock, neoplasia, septicemia, viral infections, pancreatitis) *Inherited bleeding disorders* (von Willebrand disease, factor XI deficiency; specific factor anaylsis needed for confirmation) *Causes of Epistaxis* (trauma, infectious, nasal polyps, malignant neoplasm, systemic bleeding disorder, systemic hypertension)
Cardiac arrhythmias	*Foxglove: Digitalis* sp (plant ingestion: GI signs, ventricular and/or supraventricular arrhythmias) *Lily of the valley: Convallaria majalis* (plant ingestion, GI signs, ventricular and/or supraventricular arrhythmias) *Oleander: Nerium oleander* (GI signs, ventricular and/or	*Automobile trauma* (evidence of other injuries) *Gastric dilation and volvulus* (abdominal distention, dyspnea, shock; radiographs confirmatory) *Severe anemia* (due to any cause) *Severe hypokalemia* (due to any cause) *Acidosis* (due to any cause) *Hypoxia* (due to any cause)

(continued on next page)

Table 1
(continued)

Major Clinical Abnormality	Common Toxicologic Rule Outs	Nontoxicologic Rule Outs
	supraventricular arrhythmias) *Bufo toads: Bufo* sp (endemic region; GI signs, collapse, seizures, sinus tachycardia, ventricular arrhythmias) *Azalea and other Rhododendron* plants (GI signs and possible cardiac arrhythmias) *Antidepressant toxicosis:* (CNS signs, anticholinergic effects)	*Primary heart disease* (cardiomyopathy, valvular heart disease, congenital heart problems, heartworm infestation: heart murmur, cardiomegaly, or evidence of congestive heart failure)
Dyspnea due to pulmonary edema	*Petroleum distillates:* kerosene, gasoline, and other hydrocarbons (hydrocarbon smell in the breath, salivation, vomiting, CNS depression, diarrhea, aspiration) *Zinc phosphide* (exposure to gopher bait or similar; GI and CNS signs, dyspnea due to noncardiogenic pulmonary edema) *Smoke inhalation* (dyspnea, collapse, panting, shock; smell of smoke on fur in virtually every case) *Organophosphate or carbamate* pesticides (cholinergic crisis, SLUD signs) *Paraquat herbicide* (rare; progressive dyspnea, panting, delayed onset after exposure) *Some organic arsenicals* (mainly injectable, melarsamine) *Calcium channel blockers* toxicosis, see cardiac abnormalities (noncardiogenic pulmonary edema along with cardiac signs)	*Cardiogenic* (multiple causes of left-sided congestive heart failure) *Noncardiogenic* (seizures, head trauma, electrical shock, drowning and near-drowning)
Gastrointestinal signs (vomiting, diarrhea, abdominal pain, drooling)	*Garbage poisoning* (vomiting, diarrhea, dehydration, abdominal pain) *Chocolate toxicosis* (initial stages: polydipsia, polyuria,	*Dietary discretion* (recent change in diet) *Intestinal parasites* (coccidia, roundworms, hookworms) *Foreign body* (plastic, wood,

(continued on next page)

Table 1 (continued)		
Major Clinical Abnormality	**Common Toxicologic Rule Outs**	**Nontoxicologic Rule Outs**
	vomiting, hyperactivity, tachycardia)	metal, cloth, bones; partial or complete obstruction)
	Fertilizer ingestion (NPK: vomiting, diarrhea, polydipsia)	*Infectious* (feline panleukopenia, canine distemper, canine
	NSAID toxicosis (initial stages: GI signs with or without blood in vomitus, diarrhea)	parvovirus, canine coronavirus, infectious canine hepatitis,
	Endotoxins and enterotoxins: staphylococcal, clostridial, *Escherichia coli*, salmonella (severe GI signs, progressive lethargy, dehydration, hypothermia)	leptospirosis, salmonellosis) *Gastric dilation/volvulus, intussusception* (abdominal distension, pain, dyspnea, shock)
	Zinc oxide (diaper rash ointment ingestion in dogs; mild to severe gastritis)	*Liver diseases* (secondary to gastric ulceration; evaluate serum liver parameters, pre- and postprandial bile acids)
	Iron Toxicosis (see Acute Hepatic Injury)	*Kidney diseases* (uremia secondary to either intrinsic
	Aresnical herbicides (initial stages: vomiting, abdominal pain, watery diarrhea)	renal disease or post-renal obstruction)
	Caster beans: Ricinus communis (initial GI signs within several hours)	*Endocrine disorders* (diabetic ketoacidosis, hypoadrenocorticism)
	Insoluble calcium oxalate containing plants: elephants ear (*Caladium* sp.), dumb cane (*Dieffenbachia* sp.), philodendron (*Philodendron* sp.), peace lily (*Spathiphyllum* sp.) (vomiting, diarrhea, oral swelling, salivation)	*Sudden change in the environment* (traveling, weather change, boarding, moving) *Inflammatory bowel disease*
	Zinc phosphide (GI and CNS signs, pulmonary edema; liver and kidney damage possible)	
Hypernatremia (measured serum sodium >160 mEq/L in dogs and >165 mEq/L in cats)	*Paint ball ingestion* (dogs: history of paintball ingestion, polydipsia, vomiting, diarrhea, ataxia)	*Due to pure water loss* (nephrogenic diabetes insipidus, heatstroke, fever, burns, no access to water)
	Salt toxicosis (history of inducing emesis with sodium chloride, ingestion of excessive amounts of salt-containing objects [play dough/plasticine] and foods)	*Due to hypotonic water loss* (severe diarrhea, vomiting, diabetes mellitus, polyuric kidney disease, hypoadrenocorticism
	Activated charcoal administration (can occur	

(continued on next page)

Table 1 (continued)		
Major Clinical Abnormality	**Common Toxicologic Rule Outs**	**Nontoxicologic Rule Outs**
	sporadically in some dogs, possibly due to fluid shift) *Seawater ingestion* (history of visit to a beach, lack of access to fresh water, swimming)	
Hypoglycemia	*Ingestion of xylitol-containing products* (dogs; sugar-free gum, sugar-free bakery products, etc.; hypoglycemia within 12 hours; seizures, acute hepatic damage and coagulopathy in 1–3 days) *Ingestion of oral diabetic/ hypoglycemic agents* (sulfonylureas)	Insulinoma *Acute hepatic disease,* portosystemic shunt *Functional hypoglycemia* (idiopathic in neonates, insufficient caloric intake in young puppies and kittens, severe exercise) *Intestinal parasitism* *Hypoadrenocorticism* *Leiomyosarcoma/smooth muscle tumor* Endotoxemia

2,4-D, Dichlorophenoxyacetic acid; AKI, acute kidney injury; ALT, alanine aminotransferase; aPTT, activated partial thromboplastin time; CKD, chronic kidney disease; CNS, central nervous system; CV, cardiovascular; FeLV, feline leukemia virus; FIV, feline immunodeficiency virus; GI, gastrointestinal; NPK, nitrogen, phosphorus, potassium; NSAID, nonsteroidal antiinflammatory drug; PCV, packed cell volume; PT, prothrombin time; RBC, red blood cell; SLUD, salivation, lacrimation, urination, defecation.

FURTHER READINGS

Beasley VR. Toxicology of selected pesticides, drugs, and chemicals. Vet Clin North Am Small Anim Pract 1990;20(2):554–6.

Côté E. Clinical veterinary advisor: dogs and cats. 3rd edition. St Louis (MO): Mosby; 2015.

Côté E, Khan SA. Intoxication versus acute, nontoxicologic illness: differentiating the two. In: Ettinger SJ, Feldman EC, editors. Textbook of veterinary internal medicine. 6th edition. St Louis (MO): Saunders; 2005. p. 242–5.

Fenner WR. Quick reference to veterinary medicine. 3rd edition. Baltimore (MD): Lippincott Williams and Wilkins; 2000.

Khan SA. Investigating fatal suspected poisonings. In: Poppenga RH, Gwaltney-Brant S, editors. Small animal toxicology essentials. Hoboken (NJ): John Wiley and Sons, Inc; 2011.

Volmer PA, Meerdink GA. Diagnostic toxicology for the small animal practitioner. Vet Clin North Am Small Anim Pract 2002;32:357–65.

Common Reversal Agents/ Antidotes in Small Animal Poisoning

Safdar A. Khan, DVM, MS, PhD[a,b,]*

KEYWORDS

- Reversal agents • Antidotes • Poisoning treatment • Small animal poisoning

KEY POINTS

- Various antidotes or reversal agents play a key role in the treatment of small animal poisoning.
- Along with good supportive care, antidotes can counteract the effects of a poison, shorten the time of treatment, and in many cases, certain antidotes can be life-saving for the patient.
- This article describes options available for using various antidotes in small animal poisoning cases.

Reversal Agent/Antidote	Toxicant/Main Indications	Comment(s)
N-acetylcysteine (Mucomyst)	Acetaminophen (paracetamol) overdose; may be tried for amanita mushroom toxicosis, sago palm toxicosis, xylitol toxicosis	Can be used orally; Injectable (Acetadote) available; in addition, can also use SAMe
Flumazenil (Romazicon)	Benzodiazepines (diazepam, alprazolam, lorazepam, clonazepam) overdose	Can help reverse severe central nervous system (CNS) depression/coma; short half-life; repeat in 1–3 h if needed

(continued on next page)

This article was adapted and modified from with permission from Khan SA. Clinical veterinary advisor: dogs and cats. 2nd edition. St Louis (MO): Elsevier Mosby; 2010.
The author has nothing to disclose. The views and opinions expressed in this article are those of author and do not necessarily reflect policy or position of the editors or their employer or the publisher.
[a] ASPCA Animal Poison Control Center, 1717 South Philo Road, Suite 36, Urbana, IL 61802, USA;
[b] Global Pharmacovigilance, Zoetis, 333 Portage Street, Kalamazoo, MI 49007-9970, USA
* Corresponding author: Global Pharmacovigilance, Zoetis, 333 Portage Street, Kalamazoo, MI 49007-9970.
E-mail address: Safdar.Khan@zoetis.com

Vet Clin Small Anim 48 (2018) 1081–1085
https://doi.org/10.1016/j.cvsm.2018.07.004
0195-5616/18/© 2018 Elsevier Inc. All rights reserved.

(continued)

Reversal Agent/Antidote	Toxicant/Main Indications	Comment(s)
Pamidronate (Aredia)	Cholecalciferol, calcipotriene, calcitriol	Treats hypercalcemia and hyperphosphatemia; can cause transient azotemia; may require multiple doses
Cyproheptadine (Periactin)	Serotonin syndrome caused by serotonergic substances (5-hydroxytryptophan; selective serotonin reuptake inhibitors, tricyclic antidepressants)	Can be tried per rectum in animals that cannot take it orally; can repeat once in 8–12 h
Methocarbamol (Robaxin)	For tremor control in permethrin toxicosis in cats; can also be tried in cats/dogs for tremors resulting from other pyrethrins/pyrethroids	Not an anticonvulsant; works well in permethrin, metaldehyde, tremorgens, and strychnine toxicosis; injectable preferred; oral dosing may be helpful for mild cases
Atipamezole (Antisedan)	To treat alpha-2-adrenergic agonist effects of amitraz, xylazine, clonidine, and brimonidine overdose	Atipamezole and yohimbine have alpha-2-adnergic antagonist properties; atipamezole more specific/preferred
Fomepizole (4-methyl pyrazole; Antizol-Vet)	Ethylene glycol (antifreeze) toxicosis in dogs; some benefit if used within 3 h of exposure in cats	Good safety margin; does not contribute to acidosis and CNS depression as ethanol does; can use ethanol as an alternative if fomepizole is not available
Calcium disodium EDTA (Calcium Disodium Versenate)	Lead, zinc, cadmium	Injectable; can cause gastrointestinal (GI) signs and nephrotoxicity; do not use if metal still present in GI tract
BAL (British antilewisite; Dimercaprol)	Lead, arsenic, mercury	Injection can be irritating and painful; difficult to obtain; helps remove lead from CNS
Atropine sulfate	For treating muscurinic signs in organophosphates and carbamate toxicosis, certain muscurinic mushrooms	Avoid atropinization (hyperthermia, tachycardia, mydriasis); not for treating nicotinic signs
2-PAM (Paralidoxime)	For treating nicotinic signs in organophosphate toxicosis in dogs and cats	Not useful for most carbamate toxicoses; most beneficial within 24 h of exposure but may be useful beyond this time; discontinue after 3 doses if no benefit
D-penicillamine (Cuprimine)	Zinc, cadmium, lead, copper, mercury	Used orally; can cause GI signs; do not use when metal is still present in the GI tract

(continued on next page)

(continued)

Reversal Agent/Antidote	Toxicant/Main Indications	Comment(s)
Digoxin immune Fab (Digibind)	Digitalis; cardiac glycosides	Expensive but rapid acting and efficacious; may be used in Bufo toad toxicosis
Deferoxamine (Desferol)	Iron chelator; useful in iron toxicosis	Urine may turn wine color after chelation with iron
Succimer (2-3-dimercaptosuccinic acid; Chemet)	Lead poisoning in dogs, cats, or birds	Used orally; anecdotal reports of renal failure in cats; monitor renal values when using in cats; can be used when object still present in the GI tract
Yohimbine (Yobine)	To treat alpha-2-adrenergic agonist effects of amitraz, xylazine, clonidine, and brimonidine overdose	Shorter half-life and less specific than atipamezole; use yohimbine as a second choice if atipamezole is not available
S-adenosyl-L-methionine (SAMe; Denosyl)	General hepatoprotective agent; has been suggested as a supplement	Used as an aid in hepatic damage from various causes (mushroom, xylitol, cycad, acetaminophen, and others)
Naloxone (Narcan)	Opioids/opiates	Can help reverse respiratory/CNS depression; short half-life; repeat in 1–3 h if needed
Vitamin K1 (phytonadione)	Anticoagulants (warfarin, brodifacoum, bromodiolone)	Parenteral use can cause allergic reaction; use orally for 2–4 weeks or more as needed; works better with fatty food and in divided doses
Pyridoxine (vitamin B6)	Isoniazid toxicosis in dogs	Difficult to obtain; can be used 1:1 ratio (dose of isoniazid:dose of pyridoxine); 5% to 10% intravenous infusion over 30–60 min; use in conjunction with diazepam to control CNS effects
Prussian blue	Thallium toxicosis	Used orally; difficult to obtain; thallium toxicosis no longer common
Leucovorin	Methotrexate overdose	Leucovorin is active form of folic acid; 25–250 mg/m^2 every 6 h intravenously, intramuscularly for up to 72 h
Intravenous lipid emulsion (Intralipid 10% or 20% solution)	For certain lipophilic drug toxicosis; potential for ivermectin, moxidectin and other avemectins;	Case-control studies demonstrating efficacy and safety not available; 1.5 mL/kg (20% solution) as

(continued on next page)

(continued)		
Reversal Agent/Antidote	**Toxicant/Main Indications**	**Comment(s)**
	cholecalciferol and other vitamin D_3 analogue; amlodipine; baclofen; diltiazem; lidocaine; nifedipine; verapamil; severe marijuana toxicois; permethrin toxicosis; bupropion; trazodone; phenobarbital and other barbiturates overdose; tricyclic antideprassants; propranolol	initial bolus followed by 0.25 mL/kg over 30–60 min; may have to repeat 2 or 3 times every 4–6 h provided no hyperlipemia present; lack of efficacy; hyperlipidemia; hemolysis; embolism; infection potential adverse effects
Glucagon (GlucaGen)	Used for treating hypoglycemia caused by insulin overdose and hypoglycemia agents; beta-adrenergic agents, calcium channel blockers and tricyclic antidepressant overdose for atrioventricular block, bradycardia, and hypotension	Used intravenously, bolus followed by constant rate infusion (CRI); 50 ng/kg intravenous bolus in 0.9% saline then 5–15 ng/kg/min as CRI
Methylene blue	To treat methemoglobinemia from aniline, nitrite, hydroxyurea, naphthalene, and local anaesthetic agents	1% solution injectable solution at 1.5 mg/kg intravenously; repeat once in 30 min if needed; do not give in cats as it can induce methemoblobinemia
Hydroxycobalamin (Cyanokit)	Vitamin B_{12} precursor; used to treat cyanide toxicosis	Hydroxycobalamin combines with cyanide to form cyanocobalamin, which is excreted in urine; used for treating pernicious anemia in people
Hyperbaric oxygen	Delivers 100% oxygen at pressure >1 atm; used in carbon monoxide, hydrogen sulfide toxicosis; can be helpful for cyanide toxicosis	Hyperbaric chambers may be available in veterinary schools and in some advanced veterinary clinics
Silymarin (milk thistle)	Used as a hepatoprotective agent in acetaminophen and amanita mushroom toxicosis	Used within 48 h of exposure; may have to be used for several weeks; 20–50 mg/kg/d orally
Acepromazine (PromAce)	To control hyperexcitation from amphetamine toxicosis and other similar stimulants; used for seroteneric drug overdose	Can cause hypotension; 0.02–0.1 mg/kg intravenously, intramuscularly, or subcutaneously; repeat as needed

FURTHER READINGS

Gwaltney-Brant S, Rumbeiha W. New antidotal therapies. Vet Clin North Am Small Anim Pract 2002;32(2):323–39.

Wismer T. Antidotes. In: Poppenga RH, Gwaltney-Brant S, editors. Small animal toxicology essentials. Sussex (United Kingdom): Wiley-Blackwell; 2011. p. 57–70.

Toxicology of Marijuana, Synthetic Cannabinoids, and Cannabidiol in Dogs and Cats

Ahna Brutlag, DVM, MS[a,b,]*, Holly Hommerding, DVM[a]

KEYWORDS

- Cannabis • Medical marijuana • THC • CBD • Marijuana concentrates • Poisoning
- Synthetic marijuana • Street or illicit drugs • Toxicity

KEY POINTS

- Accidental exposure to marijuana/tetrahydrocannabinol (THC)-containing products by cats and dogs is increasing in the United States. Marijuana-containing foods, many of which also contain chocolate, are the most common source reported to Pet Poison Helpline.
- Marijuana has a wide margin of safety and the prognosis following accidental exposure is good provided proper medical treatment is provided.
- Poisoning from synthetic cannabinoids may result in more severe stimulatory signs such as tremors, aggression, and seizures compared to marijuana and carries a fair prognosis.
- Exposure to large doses of cannabidiol, a nonpsychoactive cannabinoid, may still result in signs consistent with marijuana intoxication, likely due to the presence of THC in poor-quality products.

INTRODUCTION

Over the past decade, the legal landscape of marijuana has changed dramatically in both the United States and Canada. At the time of publication, all but 4 states in the United States allowed the use of cannabis (marijuana) in some form—some strictly for medical purposes and others for recreation—even though it remains illegal at a federal level. As of October, 2018, Canadian law allows for both recreational and

Disclosure: Both authors are full-time employees of Pet Poison Helpline and SafetyCall International, a 24/7 human and animal poison control center.
[a] Pet Poison Helpline, SafetyCall International, 3600 American Boulevard West, Suite 725, Bloomington, MN 55431, USA; [b] Department of Veterinary and Biomedical Sciences, College of Veterinary Medicine, University of Minnesota, 301 Veterinary Science Building, 1971 Commonwealth Avenue, St Paul, MN 55108, USA
* Corresponding author. Pet Poison Helpline, 3600 American Boulevard West, Suite 725, Bloomington, MN 55431.
E-mail address: abrutlag@petpoisonhelpline.com

Vet Clin Small Anim 48 (2018) 1087–1102
https://doi.org/10.1016/j.cvsm.2018.07.008
vetsmall.theclinics.com

medical marijuana in all provinces. In conjunction with these trends, the incidence of marijuana exposure and intoxication in pets, especially as reported to Pet Poison Helpline, an animal poison control center, has increased dramatically. This increase is presumably due to increased accessibility. Because of this, it is imperative for veterinary professionals to understand how common types of marijuana products can affect their patients following intentional or inadvertent exposure. This article reviews marijuana-containing products along with cannabidiol (CBD), a nonpsychoactive substance with a laundry list of anecdotal and increasingly supported therapeutic benefits. Finally, synthetic marijuana products (synthetic cannabinoids [SCB]), illegal substances with a much greater affinity for cannabinoid receptors than traditional marijuana that remain accessible as a "street drug," will also be covered.

DISCUSSION
A Brief History of Cannabis (Marijuana)

Cannabis (marijuana) has been widely used for centuries in the treatment of various ailments, for its psychoactive properties in recreational use, and in religious ceremony. Use of cannabis for medical purposes dates back to 2700 BCE for treatment of various maladies, including constipation, rheumatic pain, malaria, menstrual health, venereal disease, headaches, fever reduction, appetite stimulation, and as a sleep aid. Use for these ailments continued well into the 19th century, particularly in 1839 when Irish physician W.B. O'Shaughnessy began investigating its usefulness in the treatment of seizures, tetanus, rabies, and rheumatism in animal studies. He recognized its benefits as an antispasmodic agent with antianxiety and antiemetic properties, although he consequently noted side effects including catalepsy.[1]

Although marijuana faced increasing political controversy throughout the early 1900s in the United States, it was used in veterinary medicine until 1937, at which point it was effectively abolished following the passage of the Marihuana Tax Act (marihuana is an alternative spelling of marijuana)—an act that levied taxes and excessively harsh penalties on veterinarians and other health care professionals such as physicians and dentists. Mandatory criminal sentencing for recreational possession was introduced in the 1950s. In 1970, under the Controlled Substances Act, marijuana was classified as a Schedule I controlled drug, meaning "a drug with no currently accepted medical use and a high potential for abuse" per the Drug Enforcement Agency.[2] It remains a Schedule I drug to this day. Examples of other Schedule I drugs include heroin, LSD, MDMA (Ecstasy), and peyote.

Expansive knowledge has been gained over the last half century as scientists further investigate the effects of marijuana and its cannabinoid compounds in both medical and nonmedical ways. $(-)$ Δ^9-Tetrahydrocannabinol (THC) was identified as the major psychoactive cannabinoid from the cannabis plant in 1964.[3] The structure of CBD, the primary nonpsychoactive cannabinoid, was discovered in 1963.[4] The design of enantiomerically pure analogues or synthetic varieties of THC began in the 1960s in the pursuit of both analgesics and endogenous receptors presumed present in mammals at which THC, CBD, and other cannabinoids act.[3,5] Cannabinoid receptors were discovered in 1988, and specific receptors CB1 and CB2 were cloned in 1990 and 1993, respectively, at which time they were identified as G protein–coupled receptors affected by endogenous cannabinoids, termed endocannabinoids, during the early 1990s.[3]

Marijuana and SCBs have progressed to be the most widely used illicit drugs in the world, and most countries categorize them as drugs of abuse. In the United States, marijuana is one of the most commonly used drugs, just behind alcohol and ciga-rettes.[1,6] SCB varieties developed to mimic THC have also gained popularity for their psychoactive properties, most notably since 2009.[5]

Although considered a drug of abuse, the therapeutic benefits of cannabinoids have not been ignored. Since the 1980s, synthetic THC–based medications dronabinol (Marinol) and analogue nabilone (Cesamet) have been used in treatment of inappe-tence and nausea in chemotherapy patients and patients with AIDS.[3,7] Cannabis—including extracts of THC and CBD—are once again at the forefront of debate with respect to potential therapeutic benefit.[1] As of early 2018, in spite of federal law, all but 4 states in the United States legally allowed the use of medical cannabis although legislation varied considerably with respect to permissible compounds (whole plant vs THC and CBD extracts vs only allowing CBD).

DEFINITIONS OF MARIJUANA, HEMP, MEDICAL CANNABIS, AND CONCENTRATES

Marijuana is a general term that typically refers to *Cannabis sativa* and/or *cannabis ind-ica* plants, or portions of the plants, which are used for pharmacologic effects. Cannabis is a synonym for marijuana, derived from the plants' scientific names, and more commonly used in professional settings such as health care and scientific pub-lications. More than 500 chemical compounds and 100 cannabinoids, also termed phytocannabinoids, have been identified in *Cannabis sativa*. Of these, THC is the pri-mary psychoactive cannabinoid (ie, responsible for inducing a "high") and the com-pound on which the potency of marijuana products is based.[5]

Hemp is a cultivar of *Cannabis sativa* grown mainly for fiber, seeds, oil, biofuel, etc. In the United States, "industrial hemp" cannot have more than 0.3% THC on a dry weight basis.[8] Some hemp plants are being bred to have increasing concentrations of CBD and may be referred to as "medicinal hemp."

The terms "medical marijuana" or "medical cannabis" are synonymous and can accurately be used to describe any legal cannabis formulation meant for medicinal purposes, whether or not it contains THC. The legal definition of "medical cannabis" varies widely between states with respect to allowable compounds, formulations, and qualifying health conditions. Several states allow for THC to be used medically, whereas others restrict medical use to compounds such as CBD, which have no psy-choactive properties. For example, states such as California or Colorado allow human patients access to a full suite of cannabis products ranging from whole plants (live or dried) to THC-infused foods. Other states, such as Minnesota, prohibit smokable cannabis, allowing only highly purified, pharmacologic grade extracts of THC and CBD in the form of capsules, tinctures, topical creams, and oils for vaporization. In hu-man medicine, some states allow medical cannabis to be used for an exhaustive list of complaints, whereas others limit use to a range of qualifying conditions, often including chronic or intractable pain, severe nausea/vomiting/cachexia, human immu-nodeficiency virus/AIDS, amyotrophic lateral sclerosis, seizures, severe/persistent muscle spasms, posttraumatic stress disorder, Tourette syndrome, inflammatory bowel disease, and terminal illness.

The other notable category of marijuana products is "concentrates" meaning prod-ucts with high concentrations of THC (possibly >80%–90%). These may be used rec-reationally or medically and as their description implies, require smaller doses to achieve stronger and more long-lasting effects. Concentrates come in varying formu-lations and compositions, sometimes divided into "hash," concentrates made from dry or water-based extractions, and "solvent and CO_2-based processes."[9] Hashish is a sticky resin collected from the flowering buds that may be shaped or formed into a cake, ball, sticks, or slabs. Hash oil is a liquid or semisolid with a higher THC concentration than hashish. Solvent-based concentrates are increasingly common and made by soaking plant material in various solvents, which are then boiled off. Such products are generally called R-S-O as an homage to the person who popularized the technique. Other names for solvent-based concentrates include BHO, "honey oil," "honeycomb," "wax," "shatter," "budder," "errl," and "CO_2 oil." Together, these may be collectively referred to as "dabs," the act of which inhaling them is called "dabbing" or "doing a dab."[9] In addition to containing THC, concentrates may be contaminated with high concentrations of solvents, pesticides, and other chemicals.

ENDOCANNABINOID SYSTEM

Similar to opioid receptors (ie, delta, kappa, mu) that are activated by endogenous opioid peptides (eg, endorphins), mammals have cannabinoid receptors in plasma membranes that are activated by endogenous ligands called endocannabinoids. The endocannabinoid system encompasses complex intracellular signaling including enzymes for ligand biosynthesis and inactivation and plays a physiologic role in several systems primarily neurologic, inflammatory, and immune.

The two best-known and well-studied endocannabinoids are anandamide (AEA) and 2-AG, which the body produces, "on demand", to stress. These bind to G protein–coupled receptors and perform several neurotransmission functions including inhibition (mostly) of adenylate cyclase, inhibition of voltage-gated calcium channels, stimulation of protein kinases, and stimulation of potassium channels.[3]

The primary targets for endocannabinoids and THC are cannabinoid receptors 1 and 2 (CB1 and CB2). These receptors are present on the postsynaptic neuron and act via retrograde synaptic signaling mechanisms to inhibit neurotransmitter release from presynaptic neurons.[10] Endocannabinoids are synthesized, as needed, from membrane phospholipids to act in an autocrine (on the same cell) or paracrine (on nearby cells) fashion and are quickly inactivated via hydrolysis after internalization into the near-by cell.[3,11]

Endocannabinoids are 4 to 20 times less potent than THC and have a significantly shorter duration of action.[1] Administration of exogenous cannabinoids such as THC or synthetic analogues disrupt the subtle endocannabinoid signaling process and may result in the common THC tetrad of delusions, hallucinations, paranoia, and sedation.[1,11]

- CB1 receptors
  - Primarily located in the central nervous system (CNS) with lower concentrations in the peripheral nervous system (PNS).
  - In the CNS, CB1 is involved in cognitive function, emotion, motion/movement, hunger, and neuroprotection in both posttraumatic events and degenerative diseases.
  - Sensory and autonomic CB1 receptors are involved in pain perception, cardiovascular, gastrointestinal, and respiratory effects.
  - CB1 is responsible for the psychotropic effects of THC.
  - Activation inhibits retrograde release of acetylcholine, dopamine, GABA, serotonin, histamine, glutamate, and/or noradrenaline, among others.
- CB2 receptors
  - Primarily located in the PNS and are nonpsychotropic.
  - Involved in reducing inflammation and chronic pain relief.[3]
  - Activation inhibits proinflammatory cytokine production and subsequent release of antiinflammatory cytokines.[12]

Cannabinoid receptors are found in abundance within the epithelial tissues of the developing embryo with highest concentrations in the nervous system, sensory organs, and thyroid tissue. CB1 is important in the normal neuronal differentiation and axonal growth during neuronal development. The developed animal has highest CB1 concentration in the basal ganglia and cerebellum.[10] Endocannabinoid signaling is required for motor learning in the cerebellum, extinction of averse memories in the amygdala, and as an aid in memory encoding.

Although CB1 and CB2 are the most prevalent receptors in the endocannabinoid system, TRPV1 (a vanilloid receptor) may be of significant importance when activated by AEA and can play roles in motor disorders; ear/skin protection; mucosal protection of the gastrointestinal, urinary, respiratory, and circulatory tracts; and can affect cognitive processes such as emotion, learning, and satiety.[4]

MARIJUANA AND THC EXPOSURE
Product Potency

The potency of THC in the cannabis plant has increased in recent decades in the United States. The average THC concentration of marijuana in the 1960s was 1.5%, rising to 3.5% by the mid 1980s.[13] As of 1995 and 2014, concentrations increased from 4% to 12%, respectively, whereas the concentration of CBD simultaneously declined from 0.28% to less than 0.15%.[13] This increase in potency correlates with a shift in production from cannabis to the more potent sinsemilla—unpollinated, sterile flowering tops from the cultivated female cannabis plant. Sinsemilla is more potent than traditional marijuana and is gaining popularity in the United States, presumably due to demand for plants with greater psychoactive effects.[1,13]

In cannabis plants, THC is most concentrated in the flowering buds, followed by the leaves, stems, and roots. The seeds do not contain notable levels of THC.[1] Marijuana joints (cigarettes) typically contain 0.5 to 1 g of plant material with THC concentrations varying from 0.4% to 20%. The average 1 g joint contains 150 mg of THC.[9] High THC concentrations in cultivated plants are thought to be a result of cross-breeding and hydroponic year-round growing operations.[1] Hashish typically contains about 10% THC and hash oil 20% to 50%.

Exposure Scenarios in Pets

The most common route of accidental exposure to marijuana in companion animal patients is via ingestion, although some are exposed via inhalation from second-hand smoke or smoke intentionally blown in their face. Approximately 66% of the marijuana exposures reported to Pet Poison Helpline involve pets ingesting homemade or commercial edible goods.[14] The second most common source of cannabis exposures involve ingestion of plant material (~19%), followed by medical cannabis preparations and/or prescription medications such as dronabinol and nabilone (~9%).[14] Edible products are most typically brownies or cookies made using "marijuana butter" or various cooking oils that had been used to extract lipid-soluble THC from plant matter. Marijuana butter/oil can contain very high concentrations of THC and poses a greater risk for poisoning than ingestion of plant material alone. In addition, chocolate present in food may also lead to intoxication and can complicate the clinical picture. Other common food products include truffles, caramels, gummy candy, lollipops, ice cream, savory baked goods, beverages, etc. There seem to be few foods or beverages to which marijuana is *not* added.

Legalization of both recreational and medical marijuana may also increase exposure to various tinctures, vaporization liquids and associated vape pens, and oral preparations such as capsules, sublingual sprays, etc. Doses and concentrations of such products can vary widely.

Pharmacokinetics

Dogs are reported to have a larger number of cannabinoid receptors in the brain compared with humans, which may result in an increased sensitivity to the psychoactive properties of THC.[15] THC is readily and rapidly absorbed when inhaled. Absorption is slower and less predictable when ingested. Consuming THC products with a fatty meal will increase absorption due to its lipophilic nature. Most of the THC is metabolized in the liver and undergoes enterohepatic recirculation, with a small amount excreted as metabolites in the urine.[15] Because of its lipophilicity, THC is rapidly distributed into the tissues and crosses the blood-brain barrier.[6] This accounts for a short plasma but long biological half-life.[16]

The kinetic information listed pertains to dogs unless otherwise indicated.

- Minimum lethal dose greater than 3 to 9 g plant material per kilogram
- LD_{50} not established[16]
- Onset of signs: minutes (inhaled), typically within 60 min (oral)
- Excretion: 85% in feces via biliary excretion; 15% renally excreted
- Half-life (biological) 30 hours; 80% of THC is excreted within 5 days[15]
- Recovery after ingestion occurs within 24 hours in most cases, potentially up to 72 hours[14,16]
- Bioavailability (inhalation, human) 10% to 27% depending on frequency of use[6]

Clinical Signs of Poisoning

Ingestion or inhalation of THC carries a high morbidity but low mortality rate. Common signs of poisoning in dogs include lethargy, CNS depression, ataxia, vomiting (especially if plant material was ingested), urinary incontinence/dribbling, increased sensitivity to motion or sound, mydriasis, hyperesthesia, ptyalism, and bradycardia.[7,14,16] Acute onset urinary incontinence is not commonly seen with other toxin exposures and can serve as a helpful clue to veterinary staff to consider marijuana/THC exposure. Less common signs include agitation, aggression, bradypnea, hypotension, tachycardia, and nystagmus.[7,14] Rare signs include seizures or comatose conditions. Seizures may also be caused by coingestants such as chocolate or other drugs. In a 2018 study investigating the susceptibility of cannabis-induced convulsions in rats and dogs, no seizures were observed in dogs given chronic daily oral doses of cannabis extracts containing concentrations as high as 27 mg/kg THC combined with 25 mg/kg CBD (1.08:1 ratio of THC to CBD) for 56 weeks; however, other CNS signs including ataxia, tremors, and hypoactivity were observed. Because dogs were not administered THC extracts without CBD, the impact of the relatively large amount of CBD. See **Fig. 1** for signs reported to Pet Poison Helpline and **Fig. 2** for the percentage of cases in which veterinary intervention was recommended.

Fatality in pets from marijuana intoxication is extremely rare. Two canine fatalities were reported in conjunction with the ingestion of baked goods made with marijuana butter although the cases became complicated and the exact cause of death was not determined.[17] No deaths associated with marijuana have been reported to Pet Poison Helpline.[14]

CANNABIDIOL EXPOSURE

CBD is the most well-known and widely discussed nonpsychoactive phytocannabinoid with concentrations ranging from 0.3% to 4.2% in cannabis plants.[4] It is

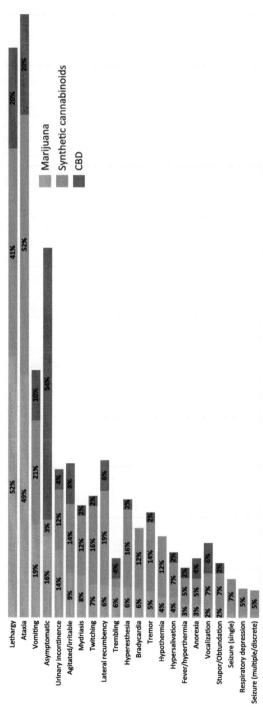

Fig. 1. Clinical signs associated with exposure to marijuana (ie, THC containing products, ~2200 cases), synthetic cannabinoids (~60 cases), and CBD (~50 cases) as reported to Pet Poison Helpline. Canines represent ~96% of the displayed data. Confirmation of exposure was not obtained in all cases, nor could co-ingestants such as chocolate or other toxicants be ruled out. Therefore, these data are meant to portray general trends only. Clinical signs reported in less than 5% of cases were excluded from this graphic.

postulated to have a variety of therapeutic benefits, such as antiseizure, antiinflammatory, analgesic, antitumor, antipsychotic, and antianxiety effects. In people, its effects may temper and counter some of the actions of THC, including reversal of THC-induced memory deficits in people.[11] Some data suggest a therapeutic synergistic effect when CBD is used in combination with THC.[4,11] For example, Sativex is a 1:1, THC:CBD oromucosal spray available in Canada for treatment of neuropathic pain in patients with multiple sclerosis (MS).[11] Likewise, many medical cannabis dispensaries offer combination CBD/THC products.

Although CBD lacks psychoactive properties, it remains a Schedule 1 controlled substance in the United States as of August, 2018. In spite of this, a rapidly increasing number of "CBD-containing" products are sold for use in both dogs and cats, including oils, treats, capsules, etc. These products can be found at some cannabis dispensaries (select states) and are readily available online. They are not approved by Food and Drug Administration (FDA), nor do they have any regulatory quality oversight. In 2015, FDA tested various "CBD-containing products," including those marketed specifically for pets, and found many did not contain the amount of CBD stated on the label (if any), whereas others also contained unlabeled THC.[18] The lack of regulation for pet products

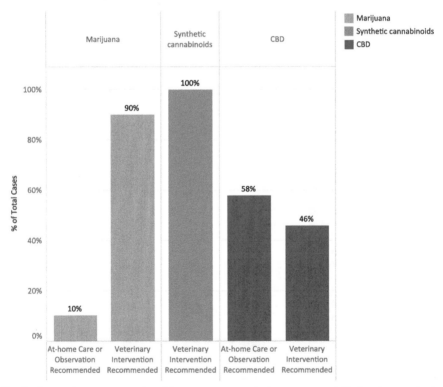

Fig. 2. Comparison amongst the ultimate recommended management site for dogs and cats exposed to marijuana (ie, THC containing products), synthetic cannabinoids, and CBD-only containing products for Pet Poison Helpline cases. Referral for veterinary intervention is based on a thorough, individual risk evaluation including but not limited to patient signalment, dose, expected or current clinical signs, current and prior medical history, and co-ingestants or concomitant medications.

leaves consumers vulnerable to unscrupulous manufacturers and poor-quality products.

Clinical Effects and Drug-Drug Interactions

There is emerging data regarding the pharmacokinetics, safety, and efficacy of CBD in pets, particularly for epilepsy and osteoarthritis (OA). In 2018, researchers at Colorado State University published a Phase I study examining the pharmacokinetics of CBD in 30 healthy, purpose bred beagle dogs.[19] Dogs received CBD via one of three formulations–transdermal cream applied to the pinnae, oral capsules containing microencapsulated CBD oil, or oral CBD infused oil at ~10 mg/kg and ~20 mg/kg daily for 6 weeks. The highest systemic absorption was observed with the infused oil product. Pharmacokinetic data is reported below. Adverse effects were not reported in this publication but are forthcoming in a subsequent paper; they included nonspecific mentions of liver enzyme elevation without corresponding clinical evidence of disease and diarrhea.[20] The investigators concluded the CBD formulation they used to be "tolerable and measureable."[20]

The first North American study investigating the efficacy of CBD for OA in client owned dogs (n = 16) demonstrated a statistically significant decrease in pain and increase in activity in dogs dosed with 2 mg/kg CBD q 12 hours for 4 weeks. While no observable adverse clinical effects were displayed, 9 of 16 dogs had a statistically significant increase in alkaline phosphatase (ALP). The reason for the increase may be due to chronic CBD dosing but other causes cannot be ruled out.[21]

CBD can inhibit certain cytochrome P450 enzymes, specifically CYP450 2C19 in people, resulting in inhibition or slowed metabolism of certain medications.[22] Dogs and cats also express CYP450 2C19 although data regarding interaction with CBD are lacking.[23]

Clinical Signs of Poisoning

Because of the lack of psychoactive properties and interaction with CB1 receptors, less severe effects are expected in case of pet exposure/overdose compared with that of THC-containing products; however, exposure can be complicated by poor-quality CBD products which may contain unlabeled THC or other agents. Of the CBD exposures reported to Pet Poison Helpline, most of the cases remained asymptomatic but those that developed signs seemed similar to marijuana exposures, including lethargy/CNS depression, ataxia, and agitation (see **Fig. 1**). See **Fig. 2** for the percentage of CBD exposure cases in which Pet Poison Helpline recommended veterinary intervention.

Other risks of accidental CBD product ingestion include exposure to carriers such as oils (aspiration), alcohols, or a massive amount of treats or novel food sources that could result in gastrointestinal upset, or other issues. Although significant systemic health effects are unlikely when ingested, intravenous (IV) dosing of 150 to 200 mg/kg in rhesus macaques did lead to tremors, hypopnea, respiratory arrest, and cardiac arrest in a dose-dependent nature.[24] Such severe signs would not be anticipated following oral exposure in small animals.

Pharmacokinetics

CBD undergoes enterohepatic recirculation but also faces extensive first-pass metabolism, which affects oral bioavailability. In spite of this, oral CBD oils appear to have better systemic uptake transdermal preparations.[19] Like other cannabinoids, CBD is highly lipophilic and rapidly distributed into the tissues.[26] Available pertinent kinetic information listed pertains to dogs:

- Cmax, median or mean (single oral dose of CBD oil): 102 ng/mL (2 mg/kg), 591 ng/mL (8 mg/kg), 625 ng/mL (~10 mg/kg), 846 ng/mL (~20 mg/kg).[19,21]
- Tmax, median (single oral dose of CBD oil): 1.5 hours (2 mg/kg), 2 hours (8 mg/kg).[19]
- Half-life, median or mean (single oral dose of CBD oil, 2-20 mg/kg): 2-4 hours.[19,21]
- Volume of distribution: 6.9 to 10.4 L/kg following 45 mg IV dose[25]

SYNTHETIC CANNABINOID EXPOSURE

SCBs manufactured for recreational purposes became popular in the United States starting in the 2000s when they were initially marketed as a "legal high." These compounds are dissolved in solvents and applied to dried plant material, intended to be smoked as an alternative to marijuana.[27] They are sold under a multitude of names including K2, Spice, Skunk, Wild Greens, Purple Haze, etc. They may also be labeled as "incense" or "potpourri" and carry a "warning" stating "not for human consumption." These products may also be laced with other chemicals/drugs such as caffeine or other stimulants. Although initially legally available in gas stations, head shops, and tattoo parlors, many of these products have been banned with the 2011 Synthetic Drug Control Act.

Clinical Effects

SCBs are designed for potent psychotropic effects and have a higher affinity for cannabinoid receptors than traditional marijuana, resulting in more severe clinical effects.[27,28] In people, SCBs are 2 to 3 times more likely to cause sympathomimetic effects including tachycardia and hypertension, 5 times more likely to cause hallucinations, and cause a higher incidence of seizures in comparison to marijuana.[29] Other signs may include cyclical agitation, aggression, and incontinence.[28] Rare but significant cases of acute kidney injury have been reported in humans as well.[29]

Clinical effect data in animals exposed to SCBs is limited, although similar signs as those seen in humans have been reported. Exposure may occur via inhalation or ingestion. A case report involving both a pet owner and a dog affected by SCBs reported hyperesthesia, tremors, miosis, hyperresponsiveness to stimuli, ataxia, seizurelike activity, aggression, and mild respiratory acidosis in the dog.[28] Similar signs were observed in the pet owner. Another case report involving presumptive SCB intoxication detailed signs of progressive ataxia, inappropriate mentation, hypothermia, stupor, and intermittent aggression with rapid progression to comatose condition, apnea, tremors, and opisthotonos.[27] Cases reported to Pet Poison Helpline are more likely to involve severe signs such as tremors and seizures, compared with marijuana, and all cases were deemed serious enough to warrant veterinary evaluation (see **Figs. 1** and **2**). These data seem to mirror the increase in severity of signs described in human medicine.

Pharmacokinetics

The pharmacokinetics of SCBs are likely similar to the non-SCBs, although limited information is available. The oral bioavailability of various SCB products is likely low and similar to that of THC and CBD, because case reports in people have indicated milder signs of shorter duration after inadvertent ingestion of baked goods laced with SCBs.[5]

- Half-life: 72 to 96 hours in dogs and people[27]
- Recovery typically occurs within 24 hours in people, perhaps shorter in duration if ingested (4–10 hours)[5,27]
- LD_{50} and minimum toxic dose have not been established[25]

CANNABINOIDS: THERAPEUTIC CONSIDERATIONS

CBD, THC, combinations thereof, and analogues have been suggested in therapy for many different disease processes and maladies. Therapeutic targets in past and recent years have included the CB receptors, fatty acid amide hydrolases (responsible for breakdown of endocannabinoids), and in encouraging an "entourage effect" to enhance effect and duration of endocannabinoids within the body. CB1 receptor agonists and even antagonists have been developed in recent years with hopes for therapeutic benefit. The 1980s brought dronabinol and nabilone to the market to aid in controlling nausea and inappetence in chemotherapy and AIDS patients. Sativex, a 1:1 THC:CBD medication, has been available since 2005 in Canada to aid in control of neuropathic pain in patients with MS. CB1 antagonists have also been developed to aid in controlling nicotine addiction in Europe, although this is not yet available in North America given concerns for side effects that include depression and suicidal thoughts.[11]

Cannabinoids have been considered in treatment or supportive care of many different medical conditions, including the following[11,12]:

- Alzheimer's disease
- Anxiety
- Arrhythmias
- Asthma
- CNS injury
- Depression
- Diabetes
- Epilepsy
- Feeding-related disorders
- Glaucoma
- Hypertension
- Inflammation, inflammatory bowel disease
- Multiple sclerosis
- Myocardial infarct
- Nausea
- Pain
- Parkinson's disease
- Rheumatoid arthritis
- Some cancers
- Tourette syndrome

The potential for therapeutic use of cannabinoids in veterinary medicine may best be supported by human medical research studies and, less commonly, in veterinary directed studies in animals. In researching antiepileptic properties, for instance, THC was investigated and found to be relatively promising in treatment of seizures in a small population of cats.[30] Perhaps some of the most promising research into use of cannabinoid-type products in veterinary medicine has been shown with use of palmitoylethanolamide (PEA), an analogue to the endocannabinoid AEA. AEA is synthesized during inflammatory processes and in instances of tissue damage. PEA is suspected to enhance function of AEA at the TRPV1 receptor and downregulate mediator release from various inflammatory cells. It has shown promise for treatment of pain, inflammation, and pruritus associated with eosinophilic granuloma complex in cats and mast cell–mediated disorders and skin disease in dogs.[31] To date there are no FDA-regulated cannabinoid products for use in pets, but nonregulated CBD supplements or nutraceuticals can be purchased from several companies in the form of treats, oils, capsules, and liquids for use in dogs and cats.

DIAGNOSIS
Specific Diagnostics

There is no reliable patient-side test available for diagnosis of cannabis or SCB exposure in veterinary patients. The readily available human urine drug screen immune assays designed to detect marijuana exposure are ineffective for SCB detection in both people and animals and often yield false negatives in veterinary patients exposed to marijuana/THC.[32] Liquid chromatography mass spectrometry (LC/MS) remains the gold standard for drug screening in both humans and animals. Because of the wide variability of SCBs, clinicians wishing to submit samples for testing are advised to consult with the diagnostic laboratory before sending.

Potential reasons for false-negative results using urine drug screens:
- Sample run too soon after exposure
- Large number of nondetectable metabolites of THC unique to dog urine
- Secondary to poor handling (THC binds to glass and rubber stoppers)[15]
- Increased patient water consumption resulting in dilute urine[16]
- SCB exposure, because these do not test positive[5,28]

Potential reasons for false-positive results using urine drug screens:
- In people, nonsteroidal antiinflammatory drugs, such as ibuprofen, naproxen, and niflumic acid, and efavirenz (antiviral drug) may cause false positives depending on the brand of test. Whether or not these agents could affect testing with dog or cat urine is unknown.[33]

Nonspecific Diagnostics

The following routine diagnostics can guide supportive care and alert clinicians to secondary intoxications or unrelated medical problems.

- Radiographs: monitor for evidence of ingested foil, other packaging materials, or batteries in the instance of a vaporizer pen ingestion and the rare risk for foreign body obstruction if baggies, pipes, or vape pens are consumed.
- CBC/chemistry/prefluid urinalysis: rule out primary underlying causes and establish normal baselines.
- Minimally: packed cell volume/total protein to monitor hydration status, electrolytes (monitor sodium if multidose-activated charcoal is given and monitor potassium if severely symptomatic), blood glucose (monitor intermittently in severely affected patients), and renal profile (in the event hypotension occurs and causes perfusion concerns).

DIFFERENTIAL DIAGNOSES

The clinical signs for marijuana and SCBs are nonspecific and differential diagnoses must be considered if exposure cannot be confirmed. Differentials may include but are not limited to alcohols (ethanol, methanol, ethylene glycol, diethylene glycol, propylene glycol), opiates, benzodiazepines, muscle relaxants, tranquilizers, bromethalin (rodenticide), macrocyclic lactones (ivermectin, milbemycin), and other illicit drugs (LSD, PCP, and hallucinogenic mushrooms).

GENERAL TREATMENT PLAN
Decontamination

A. Emesis can be performed if a toxic dose was ingested, exposure was within the last 30 to 60 minutes or a significant amount of material remains in the stomach, the patient is asymptomatic and thus low risk for aspiration, and spontaneous vomiting has not occurred.
   a. The preferred emetics in dogs are apomorphine (0.03 mg/kg IV) or hydrogen peroxide, 3% (1–2 mL/kg PO, food in the stomach increases chance of success).
   b. The preferred emetics in cats are dexmedetomidine (7–10 mcg/kg intramuscularly [IM]) or xylazine (0.44 mg/kg IM). Reverse as needed with atipamezole.
B. Multidose activated charcoal may be considered in asymptomatic patients who are at low risk for aspiration.
   a. Administer one dose of activated charcoal (1–4 g/kg PO) with sorbitol to start the series
   b. Administer a half dose of activated charcoal (or 0.5–1 g/kg PO) without sorbitol every 6 to 8 hours × 1 to 2 additional doses
   c. Do not administer if the patient is at increased risk for aspiration, hypernatremic, dehydrated, or not passing stool before redosing.
C. Massive ingestions may benefit from gastric lavage with the patient under anesthesia and airway secured. A dose of activated charcoal with sorbitol may be placed through the stomach tube.
D. If suspect material is noted on rectal examination, enemas may expedite clearance.

Supportive Care

A. Antiemetics as needed. Do not use maropitant or antiemetics with a prokinetic effect if the patient is at risk for a foreign body obstruction.
B. IV fluids 1 to 1.5 x maintenance, adjust as needed for perfusion changes. IV fluids are not expected to expedite or enhance excretion of cannabinoids to a great degree.
C. Thermoregulation and nursing care
   a. Warming or cooling therapy as needed. Hypothermia is more common with marijuana exposure, whereas hyperthermia is more commonly associated with SCB exposure.
   b. Generalized nursing care should be provided to obtunded or profoundly sedate patients including body rotation, ocular lubrication q 4 to 6 hours, etc.
   c. Keep the patient clean and dry. Although rarely necessary, an incontinent patient may benefit from a temporary urinary catheter.

Monitoring

A. Mildly affected cases may be monitored at home if kept in a safe environment with no fall risk.
B. Monitor vitals and blood pressure q 1 to 6 hours depending on patient status.

Medications

A. For agitation: butorphanol (0.1–0.4 mg/kg IM or IV) +/− acepromazine (0.01–0.2 mg/kg slow IV, IM, or subcutaneous, titrate dose for effect). Avoid acepromazine in hypotensive patients.
B. Tremors: methocarbamol (44–220 mg/kg slow IV to effect, select dose based on severity of signs). Re-dose PRN.

C. Seizures: diazepam (0.5–1.0 mg/kg IV), phenobarbital, propofol, levetiracetam
D. Bradycardia: atropine

Intravenous lipid emulsion
Intravenous lipid emulsion (ILE) has been suggested for marijuana and SCB intoxications in pets and used with varied success.[15,17,27] The potential therapeutic benefit of ILE is based on the knowledge that THC and cannabinoids are extremely lipophilic. All pharmacologically active cannabinoid compounds have a LogP greater than 4.5.[34] Please see Sharon Gwaltney-Brant and Irina Meadows's article, "Intravenous Lipid Emulsions in Veterinary Clinical Toxicology," in this issue for additional information on ILE.

- THC[35]:
  - LogP = 7.68
  - LogD at pH 7.4 = 7.25
- CBD[36]:
  - LogP = 7.03
  - LogD at pH 7.4 = 6.43

The veterinary toxicologists at Pet Poison Helpline do not routinely recommend the use of ILE in cases of marijuana or SCB exposure, in part because of scant supportive data, both in the literature and from the Pet Poison Helpline database, but also because ILE may negatively affect the effect of therapies such as sedatives or anticonvulsants.

PROGNOSIS

Most companion animals recover from marijuana exposures within 24 to 36 hours. Severe cases may be affected for up to 72 hours. Prognosis is generally good with supportive care.

SUMMARY

Marijuana, THC, CBD, and SCB exposures and intoxications have been increasing in frequency in both human and veterinary medicine. As therapeutic benefits of cannabinoids come to light and societal perceptions change, veterinary professionals are likely to see a continued increase in legalization and decriminalization of marijuana and individual cannabinoids and thus likely to see an increase in inadvertent companion animal exposure and intoxication. Vigilant and careful physical examinations with attentive and empathetic history taking skills devoid of judgment are imperative to help in diagnosing and best treating our companion animal patients.

ACKNOWLEDGMENTS

The authors would like to express their sincere gratitude to Amanda Poldoski, DVM, at Pet Poison Helpline for her data interpretation and creation of the figures in this text, and to Morgan Maisel, DVM/MPH candidate 2019, for her work on analyzing Pet Poison Helpline's CBD and synthetic cannabinoid cases.

REFERENCES

1. Adams IB, Martin BR. Cannabis: pharmacology and toxicology in animals and humans. Addiction 1996;91:1585–614.

2. Anon. DEA/Drug Scheduling. Available at: https://www.dea.gov/druginfo/ds. shtml. Accessed June 19, 2018.

3. Marzo VD, Bifulco M, Petrocellis LD. The endocannabinoid system and its therapeutic exploitation. Nat Rev Drug Discov 2004;3:771–84.

4. Long EL, Malone D, Taylor D. The pharmacological effects of cannabidiol. Drugs Future 2005;30:747.

5. Obafemi AI, Kleinschmidt K, Goto C, et al. Cluster of acute toxicity from ingestion of synthetic cannabinoid-laced brownies. J Med Toxicol 2015;11:426–9.

6. Sharma P, Murthy P, Bharath MMS. Chemistry, metabolism, and toxicology of cannabis: clinical implications. Iran J Psychiatry 2012;7:149–56.

7. Janczyk P, Donaldson CW, Gwaltney S. Two hundred and thirteen cases of marijuana Toxicoses in Dogs. Vet Hum Toxicol 2004;46:19–21.

8. Anon. Statement of Principles on Industrial Hemp. 2016. Available at: https://www. federalregister.gov/documents/2016/08/12/2016-19146/statement-of-principles-on-industrial-hemp. Accessed June 24, 2018.

9. Raber JC, Elzinga S, Kaplan C. Understanding dabs: contamination concerns of cannabis concentrates and cannabinoid transfer during the act of dabbing. J Toxicol Sci 2015;40:797–803.

10. Pirone A, Lenzi C, Coli A, et al. Preferential epithelial expression of type-1 cannabinoid receptor (CB1R) in the developing canine embryo. SpringerPlus 2015;4: 804. Available at: http://www.springerplus.com/content/4/1/804. Accessed June 19, 2018.

11. Murray RM, Morrison PD, Henquet C, et al. Cannabis, the mind and society: the hash realities. Nat Rev Neurosci 2007;8:885–95.

12. Landa L, Sulcova A, Gbelec P. The use of cannabinoids in animals and therapeutic implications for veterinary medicine: a review. Veterinární Medicína 2016;61: 111–22.

13. ElSohly MA, Mehmedic Z, Foster S, et al. Changes in cannabis potency over the last 2 decades (1995–2014): analysis of current data in the United States. Biol Psychiatry 2016;79:613–9.

14. Pet Poison Helpline case database. Bloomington (MN): Pet Poison Helpline & SafetyCall International, PLLC; 2004. 2018.

15. Fitzgerald KT, Bronstein AC, Newquist KL. Marijuana poisoning. Top Companion Anim Med 2013;28:8–12.

16. Donaldson CW. Marijuana exposure in animals. Vet Med 2002;437–9.

17. Meola SD, Tearney CC, Haas SA, et al. Evaluation of trends in marijuana toxicosis in dogs living in a state with legalized medical marijuana: 125 dogs (2005-2010): THC toxicosis. J Vet Emerg Crit Care 2012;22:690–6.

18. US Food & Drug Administration. Warning Letters and Test Results for Cannabidiol-Related Products. Available at: https://www.fda.gov/NewsEvents/ PublicHealthFocus/ucm484109.htm. Accessed June 27, 2018.

19. Bartner LR, McGrath S, Rao S, et al. Pharmacokinetics of cannabidiol administered by 3 delivery methods at 2 different dosages to healthy dogs. Can J Vet Res 2018;82:178–83.

20. Rumple S. High Time for cannabis research. Trends Magazine, American Animal Hospital Association 2018;29–34.

21. Gamble L, Boesch JM, Frye CW, et al. Pharmacokinetics, safety, and clinical efficacy of cannabidiol treatment in osteoarthritic dogs. Front Vet Sci 2018;5:165.

22. Narimatsu S, Watanabe K, Matsunaga T, et al. Inhibition of hepatic microsomal cytochrome P450 by cannabidiol in adult male rats. Chem Pharm Bull 1990;38: 1365–8.

23. Greb A, Puschner B. Cannabinoid treats as adjunctive therapy for pets: gaps in our knowledge. Toxicol Commun 2018;2:10–4.

24. Rosenkrantz H, Fleischman RW, Grant RJ. Toxicity of short-term administration of cannabinoids to rhesus monkeys. Toxicol Appl Pharmacol 1981;58:118–31.

25. Harvey DJ, Samara E, Mechoulam R. Comparative metabolism of cannabidiol in dog, rat and man. Pharmacol Biochem Behav 1991;40:523–32.

26. Samara E, Bialer M, Mechoulam R. Pharmacokinetics of cannabidiol in dogs. Drug Metab Dispos 1988;16:469–72.

27. Williams K, Wells RJ, McLean MK. Suspected synthetic cannabinoid toxicosis in a dog. J Vet Emerg Crit Care 2015;25:739–44.

28. Gugelmann H, Gerona R, Li C, et al. 'Crazy Monkey' poisons man and dog: human and canine seizures due to PB-22, a novel synthetic cannabinoid. Clin Toxicol 2014;52:635–8.

29. Murphy TD, Weidenbach KN, Houten CV, et al. Acute kidney injury associated with synthetic cannabinoid use - Multiple States, 2012. MMWR Morb Mortal Wkly Rep 2012;62:93–8.

30. Wada JA, Sato M, Corcoran ME. Antiepileptic properties of Δ9-tetrahydrocannabinol. Exp Neurol 1973;39:157–65.

31. Re G, Barbero R, Miolo A, et al. Palmitoylethanolamide, endocannabinoids and related cannabimimetic compounds in protection against tissue inflammation and pain: Potential use in companion animals. Vet J 2007;173:21–30.

32. Teitler JB. Evaluation of a human on-site urine multidrug test for emergency use with dogs. J Am Anim Hosp Assoc 2009;45:59–66.

33. Saitman A, Park H-D, Fitzgerald RL. False-positive interferences of common urine drug screen immunoassays: a review. J Anal Toxicol 2014;38:387–96.

34. Thomas BF, Compton DR, Martin BA. Characterization of the lipophilicity of natural and synthetic analogs of delta 9-tetrahydrocannabinol and its relationship to pharmacological potency. J Pharmacol Exp Ther 1990;255:624–30.

35. Anon. CSID:15266. Available at: http://www.chemspider.com/Chemical-Structure.15266.html. Accessed June 24, 2018.

36. Anon. CSID:559095. Available at: http://www.chemspider.com/Chemical-Structure.559095.html; http://www.chemspider.com/Chemical-Structure.559095.html?rid=79a89166-d9cf-41ea-9313-8366b7493a83. Accessed June 24, 2018.

Radiation Emergencies
Dogs and Cats

Stephen B. Hooser, DVM, PhD

KEYWORDS

- Radiation • Emergencies • Incidents • Preparedness • Dogs • Cats

KEY POINTS

- Exposure of companion animals to large, clinically significant amounts of ionizing radiation is unlikely; however, accidental release of large amounts of radiation has occurred in the past, and nuclear terrorism is possible.
- If an incident occurs, early reaction to the emergency will be by traditional first responders, followed rapidly by responses from state and federal emergency personnel.
- In some circumstances, it is possible that veterinarians may be called upon to assist by helping to evaluate animals for contamination and/or exposure, perform initial lifesaving tasks, and decontaminate people's pets.
- Veterinarians and other veterinary professionals should have a basic understanding of how radiation exposure may occur, the possible effects on companion animals, and how to provide veterinary care and assistance in a radiation emergency.

BACKGROUND RADIATION; RADIATION IS ALL AROUND US (AND IN US)

Companion animals and people are continually exposed to low levels of ionizing radiation from the environment, the cosmos, and man-made sources. The majority of background ionizing radiation comes from naturally-occurring radioactive minerals outside and inside our bodies, cosmic radiation from space, and some from man-made sources such as radiographs. Known radiation hazards are generally denoted with a yellow and black warning symbol (**Fig. 1**). The closer one gets to space in elevation or an airplane, the greater the cosmic radiation. The more radiographic procedures, the greater the exposure to x-rays. The background ionizing radiation for a US citizen averages 620 mrem (equivalent to 6.2 millisieverts) per year. An estimate of one's background radiation exposure can be calculated at the US Environmental Protection Agency's (EPA's) Radiation Protection, Calculate Your Radiation Dose Web site by entering home, work, medical (radiographs), environmental (flying and

The author has nothing to disclose.

Department of Comparative Pathobiology, Animal Disease Diagnostic Laboratory, College of Veterinary Medicine, Purdue University, 406 South University Street, West Lafayette, IN 47907, USA

E-mail address: Shooser1@purdue.edu

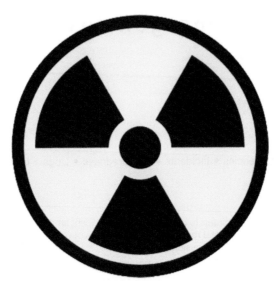

Fig. 1. Radiation warning symbol. (*From* Wikimedia commons. Available at: https://commons.wikimedia.org/wiki/File:Radiation_warning_symbol.png. Accessed August 5, 2018.)

home altitude), and personal lifestyle variables. Using the calculator for an extremely rough estimate (as it is designed for an average person rather than for an average dog or cat), the estimate for a household pet can be lower than that of its owner. For example, the total yearly dose for my dog is 115 mrem (mrem), whereas mine is 128 mrem per year, because I have had a dental radiograph, fly occasionally (both flight altitude and airport security screening), and work in a brick/concrete building.

WHY EXCESSIVE EXPOSURE TO IONIZING RADIATION IS BAD

Radioactivity is the process of spontaneous transformation of the nucleus of an unstable atom with the emission of high-energy rays and particles (alpha or beta particles), whereas radiation is energy moving in the form of particles or waves that can be absorbed by an organism's body, tissues, cells, and macromolecules such as proteins and DNA.[1] Animals exposed to a source of ionizing radiation can suffer radiation sickness if the dose is high, but do not become radioactive themselves. For example, animals undergoing a radiographic procedure are exposed to x-rays (similar to gamma rays), but do not become radioactive.

Ionizing radiation is energy in the form of rays or particles, primarily gamma rays, alpha particles, and beta particles, which transfer some of their energy to matter as they move through it. The transfer of energy can remove electrons from the orbits of atoms, leading to the formation of ions in that matter, hence the term, ionizing radiation. In companion animals, if the matter that is being ionized includes molecules in the cells and tissues of an animal, excessive amounts are obviously bad for that animal. As with chemical toxicants, radiation exposure to living organisms displays a dose response. The greater the dose, the greater the response. In the case of ionizing radiation, dose is the amount of radiant energy absorbed by the body, organ, or specific tissue, from either external sources or internally deposited radioactivity.[1]

An animal can receive an external dose by standing near a gamma- or high-energy beta-emitting source (alpha particles penetrate skin poorly, **Fig. 2**). They can receive an internal dose by ingesting or inhaling radioactive material. Alpha, beta, and gamma radiation are all capable of eliciting damage when inside the animal. External exposure stops when the animal leaves the area of the source, or it is removed from their fur or skin by decontamination processes. Internal exposure continues until the radioactive material is flushed from the body by natural elimination or by radioactive decay.[2] In general, contamination results when a radioisotope (as gas, liquid, or solid) is released into the environment. External contamination occurs when loose bits of radioactive material are deposited on surfaces such as the fur and skin. Internal contamination occurs when the radioactive bits are inhaled, ingested, or lodged in a wound. If contaminated, animals should be decontaminated as soon as possible. Animals that have been exposed to radiation, but not contaminated with radioactive material, do not need to be decontaminated. However, because radiation cannot be seen, smelled, heard, or tasted, radiological testing with the appropriate instruments is the only way to detect the presence of radioactive material.[3]

The deleterious effects of excessive doses of ionizing radiation to tissues begin with transfer of energy to atoms, leading to ionization of cellular molecules. Numerous unchecked ionizations directly affect cellular macromolecules including DNA and proteins. In addition, transfer of radiant energy can ionize water, resulting in the formation of highly reactive free radicals, which can also damage DNA, proteins, and lipids in cell membranes. Given that 55% to 60% of the body is water, formation of, and damage by, free radicals can be severe. This damage compromises cellular function and can lead to cell death. Ionization of macromolecules or water is an initial step in tissue damage caused by radiation. Ionization-induced damage can therefore result in cell death, DNA mutations, or other alterations in cellular function. Damage can manifest itself acutely and follow a predictable dose response (ie, increasing dose results in increasing damage, such as increasing skin reddening with increasing exposure to gamma radiation), or it can produce delayed effects such as those related to formation of DNA mutations and initiation of carcinogenesis. In the animal as a whole, acute exposure to large amounts of ionizing radiation has a pronounced effect on rapidly dividing cells such as those in skin and hair, the gastrointestinal (GI) tract, and the bone marrow, resulting in some of the clinical signs seen in radiation

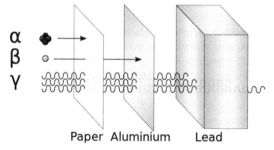

Fig. 2. Alpha, beta and gamma radiation penetration. Alpha particles are stopped by a sheet of paper, while beta particles can be stopped by an aluminum plate. Gamma radiation is dampened when it penetrates matter. Gamma rays can be stopped by 4 m of lead. (*From* Wikimedia commons; Alfa_beta_gamma_radiation.svg: user: stannered. Available at: https://commons.wikimedia.org/wiki/File:Alfa_beta_gamma_radiation_penetration.svg. Accessed August 5, 2018.)

poisoning. This is also the basis for using radiation therapy to kill rapidly dividing cancer cells.[1]

RADIATION EMERGENCIES

According to the Harvard-Kennedy, Belfer Center 2011 report, The US-Russia Joint Threat Assessment on Nuclear Terrorism, "Nuclear terrorism is a real and urgent threat."[4] In light of this continuing threat, the US Department of Agriculture (USDA) Animal and Plant Health Inspection Service (APHIS) has been part of 2 federal/state/local planning exercises involving large-scale radiation emergencies, one in 2014 and one as recently as 2017, in which radiological exposure and decontamination of pets were integral parts.[5,6] Worldwide over the past 50 years, accidents have occurred that released radioactive material into the environment with varying amounts of human and animal exposure. Fortunately, 2 of the earlier accidents at nuclear power plants, those at Windscale in the United Kingdom in 1957 and at Three Mile Island in 1979 in the United States, were contained and released relatively small amounts of radioactivity.[1] However, the 1986 accident at the Chernobyl nuclear power plant in Ukraine released considerable radiation locally and into the environment as nuclear fallout. Winds carried radioactivity around the world, but radioactive fallout was deposited primarily in northern Europe, causing environmental contamination in pastures, forages, livestock, and wildlife. The 2011 earthquake and tsunami that resulted in damage to the Fukushima Daiichi nuclear power plant in Japan resulted in contamination in the 20 km restricted zone around the plant, but released far less radioactive material into the environment than Chernobyl. Companion animals were among those exposed in at Chernobyl and Fukushima, with only small numbers of dogs and cats found to be contaminated around the Fukushima site.[7]

TYPES OF RADIATION EMERGENCES

Exposure of companion animals to excessive sources of radiation could occur in several ways. This could be through the use of an improvised nuclear device, a radiological dispersal device (dirty bomb), or a radiological exposure device by terrorist groups, or it could result from an accident associated with a nuclear power plant, transportation of nuclear material, or an occupational accident.

Improvised Nuclear Device

There are terrorist groups that actively seek out nuclear weapons or enough nuclear material to make a device capable of a nuclear explosion (an improvised device). If detonated, such a device would produce an intense pulse of heat, light, air pressure, and radiation (**Fig. 3**). The explosion would distribute highly radioactive materials that would be deposited locally and could be carried long distances by the wind and deposited as fallout. Animals close to the blast site could experience severe injury or death. Contamination of animals and the environment would occur as a result of fallout of nuclear particulates.

Dirty Bomb or Radiological Dispersal Device

A dirty bomb is a mix of explosives with radioactive powder or pellets. It is also known as a radiological dispersal device (RDD). It cannot create an atomic blast like an improvised nuclear device or nuclear weapon. When a dirty bomb explodes, the force of the blast carries radioactive material into the surrounding area and can cause injury to animals and people in the vicinity. The initial and potentially greatest source of injury

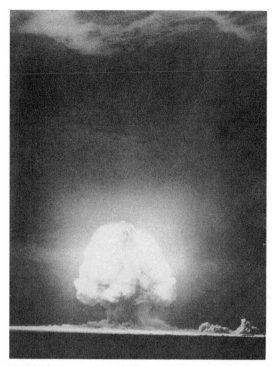

Fig. 3. Trinity test. World's first atomic bomb detonated by the United States at Trinity site in southern New Mexico on July 16, 1945. Fast-rising incandescent cloud produced by explosion. (*From* Wikimedia commons. Available at: https://commons.wikimedia.org/wiki/File: Trinity_atmospheric_nucleat_test_-_July_1945_-_Flickr_-_The_Official_CTBTO_Photostream. jpg. Accessed August 5, 2018.)

comes from the explosion, not the radiation. Only animals very close to the blast site would be exposed to enough radiation to cause immediate serious illness. However, the radioactive dust and smoke could spread farther away and would be dangerous when breathing in the dust, eating contaminated food, or drinking contaminated water.

Radiological Exposure Device

Radioactive material could be hidden from sight in a public place to stealthily expose animals and people to radiation. Those who passed close to the sight, or were housed near it, would be exposed.

Nuclear Power Plant Accident

Radioactive material ejected in a plume from a power plant accident could settle on animals that are outdoors, on buildings, or in food and water. In the event of a tsunami or flood waters, radioactive materials could be washed from the plant into the immediate environment. In either of these circumstances, radioactive contamination could be external, on skin and fur, or internal if inhaled or ingested in food and water. From these types of radiation exposures, both short-term and long-term health effects could occur.

Transportation Accidents

Radioactive material can be transported by trucks, rail, or other shipping methods. Shipments involving significant amounts of radioactive material are required to have documentation, labels, and placards identifying the cargo as radioactive. Accidents could release radioactive material into the environment and expose animals that come in contact.

Occupational Accidents

The health effects from an occupational accident involving radiation could range from no health effects to very serious health effects based on several factors:

1. The type and amount of radioactive materials
2. How long the animals were near the radioactive material or how long the radioactive material was in, or on their bodies
3. How close they were to the radioactive material
4. What parts of their bodies were exposed (ie, internal or external exposure)[8]

PREPARATIONS

Experience from past disasters has shown that when people have to evacuate their homes, they often want to take their pets or service animals with them. In fact, the federal government advises pet owners against leaving pets behind if they ever have to evacuate their homes. It is reported that most animal owners want to save their animals and are willing to take risks in order to do so. Pet owners often are willing to put themselves in danger in order to save their pets, and farmers also try to save their animals. Therefore, in order to avoid increasing the risks during the crisis period and to help the local community recover quickly afterward, animals need to be saved together with their owners. In a nuclear emergency, the pets accompanying their owners will present a challenge to response and relief organizations as pet evacuation, decontamination, and sheltering have to be considered along with evacuation, decontamination, and sheltering of people. The federal Pet Evacuation and Transportation (PETS) Act of 2006 requires that state and local emergency plans address the needs of people with household pets or service animals. Therefore, as resources permit, animal issues will be managed as an element of protecting public health and safety.[9,10] For veterinarians and the public, recommendations and guides help prepare for many types of emergencies and disasters, including nuclear disasters (**Fig. 4**), are available from the American Veterinary Medical Association (AVMA), US Department of Health and Human Services (HHS), US Centers for Disease Control and Prevention (CDC), Radiation Emergency Medical Management (REMM), the US Department of Homeland Security (DHS), and the Federal Emergency Management Agency (FEMA).[11–15]

Radiation emergencies require a coordinated effort among local, state, and federal agencies. At the state level, governors would request a national disaster declaration, which must be approved at the presidential level. When declared a national disaster, medical resources from the federal government become available. The National Disaster Medical System (NDMS) is a federal resource organized under HHS. The NDMS coordinates several disaster response teams, which can include National Veterinary Response Teams (NVRTs) added to Disaster Medical Assistance Teams (DMATs).[16] NVRT members include veterinarians, animal health technicians, epidemiologists, safety specialists, logisticians, communications specialists, and other support personnel.[17]

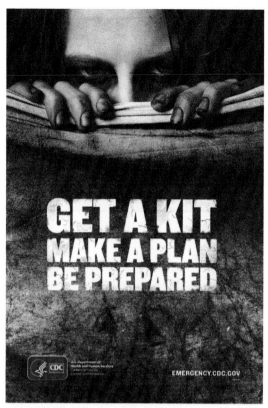

Fig. 4. Recommendations and guides are available to help prepare for many types of emergencies and disasters including nuclear incidents. (*From* CDC Office of Public Health Preparedness and Response. Available at: https://www.cdc.gov/phpr/zombie/posters.htm. Accessed August 5, 2018.)

In the event of a radiation emergency, traditional first responders (firefighting, emergency medical and law enforcement) will typically establish control zones around contaminated areas. Within control zones, tasks will be assigned to individuals trained and certified for them. The initial local response can typically occur within minutes. State/regional level of response may take hours. Federal response with DMAT teams can take days. In addition to the National Disaster System of the Federal government, all states have emergency response plans in which the response for animal health emergencies is frequently overseen by state departments of agriculture or boards of animal health.[15,16] Although work remains to be done at all levels, a recent study has found that disaster planning for animals has increased over the past decade.[9]

IN THE EVENT OF A RADIOLOGICAL EMERGENCY

Response to a radiological emergency depends upon the type of incident. As already described, some incidents could require immediate evacuation from the area; others could involve sheltering in place, and others could also involve long-term monitoring of the situation with appropriate actions taken as needed.

In general, in the event of a radiological emergency, the recommendation would be to listen to local first responders, get to a place of safety, stay inside, and stay tuned for updated instructions from emergency response officials (**Fig. 5**).[3,13,18–21]

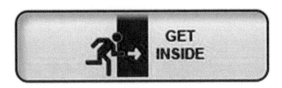

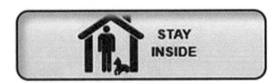

Fig. 5. Centers for Disease Control and Prevention. What to do during a radiation emergency: get inside, stay inside, stay tuned. (*From* Center for Disease Control and Prevention. Available at: https://emergency.cdc.gov/radiation/stayinside.asp. Accessed August 5, 2018.)

If it is necessary to evacuate with pets, the CDC has provided general guidance:

1. Listen for instructions and information on pet evacuation and the location of available pet shelters.
2. Pets will not be allowed into any shelter until they have been washed to remove radioactive material (see section on decontamination).
3. If evacuating with a pet, bring a cage, leash, food, medication, and veterinary records, including immunization records.[21]

Patient Care

Triage and treatment of patients in a radiation incident depend on the type of incident, and the possible scenarios are complex. If in the initial stages of a suspected radiation incident, the REMM site of HHS provides a basic algorithm applicable to people or companion animals to quickly evaluate patients for contamination or exposure to radiation, and medically stabilize them for subsequent appropriate treatment and decontamination (**Fig. 6**).

The major decisions points of the algorithm are

1. Evaluate for contamination and/or exposure
    Is it a radiological incident (radiation without a nuclear blast) or a nuclear incident (nuclear blast)? In addition to the bright light and explosion, a nuclear blast produces many different types of radioisotopes and spreads them further than a radiological incident.
    How do you know a radiation incident has occurred? A radiological incident may not be as obvious as a nuclear incident.

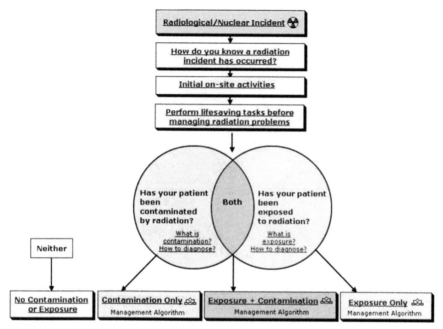

Fig. 6. Algorithm to evaluate for radiation contamination or exposure. (*From* US Dept. Health & Human Services Radiation Emergency Medical Management (U.S. Health & Human Services REMM). Available at: https://www.remm.nlm.gov/newptinteract.htm#skip. Accessed August 5, 2018.)

2. Initial on-site activities: perform lifesaving tasks before managing radiation problems
3. Has your patient been contaminated by radiation (radioactive particles externally or internally) or has your patient been exposed to radiation (exposure to ionizing radiation)?
   Contamination only management algorithm
   Exposure only management algorithm
   Both contamination and exposure algorithm
   Neither contamination nor exposure

Decontamination

Decontamination of pets should only be performed if it is possible to minimize the potential for injury to the animals and the owners. Within emergency control zones, decontamination of animals will be performed by trained personnel. Outside of the control zone, if the owners are instructed to stay inside, their pets should be inside also.[22]

When decontaminating, thorough cleaning of animals can present a challenge, because there is no layer of clothing to take off, and animals with long hair are more difficult to clean. As with people, any action to dust off and partially remove contamination is helpful. When brushing animals, care should be taken to avoid inhaling any particulates. Using a dust mask and brushing the animals outside and upwind from the animal may be appropriate. When possible, bathing and grooming thoroughly will be useful in removing additional contamination (**Fig. 7**).

An important health and safety consideration is the possibility for the animals to recontaminate themselves and bring that contamination inside the home or shelter. Animals cross-contaminating the owners, especially children who pet them, present

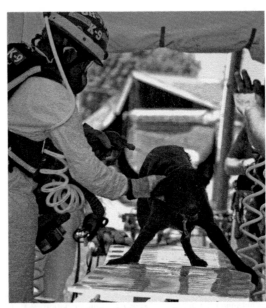

Fig. 7. Rescue dog gets decontaminated after conducting search and rescue at Vibrant Response Exercise, August, 2014. (*From* Wikimedia commons. Available at: https://commons.wikimedia.org/wiki/File:Rescue_Dogs_get_decontaminated_after_conducting_search_and_rescue_at_Vibrant_Response_2014_140804-A-PC120-058.jpg. Accessed August 5, 2018.)

a health risk. For people sheltering at home, communication messages should address the need for placing pets in cages or on a leash as appropriate if there is any risk of animals becoming contaminated again after washing.[10]

If needed, the CDC has guidance for self-decontamination of pets:[23]

1. If your pet was outside, bring your pet inside.
    Wash your pet carefully with shampoo or soap and water and rinse completely.
    Wear waterproof gloves and a dust mask (or other material to cover your mouth) if you can.
    Keep cuts and abrasions (both yours and your pets) covered when washing your pet to keep radioactive material out of the wound.
    Wash your hands and face after washing your pet.
2. Pet food in sealed containers (cans, bottles, boxes) will be safe for animals to eat.
    Wipe off pet food containers with a damp cloth or clean towel before opening them. Wipe off pet bowls, dishes, and mats as well. Put the used cloth or towel in a plastic bag or other sealable container and place the bag in an out-of-the-way place, away from other people and pets.
3. For pet sanitation, put newspapers or other absorbent material in your pet's area so your pet can relieve itself indoors.
    Do not touch soiled material with your bare hands.
    Place soiled material into a plastic bag or other sealable container.
    Place the bag in an out-of-the-way place, away from other people and pets.

SUMMARY

Exposure of companion animals to large, clinically significant amounts of ionizing radiation is unlikely. If it occurs, early reaction to the situation will be by traditional first responders, followed rapidly by responses from state and federal emergency personnel. However, accidental release of large amounts of radiation has occurred, and nuclear terrorism is possible. In these events, it is possible that veterinarians will be called upon to assist by helping to evaluate animals for contamination and/or exposure, perform initial lifesaving tasks, and decontaminate people's pets. Therefore, veterinarians and other veterinary professionals should have a basic understanding of how radiation exposure may occur, what is happening, the possible effects on companion animals and how to provide veterinary care and assistance in a radiation emergency.

TERMINOLOGY FOR MEASUREMENT OF RADIATION

Activity or radioactivity is measured by the number of atoms disintegrating per unit time.[2] A becquerel is 1 disintegration per second. A curie is 37 billion disintegrations per second, which is the number of disintegrations per second in 1 g of pure radium. A disintegrating atom can emit a beta particle, an alpha particle, a gamma ray, or some combination of all these, so becquerels or curies alone do not provide enough information to assess the risk to a person or animal from a radioactive source.

Disintegrating atoms emit different forms of radiation (ie, alpha particles, beta particles, gamma rays, or x-rays). As radiation moves through the body, it dislodges electrons from atoms, disrupting molecules. Each time this happens, the radiation loses some energy until it escapes from the body or disappears. The energy deposited indicates the number of molecules disrupted. The energy the radiation deposits in tissue is called the dose, or more correctly, the absorbed dose. The units of measure for absorbed dose are the gray (1 J per kilogram of tissue) or the rad (1/100 of a gray). The cumulative dose is the total absorbed dose or energy deposited by the body or a region of the body from repeated or prolonged exposures.

Alpha particles, beta particles, gamma rays, and x-rays affect tissue in different ways. Alpha particles disrupt more molecules in a shorter distance than gamma rays, but gamma rays are more penetrating. A measure of the biologic risk of the energy deposited is the dose equivalent. The units of dose equivalent are sieverts or rem. Dose equivalent is calculated by multiplying the absorbed dose by a quality factor.

GLOSSARY
Absorbed Dose

Absorbed dose describes the amount of radiation absorbed by an object or person.[2,24] The unit for absorbed dose is the rad (US unit) or the gray. One gray is equal to 100 rad.

Alpha Particle

The nucleus of a helium atom, made up of 2 neutrons and 2 protons with a charge of +2. Certain radioactive nuclei emit alpha particles. Alpha particles generally carry more energy than gamma or beta particles, and deposit that energy quickly while passing through tissue. Alpha particles can be stopped by a thin layer of light material, such as a sheet of paper, and cannot penetrate the outer, dead layer of skin. Therefore, they do not damage living tissue when outside the body. When alpha-emitting atoms are inhaled or swallowed, however, they are especially damaging, because they transfer relatively large amounts of ionizing energy to living cells.

Becquerel

Becquerels are the international unit used to measure radioactivity. One becquerel is the amount of a radioactive material that will undergo 1 transformation per second. Becquerels are not used to measure radiation dose or radiation exposure. The US unit is the Curie (Ci).

Beta Particles

Electrons ejected from the nucleus of a decaying atom. Although they can be stopped by a thin sheet of aluminum, beta particles can penetrate the dead skin layer, potentially causing burns. They can pose a serious direct or external radiation threat and can be lethal depending on the amount received. They also pose a serious internal radiation threat if beta-emitting atoms are ingested or inhaled.

Biological Half-Life

Biological half-life is defined as the time required for one-half of the amount of a substance, such as a radionuclide, to be expelled from the body by natural metabolic processes, not counting radioactive decay, once it has been taken in through inhalation, ingestion, or absorption.

Contamination (Radioactive)

Radioactive contamination is the deposition of unwanted radioactive material on the surfaces of structures, areas, objects, animals or people where it may be external or internal.

Curie

The curie is US unit used to measure radioactivity. One curie is roughly the activity of 1 g of Radium-226. Curies are not used to measure radiation dose. The international unit is the becquerel.

Dirty Bomb

A dirty bomb is a device designed to spread radioactive material by conventional explosives when the bomb explodes. A dirty bomb kills or injures people through the initial blast of the conventional explosive and spreads radioactive contamination over possibly a large area, hence the term "dirty." Such bombs could be miniature devices or large truck bombs. A dirty bomb is much simpler to make than a true nuclear weapon.

Effective Dose

Effective dose describes the amount of radiation absorbed by a person, adjusted to account for the type of radiation received and the effect on particular organs. The unit used for effective dose is rem (US unit) or sievert (international unit).

Effective Half-Life

Effective half-life is the time required for the amount of a radionuclide deposited in a living organism to be diminished by 50% as a result of the combined action of radioactive decay and biologic elimination.

Exposure

Exposure describes the amount of radiation traveling through the air. Many types of radiation monitors measure exposure. The units for exposure are the roentgen (R, US unit) and coulomb/kilogram (C/kg, international unit).

External Exposure

External exposure is defined as exposure to radiation outside of the body.

Gamma Rays

Gamma rays are high-energy electromagnetic radiation emitted by certain radionuclides when their nuclei transition from a higher to a lower energy state. These rays have high energy and a short wavelength. All gamma rays emitted from a given isotope have the same energy, a characteristic that enables scientists to identify which gamma emitters are present in a sample. Gamma rays penetrate tissue farther than do beta or alpha particles, but leave a lower concentration of ions in their path to potentially cause cell damage. Gamma rays are very similar to x-rays.

Gray

Gray is the international unit used to measure absorbed dose (the amount of radiation absorbed by an object or person). The US unit for absorbed dose is the rad. One gray is equal to 100 rad. It does not describe the biological effects (effective dose) of different types of radiation.

One sievert is equal to 100 rem. More commonly, dose is measured in much smaller units: millirems or millisieverts. A millirem is one-thousandth of a rem. A millisievert is one-thousandth of a sievert.

Internal Exposure

Internal exposure is defined as exposure to radioactive material taken into the body.

Nuclide

The term nuclide is a general term applicable to all atomic forms of an element. Nuclides are characterized by the number of protons and neutrons in the nucleus, as well as by the amount of energy contained within the atom.

Rad (Radiation Absorbed Dose)

Rad is defined as a basic unit of absorbed radiation dose. It is a measure of the amount of energy absorbed by the body. The rad is the traditional unit of absorbed dose. It is being replaced by the unit gray, which is equivalent to 100 rad. One rad equals the dose delivered to an object of 100 erg of energy per gram of material. It does not describe the biological effects (effective dose, measured in rem or sievert) of the different types of radiation.

Radiation

Radiation is defined as energy moving in the form of particles or waves. Familiar types of radiation are heat, light, radio waves, and microwaves. Ionizing radiation is a very high-energy form of electromagnetic radiation.

Radioactive Half-Life

Radioactive half-life is the time required for a quantity of a radioisotope to decay by half. For example, because the half-life of iodine-131 (I-131) is 8 days, a sample of I-131 that has 10 mCi of activity on Jan. 1, will have 5 mCi of activity 8 days later, on Jan. 9.

Radioactivity

Radioactivity is the process of spontaneous transformation of the nucleus, generally with the emission of alpha or beta particles and often accompanied by gamma rays. This process is related to the decay or disintegration of an atom. Radioactivity refers to the amount of ionizing radiation released by a material. Whether it emits alpha or beta particles, gamma rays, x-rays, or neutrons, a quantity of radioactive material is expressed in terms of its radioactivity (or simply its activity). This represents how many atoms in the material decay in a given time period. The units of measurement for radioactivity are the curie (US unit) and becquerel (international unit).

Radiological Dispersal Device

An RDD is a device that disperses radioactive material by conventional explosive or other mechanical means, such as a spray.

Radionuclide

A radionuclide is an unstable and therefore radioactive form of a nuclide.

Rem (Roentgen Equivalent, Man)

Rem is the US unit to measure effective dose. This relates the absorbed dose in human tissue to the effective biological damage of the radiation.

Not all radiation has the same biological effect, even for the same amount of absorbed dose. It is determined by multiplying the number of rads by the quality factor, a number reflecting the potential damage caused by the particular type of radiation. The rem is the traditional unit of equivalent dose, but it is being replaced by the sievert, which is equal to 100 rem.

Sievert

Sievert is an international unit used to measure effective dose. This relates the absorbed dose in human tissue to the effective biological damage of the radiation. Not all radiation has the same biological effect, even for the same amount of absorbed dose. The US unit is rem.

Terrestrial Radiation

Terrestrial radiation is radiation emitted by naturally occurring radioactive materials, such as uranium, thorium, and radon in the earth.

Thermonuclear Device

A thermonuclear device or nuclear bomb is a device with explosive energy that comes from fusion of small nuclei, or fission of large nuclei.

REFERENCES

1. McClellan RO. Radiation toxicity. In: Hayes AW, Kruger CL, editors. Hayes' principles and methods of toxicology. 6th edition. Boca Raton (FL): CRC Press, Taylor & Francis Group; 2014. p. 883–955.
2. US Department of Health & Human Services, Centers for Disease Control and Prevention, Emergency Preparedness and Response, Radiation Dictionary. Available at: https://emergency.cdc.gov/radiation/glossary.asp. Accessed June 10, 2018.
3. US Department of Health & Human Services, Radiation Emergency Medical Management. Veterinarians. Available at: https://www.remm.nlm.gov/remm_PetOwners.htm. Accessed June 10, 2018.
4. Bunn M, Morozov Y, Mowatt-Larssen R, et al. The US-Russia Joint Threat Assessment on Nuclear Terrorism. Belfer Center for Science and International Affairs,

Institute for US and Canadian Studies, Harvard University. 2011. Available at: https://www.belfercenter.org/publication/us-russia-joint-threat-assessment-nuclear-terrorism. Accessed June 10, 2018.

5. United States Department of Agriculture, Animal and Plant Health Inspection Service, Emergency Response, Emergency Support Function #11, Reports. Vibrant Response Exercise 2014, After Action Report (AAR), July 21-25, 2014, ESF #11. Available at: https://www.aphis.usda.gov/emergency_response/downloads/hazard/AAR_Vibrant_Response_Exercise_2014.pdf. Accessed June 16, 2018.

6. United States Department of Agriculture, Animal and Plant Health Inspection Service, Emergency Response, Emergency Support Function #11, Reports. Gotham Shield Exercise, FEMA Region II, 2017, Emergency Support Function, (ESF) #11, After Action Report (AAR), Apr 24 -28, 2017. Available at: https://www.aphis.usda.gov/emergency_response/downloads/hazard/AAR-Gotham-Shield-EX-RII2017.pdf. Accessed June 16, 2018.

7. Wada S, Ito N, Watanabe M, et al. Whole body counter evaluation of internal radioactive cesium in dogs and cats exposed to the Fukushima nuclear disaster. PLoS One 2017;12(1):e0169365.

8. US Department of Health & Human Services, Centers for Disease Control and Prevention, Emergency Preparedness and Response, Radiation Emergencies, Types of Radiation Emergencies. Available at: https://emergency.cdc.gov/radiation/moretypes.asp. Accessed June 5, 2018.

9. Nolen R. Study finds gains in disaster planning for animals. J Am Vet Med Assoc 2017;251:1366–7.

10. U.S. Department of Homeland Security, Federal Emergency Management Agency. Planning guidance for response to a nuclear detonation. 2nd edition. National Security Staff Interagency Policy Coordination Subcommittee for Preparedness & Response to Radiological and Nuclear Threats; 2010. Available at: https://www.fema.gov/media-library/assets/documents/24879. Accessed June 13, 2018.

11. American Veterinary Medical Association, Disaster Preparedness for Veterinarians. Available at: https://www.avma.org/KB/Resources/Reference/disaster/Pages/default.aspx. Accessed June 10, 2018.

12. US Department of Health & Human Services, Centers for Disease Control. Zombie preparedness. Available at: https://www.cdc.gov/phpr/zombie/index.htm. Accessed June 12, 2018.

13. US Department of Health & Human Services, Radiation Emergency Medical Management. Available at: https://www.remm.nlm.gov/. Accessed June 16, 2018.

14. US Department of Homeland Security, Federal Emergency Management Agency. Prepare for emergencies now: information for pet owners. Available at: https://www.fema.gov/media-library/assets/documents/90356. Accessed June 13, 2018.

15. Wenzel J. Awareness-level information for veterinarians on control zones, personal protective equipment, and decontamination. J Am Vet Med Assoc 2007;231:48–51.

16. Wanner GK, Bhimji SS. EMS, care teams in disaster response. In: StatPearls. Treasure Island (FL): StatPearls Publishing; 2018. Available at: https://www.ncbi.nlm.nih.gov/books/NBK482333/. Accessed June 6, 2018.

17. US Department of Health & Human Services, Public Health Emergency, National Veterinary Response Teams. Available at: https://www.phe.gov/Preparedness/responders/ndms/ndms-teams/Pages/nvrt.aspx. Accessed June 6, 2018.

18. US Department of Health & Human Services, Centers for Disease Control and Prevention. Emergency preparedness, shelter in place. Available at: https://emergency.cdc.gov/shelterinplace.asp. Accessed June 16, 2018.

19. US Department of Health & Human Services, Centers for Disease Control and Prevention. Radiation Emergency Preparedness and Response. Radiation emergencies – what should I do? Available at: https://emergency.cdc.gov/radiation/whattodo.asp. Accessed June 16, 2018.

20. US Department of Health & Human Services, Centers for Disease Control and Prevention. Radiation emergency preparedness and response. What about my pets? Available at: https://emergency.cdc.gov/radiation/pets.asp. Accessed June 10, 2018.

21. US Department of Health & Human Services, Centers for Disease Control and Prevention. Radiation emergency preparedness and response. Stay tuned to learn how to evacuate. Evacuating with pets. Available at: https://emergency.cdc.gov/radiation/evacuation.asp#pets. Accessed June 10, 2018.

22. Murphy LA. Basic veterinary decontamination: who, what, what?. In: Wingfield WE, Palmer SB, editors. Veterinary disaster response. 1st edition. Ames (IA): Wiley-Blackwell; 2009. p. 231–8.

23. US Department of Health & Human Services, Centers for Disease Control and Prevention, Emergency Preparedness and Response, Decontamination - Pets? Available at: https://emergency.cdc.gov/radiation/selfdecon_pets.asp. Accessed June 5, 2018.

24. EPA Radiation Protection, Radiation Terms and Units. Available at: https://www.epa.gov/radiation/radiation-terms-and-units. Accessed June 5, 2018.

UNITED STATES POSTAL SERVICE® Statement of Ownership, Management, and Circulation
(All Periodicals Publications Except Requester Publications)

1. Publication Title	2. Publication Number	3. Filing Date
VETERINARY CLINICS OF NORTH AMERICA: SMALL ANIMAL PRACTICE	003 – 150	9/18/2018

4. Issue Frequency	5. Number of Issues Published Annually	6. Annual Subscription Price
JAN, MAR, MAY, JUL, SEP, NOV	6	$325.00

7. Complete Mailing Address of Known Office of Publication (Not printer) (Street, city, county, state, and ZIP+4®)

ELSEVIER INC.
230 Park Avenue, Suite 800
New York, NY 10169

Contact Person
STEPHEN R. BUSHING

Telephone (Include area code)
215-239-3688

8. Complete Mailing Address of Headquarters or General Business Office of Publisher (Not printer)

ELSEVIER INC.
230 Park Avenue, Suite 800
New York, NY 10169

9. Full Names and Complete Mailing Addresses of Publisher, Editor, and Managing Editor (Do not leave blank)

Publisher (Name and complete mailing address)

TAYLOR E BALL, ELSEVIER INC.
1600 JOHN F KENNEDY BLVD. SUITE 1800
PHILADELPHIA, PA 19103-2899

Editor (Name and complete mailing address)

COLLEEN DIETZLER, ELSEVIER INC.
1600 JOHN F KENNEDY BLVD. SUITE 1800
PHILADELPHIA, PA 19103-2899

Managing Editor (Name and complete mailing address)

PATRICK MANLEY, ELSEVIER INC.
1600 JOHN F KENNEDY BLVD. SUITE 1800
PHILADELPHIA, PA 19103-2899

10. Owner (Do not leave blank. If the publication is owned by a corporation, give the name and address of the corporation immediately followed by the names and addresses of all stockholders owning or holding 1 percent or more of the total amount of stock. If not owned by a corporation, give the names and addresses of the individual owners. If owned by a partnership or other unincorporated firm, give its name and address as well as those of each individual owner. If the publication is published by a nonprofit organization, give its name and address.)

Full Name	Complete Mailing Address
WHOLLY OWNED SUBSIDIARY OF REED/ELSEVIER, US HOLDINGS	1600 JOHN F KENNEDY BLVD. SUITE 1800 PHILADELPHIA, PA 19103-2899

11. Known Bondholders, Mortgagees, and Other Security Holders Owning or Holding 1 Percent or More of Total Amount of Bonds, Mortgages, or Other Securities. If none, check box ▶ ☐ None

Full Name	Complete Mailing Address
N/A	

12. Tax Status (For completion by nonprofit organizations authorized to mail at nonprofit rates) (Check one)
The purpose, function, and nonprofit status of this organization and the exempt status for federal income tax purposes:
☒ Has Not Changed During Preceding 12 Months
☐ Has Changed During Preceding 12 Months (Publisher must submit explanation of change with this statement)

PS Form 3526, July 2014 [Page 1 of 4 (see instructions page 4)] PSN: 7530-01-000-9931   PRIVACY NOTICE: See our privacy policy on www.usps.com.

---

13. Publication Title			14. Issue Date for Circulation Data Below
VETERINARY CLINCS OF NORTH AMERICA: SMALL ANIMAL PRACTICE			JULY 2018

15. Extent and Nature of Circulation			Average No. Copies Each Issue During Preceding 12 Months	No. Copies of Single Issue Published Nearest to Filing Date
a. Total Number of Copies (Net press run)			590	740
b. Paid Circulation (By Mail and Outside the Mail)	(1)	Mailed Outside-County Paid Subscriptions Stated on PS Form 3541 (Include paid distribution above nominal rate, advertiser's proof copies, and exchange copies)	354	445
	(2)	Mailed In-County Paid Subscriptions Stated on PS Form 3541 (Include paid distribution above nominal rate, advertiser's proof copies, and exchange copies)	0	0
	(3)	Paid Distribution Outside the Mails Including Sales Through Dealers and Carriers, Street Vendors, Counter Sales, and Other Paid Distribution Outside USPS®	134	183
	(4)	Paid Distribution by Other Classes of Mail Through the USPS (e.g. First-Class Mail®)	0	0
c. Total Paid Distribution (Sum of 15b (1), (2), (3), and (4))		▶	488	628
d. Free or Nominal Rate Distribution (By Mail and Outside the Mail)	(1)	Free or Nominal Rate Outside-County Copies included on PS Form 3541	82	96
	(2)	Free or Nominal Rate In-County Copies Included on PS Form 3541	0	0
	(3)	Free or Nominal Rate Copies Mailed at Other Classes Through the USPS (e.g. First-Class Mail)	0	0
	(4)	Free or Nominal Rate Distribution Outside the Mail (Carriers or other means)	0	0
e. Total Free or Nominal Rate Distribution (Sum of 15d (1), (2), (3) and (4))		▶	82	96
f. Total Distribution (Sum of 15c and 15e)		▶	570	724
g. Copies not Distributed (See Instructions to Publishers #4 (page #3))		▶	20	16
h. Total (Sum of 15f and g)		▶	590	740
i. Percent Paid (15c divided by 15f times 100)			85.61%	86.74%

* If you are claiming electronic copies, go to line 16 on page 3. If you are not claiming electronic copies, skip to line 17 on page 3.

16. Electronic Copy Circulation		Average No. Copies Each Issue During Preceding 12 Months	No. Copies of Single Issue Published Nearest to Filing Date
a. Paid Electronic Copies	▶	0	0
b. Total Paid Print Copies (Line 15c) + Paid Electronic Copies (Line 16a)	▶	488	628
c. Total Print Distribution (Line 15f) + Paid Electronic Copies (Line 16a)	▶	570	724
d. Percent Paid (Both Print & Electronic Copies) (16b divided by 16c × 100)	▶	85.61%	86.74%

☒ I certify that 50% of all my distributed copies (electronic and print) are paid above a nominal price.

17. Publication of Statement of Ownership

☒ If the publication is a general publication, publication of this statement is required. Will be printed   ☐ Publication not required.
in the   NOVEMBER 2018   issue of this publication.

18. Signature and Title of Editor, Publisher, Business Manager, or Owner

Stephen R. Bushing   Date 9/18/2018

STEPHEN R. BUSHING - INVENTORY DISTRIBUTION CONTROL MANAGER

I certify that all information furnished on this form is true and complete. I understand that anyone who furnishes false or misleading information on this form or who omits material or information requested on the form may be subject to criminal sanctions (including fines and imprisonment) and/or civil sanctions (including civil penalties).

PS Form 3526, July 2014 (Page 3 of 4)   PRIVACY NOTICE: See our privacy policy on www.usps.com

Moving?

Make sure your subscription moves with you!

To notify us of your new address, find your **Clinics Account Number** (located on your mailing label above your name), and contact customer service at:

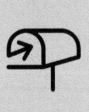

Email: journalscustomerservice-usa@elsevier.com

800-654-2452 (subscribers in the U.S. & Canada)
314-447-8871 (subscribers outside of the U.S. & Canada)

Fax number: 314-447-8029

**Elsevier Health Sciences Division
Subscription Customer Service
3251 Riverport Lane
Maryland Heights, MO 63043**

*To ensure uninterrupted delivery of your subscription, please notify us at least 4 weeks in advance of move.

Printed and bound by CPI Group (UK) Ltd, Croydon, CR0 4YY

03/10/2024

01040398-0006